Field trials of health i
in developing countri

2nd editio

C000097388

Macmillan Education
Between Towns Road, Oxford OX4 3PP
A division of Macmillan Publishers Limited
Companies and representatives throughout the world

www.macmillan-africa.com

ISBN 0 333 64058 6

First published 1991 by Oxford University Press

This edition published 1996

Printed in China

2005 2004 2003 2002
12 11 10 9 8 7 6

Foreword to the first edition, 1991

Tore Godal, Director of UNDP/World Bank/WHO Special
Programme for Research and Training.

The United Nations Development Programme/World Bank/
World Health Organization Special Programme for Research and
Training in Tropical Diseases (the TDR Programme) was set up 15
years ago, with the aim of exploiting the rapid advances that were
being made in immunology, biochemistry and molecular biology
to develop new drugs, vaccines, and diagnostic and vector control
products against six of the major tropical diseases. Much of the
work supported by TDR has been laboratory based and from this
investment a range of promising new products have emerged with
potential for use against tropical diseases. Before these products
can be introduced into disease control programmes they must go
through a series of investigations which may include studies *in
vitro*, in animal test systems, and in human volunteers to assess
safety, toxicity, and potency, and to determine the appropriate
dosage for human use. After these stages it is essential that the
products be evaluated under field conditions, often in the form of
large-scale randomized controlled trials. Only when the results of
all these forms of study are available is it possible to estimate the
potential beneficial effect of the intervention for disease control in
routine programmes.

None of the investigational stages is without difficulty and the
last, the conduct of large-scale trials, poses special problems. From
early in the evolution of the TDR programme it was appreciated
that the capacity to carry out field research in the tropical disease
endemic countries was generally weak due to the shortage of
personnel with the necessary research training and experience.
The Programme has sought to strengthen capacity in this respect in
various ways, through sponsoring postgraduate training, workshops and recently by promoting regional networks to link field
researchers in the developing countries (the FIELDLINCS programme) through regular workshops, exchanges and short course
training.

Since the first edition of the manual was published, several improvements have been suggested, and we have tried to incorporate the most important of these into the second edition. The first edition had the title *Methods for Field Trials of Interventions against Tropical Diseases: a Toolbox* and we hope that the change of title for the second edition does not create too much confusion. It was pointed out that many issues discussed in the manual were relevant to the conduct of field epidemiological studies in developing countries, not only on diseases that are considered as 'tropical', and not only for intervention studies. Though some sections have wider relevance, we have preserved intervention studies in the title because they are the main orientation of the manual.

The changes in the second edition are as follows. The chapter on study size has been revised to take account of recent work on the sample size computations for cluster-randomized trials. A section on geographical position systems has been added to Chapter 6. The chapter on social research methods was redrafted by Joel Gittelsohn and the chapter on data processing was updated to take account of advances in computing software and hardware. A chapter has been added on writing grant applications and the final chapter on the dissemination of results has been expanded.

It is our intention that, over time, the manual will be refined and improved further as experience is gained with its practical use. We encourage those who use the manual to write to the editors if there are aspects of the manual they think are in need of improvement or change.

Responsibility for producing initial drafts of the different chapters of the manual were assigned among the participants listed at the front of the book. The initial drafts were reviewed by the participants during a week-long meeting and were modified as a consequence of the extensive discussions that took place. In this way many different persons contributed to the different chapters and it seemed inappropriate, therefore, to attribute responsibility for the final form of any one chapter to individuals, as each chapter owes its final form to the collective contributions of those listed.

The text was edited by the two of us to try to maintain a uniform style. The manual was also circulated to other field research scientists for their suggestions for any changes. We gratefully acknowledge the valuable contributions from Astier Almedon, Steve Bennett, Fred Binka, Boachie Boatin, Loretta Brabin, David Brandling-Bennett,

Gilbert Burnham, Peter Byass, Andreas de Francisco, Tony Degremont, Aime de Muynck, Don de Savigny, Isabelle de Zoysa, Anne Dick (to Chapter 15), Nicola Dollimore, Herbert Gillies, Brian Greenwood, Hazel Inskip, Japhet Killewo, Sarah Macfarlane, Bruce Macleod, Gilly Maude, Daan Mulder, Andrzej Radalowicz, Brian Southgate, Malcolm Pike, Roger Webber, Jimmy Whitworth, Andrew Wilkins and Fabio Zicker. We have incorporated many of their suggestions and those of others who we have undoubtedly omitted to acknowledge (and to whom we apologise!).

We are grateful to the literary executor of the late Sir Ronald A. Fisher FRS, to Dr Frank Yates FRS and the Longman Group UK Ltd, London, for permission to reprint Table 33 from their book *Statistical tables for biological, agricultural and medical research*, 6th ed. (1974).

London and Baltimore P.G.S.
March 1996 R.H.M.

Contributors

The following persons were responsible for producing a first draft of the manual and for the subsequent revisions, including those in the second edition.

J. Cattani	UNDP/World Bank/WHO Special Programme for Research and Training in Tropical Diseases, World Health Organization, 1211 Geneva 27, Switzerland.
J. Cleland	Centre for Population Studies, London School of Hygiene and Tropical Medicine, Keppel Street, London WC1E 7HT, UK.
N.E. Day	Medical Research Council Biostatistics Unit, 5 Shaftesbury Road, Cambridge CB2 2BW, UK.
J. Gittelsohn	Department of International Health, The Johns Hopkins University School of Hygiene and Public Health, 615 North Wolfe Street, Baltimore, MD 21205, USA.
A.J. Hall	Communicable Diseases Epidemiology Unit, London School of Hygiene and Tropical Medicine, Keppel Street, London WC1E 7HT, UK.
R.J. Hayes	Tropical Health Epidemiology Unit, London School of Hygiene and Tropical Medicine, Keppel Street, London WC1E 7HT, UK.
B. Hogh	Epidemiology Research Unit, Statens Seruminstitut, 5 Artillerivej, DK-2300, Copenhagen S, Denmark.
B.R. Kirkwood	Maternal and Child Epidemiology Unit, London School of Hygiene and Tropical Medicine, Keppel Street, London WC1E 7HT, UK.
E.L. Makubalo	Medical Research Council, University of Natal Medical School, Umbilo Road, Durban, South Africa.
T.F. de C. Marshall	Maternal and Child Epidemiology Unit, London School of Hygiene and Tropical Medicine, Keppel Street, London WC1E 7HT, UK.
L. Molineaux	46 Route Peney-Dessus, Peney-Dessus, 1242 Satigny, Geneva, Switzerland.
R.H. Morrow	Department of International Health, The Johns Hopkins University School of Hygiene and Public Health, 615 North Wolfe Street, Baltimore, MD 21205, USA.

2 DIFFERENT KINDS OF INTERVENTION TO BE EVALUATED

Interventions may be divided into two broad categories, those that are used to treat a disease process already underway and those that are used to prevent the initiation of the disease process. Some interventions fall into both categories. The primary effect of preventive strategies is to reduce the incidence of new cases of disease whereas that of treatment strategies is to interfere with the natural history of the disease process by curing or alleviating the disease or preventing the development of more severe disease or death.

The basic unit to which an intervention is applied will depend upon the nature of the intervention and the strategy for its use. The unit may be the individual, the family or household, or the community.

2.1 Drugs for treatment of disease

The way in which a drug is to be used for disease control will influence the design of field trials to evaluate its impact. Most drugs employed in tropical disease control programmes are used to kill or inhibit the pathogen in the host. Strategies for disease control that use such agents involve case detection (which requires an appropriate case definition and diagnostic method) followed by treatment designed to reduce morbidity and mortality. Often the success of this approach depends critically upon case finding, and for diseases such as tuberculosis and leprosy it depends also on case holding, i.e. being able to follow and treat each patient at regular intervals over a long period of time. Case finding and treatment may also reduce transmission of an agent if cases are the main reservoirs of infection, if case detection methods locate a high proportion of prevalent cases, and if the treatment is sufficiently effective.

2.2 Treatments for prevention of infection or disease

Drugs or other interventions may also be used for prevention of infection or disease. Generally, the use of drugs for prophylaxis does not require individual diagnosis, but community or group diagnosis is needed to identify groups that should receive the prophylaxis. Whether requiring specific diagnosis or not, therapeutic or preventative agents are usually taken on an individual basis, though sometimes interventions to be applied on a mass basis can be distributed to a community through the water supply (for example, fluoride against dental caries) or in food (for example, diethylcarbamazine for filariasis and chloroquine for malaria in medicated salt, and vitamins in fortified bread).

Prophylaxis is usually aimed at preventing or limiting infection, particularly in those at high risk for a limited period of time (for example, antimalarials taken by those visiting malarious areas). The value of such an approach is limited by the duration of action of the intervention, by adverse reactions to the prophylactic agent, and possibly by the role of the intervention in stimulating the development of drug resistant organisms. For some purposes prophylaxis may be used by those who are permanent residents of tropical disease endemic areas (for example, antimalarials in pregnancy, and vitamin A supplementation in areas of deficiency).

Drugs also may be used prophylactically for treatment of pre-clinical infection (for example, during the incubation period before onset of symptoms, as for *gambiense* type of trypanosomiasis), or for treatment of subclinical infection (for example, ivermectin against onchocerciasis, and praziquantel against schistosomiasis).

Strategies for the use of such interventions include the mass treatment of entire populations or the targeted treatment of identifiable subgroups (such as school-age children) in areas where the infection is sufficiently prevalent. In some cases the objective of such treatment is to reduce the transmission of the agent in the community; in others it is applied only for the benefit of the individual treated. Treating all those in a defined group may be more cost-effective than screening the whole group and only treating those found to be infected.

2.3 Vaccines for prevention

Vaccines protect individuals at risk of acquiring infection by inducing a variety of immune mechanisms. These immunological reactions may lead to protection from infection, reduction of parasitic proliferation within the host after invasion (and hence curtailment of disease) and/or reduction of transmission from the host. Vaccines may be administered to protect individuals at risk of acquiring

disease. Classic vector control measures include drainage of swamps, elimination of casual water (for control of the *Aedes* mosquito), clearing of bush (for tsetse fly control), control of water levels in irrigation schemes, and urban water drainage systems. Means to reduce human faecal and urine contamination have included latrine construction, provision of sewage systems, clean water supplies, and protected food storage. Nearly all require substantial educational efforts and some lifestyle changes.

3 BIOMEDICAL–BEHAVIOURAL CONTINUUM OF INTERVENTIONS

As noted in Section 2, field trials of interventions against tropical diseases will usually involve aspects of human behaviour and this may have important implications for the trial design. Interventions can be classified along a biomedical–behavioural continuum. At one extreme is the purely biomedical intervention which requires no behavioural change, for example, insecticide spraying of river rapids against *Simulium damnosum* larvae. At the other extreme are behavioural interventions which have a biomedical rationale but no biomedical element or agent, for example, boiling of drinking water. Trials of interventions that have a large behavioural component typically require a greater emphasis on social research than do purely biomedical interventions, but there are few interventions for which some kind of social research is not appropriate.

The intervention to be evaluated in a trial must be defined precisely, not only in terms of the biological and chemical composition of the agent, but also in terms of any health education or promotion that is a component part of the intervention strategy. Both may influence the measured impact on disease, sometimes independently, and it will be important to take this into account when designing the appropriate 'control' intervention. For example, if it is important to assess the impact of the biomedical intervention, independent of a health education component, it may be necessary to include the health education component for those in the 'control' group also.

The co-operation required from the study subjects to ensure effective application of an intervention ranges from passive acquiescence to active change of behavioural patterns. Change may involve innovative behaviour or alteration of existing habits. If an intervention involves behavioural alterations, prior social research into the reasons for existing behaviour is likely to be required. Such enquiries may indicate the intensity and levels of educational effort (community or individual) required to ensure co-operation.

4 EVOLUTION OF NEW INTERVENTIONS AND DISEASE CONTROL STRATEGIES

Many intervention products, and especially drugs and vaccines, are likely to originate from basic research in laboratories. Such products must go through a long series of tests before they can be considered for use in the kinds of field trials which are the focus of this manual. Before any human use, a new product will be tested in the laboratory for its activity and toxicity in various *in vitro* and animal test systems. If it successfully passes through these stages, studies of safety, toxicity, and activity may be conducted in a small number of human volunteers with careful clinical monitoring. A series of further studies, each including increasing numbers of subjects, must be carried out before a new product can be introduced for widespread use. Careful monitoring, often in a clinical setting for possible adverse reactions, is characteristic of early studies. The optimal dose and frequency of application must be worked out. Early investigations will include some measures of effects which often are intermediate to the outcome of principal interest. For example, with a vaccine, the induction of an immune response may be assessed, which it is hoped will correlate with protection or activity against the disease of interest. To determine efficacy, trials are always required that include a comparison intervention (which may be a placebo if there is no effective equivalent intervention against the disease under study), in which the interventions are allocated between subjects or groups of subjects on a random basis. Legal registration procedures are mandated in most countries before a drug or vaccine can be put into general use, and these procedures normally require documentation of safety and efficacy of the intervention based on randomized controlled trials involving many hundreds of subjects. Registration issues are not

2
Study design

1 Introduction

    1.1 The study plan
    1.2 Ethical considerations

2 Definition of study objectives
    2.1 The idea for a study
    2.2 Purpose
    2.3 Specific objectives
    2.4 Subsidiary objectives

3 Selection of interventions
    3.1 Characteristics required
    3.2 Number of interventions compared
    3.3 Combined interventions
    3.4 Choice of comparison intervention

4 Allocation of interventions
    4.1 Randomization and 'blindness'
    4.2 Unit of application
    4.3 'Stepped-wedge' design
    4.4 Other approaches to allocation

5 Choice of outcome measures

6 Study population
    6.1 Criteria for selection of trial population
    6.2 Inclusion and exclusion criteria
    6.3 Size
    6.4 Compliance

7 Implementation
    7.1 Community acceptance
    7.2 Staff recruitment and training
    7.3 Field organization

8 Data handling
    8.1 Data collection
    8.2 Data processing

1 INTRODUCTION

Intervention studies should be designed to produce unambiguous evaluations of the effects of interventions which are precise enough for the purpose of public health planning. A common goal of an intervention study is to evaluate the effect of a specific intervention applied in a specific manner to a well-defined population. In the design the major issues will be; first, the nature of the intervention, the strategy for its use and the natural size of the unit at which intervention operates (for example, individual, household, village, geographical area); second, the effects and how they should be measured; and third, the comparisons that need to be made with other interventions.

In most developing countries disease control is the direct responsibility of the Ministry of Health. Therefore, wherever possible, the Ministry should be involved in, if not directly responsible for, the planning and conduct of trials, and the results must be made available in such a way that they are of direct relevance to national disease control activities.

1.1 The study plan

This chapter gives an overview of the factors to consider in the planning of field trials of interventions against tropical diseases. The planning process is a major exercise which starts, and which should be largely completed, before any substantial field activities have taken place, other than initial feasibility studies and small-scale pilot investigations. The study plan encompasses all aspects of an investigation, from formulation of detailed objectives based on the initial idea, through preparation for all field activities, through collection of data and analysis of results, to their publication, dissemination, and use in disease control. The plan should also take account of the form of any studies that will follow, depending on the possible different outcomes of the study in hand.

Detailed planning is necessary for several purposes. First, details of the plan of investigation will be required by local and national administrations to review for approval. A similar description will be required by the agency that is going to review the proposal for funding or support. The detail required in such grant applications varies greatly from agency to agency. Some require a thick document with full details of all study procedures, while others put quite a small upper limit on the size of any application they are prepared to review (for example, six pages). It is usually more time-consuming to prepare the former kind of application, but the latter kind may present a more formidable challenge, because in relatively few words the investigators have to present convincing evidence that they have considered and worked out all issues to be included in the longer application.

A second reason for detailed planning at the start of an investigation is that possible problems must be anticipated in advance and solutions thought through in order to reduce the likelihood of the study falling behind schedule, or having to be abandoned, due to unexpected problems. It is rare to be able to predict all potential problems, but the more that have been considered in advance then the smaller the chance of catastrophe.

A good estimate of the resources needed (for example, for transport, staff, allowances, items of equipment) must be made in order to be able to calculate the level of funding to be requested in any grant application. Underestimating the support needed may jeopardize some of the objectives, which may have to be revised or abandoned in the middle of the study, whereas overestimating the cost may prejudice the funding agency against agreeing to support the study. Sufficient time must also be allocated for the various stages of a trial.

In this chapter the steps to be encompassed in the study plan are discussed in the approximate order that they would arise, from the formulation of objectives through to the eventual publication, dissemination, and use of the findings. In the remaining chapters, specific issues relevant to the planning process are reviewed in greater detail and cross-references are given in this chapter, where appropriate.

1.2 Ethical considerations

Ethical considerations impinge on many aspects of the design and conduct of intervention studies. Any research investigation on human subjects should be submitted for ethics committee review. The submission must make clear that the ethical implications of all aspects of a study have been given full consideration by the investigator. Intervention trials against tropical diseases in communities whose residents are often poor and deprived in many ways may pose difficult ethical dilemmas for an investigator and for the bodies that must review the research proposals. The dogma that an investigator should treat everyone in an investigation as though they were a member of his or her own family is both difficult to apply and probably inappropriate in the situations of extreme poverty in which many tropical diseases flourish. A related issue concerns the responsibility that an investigator has to those who live in the same community as the study subjects but who, for whatever reason, are not included in the study. Very commonly an investigator must walk a tightrope, balancing his or her responsibilities to the individual with those related to the improvement of the public health. The Ministry of Health knows these problems well as they are implicit in any allocation of the health budget between preventive and curative care, but, commonly, allocation of the routine health budget is regarded as one step removed from that encountered by the public health research worker in the community, who may have to face these issues directly in the context of a specific research investigation. There are no simple solutions to these problems. It is important that each research study is subject to strict ethical review, with due attention to the specific conditions in and under which it will be conducted. A discussion of the issues involved is given in Chapter 4.

2 DEFINITION OF STUDY OBJECTIVES

Once an idea for a study has been formulated, it will be necessary to detail the objectives of the study. To do this the researcher will need to find out what has already been done regarding the evaluation of the intervention or interventions of a similar kind. This may involve meeting or corresponding with those undertaking similar studies and it will certainly involve conducting a literature review to find out what has been published that is relevant.

With this background information the objectives of the study can be formulated. These will include the purpose, which is a general statement regarding the role that the intervention to be evaluated might have for the control of disease. The specific objectives give more detailed statements of the magnitude and nature of any effects of the intervention on disease that the study has been designed to detect. Finally, a list of subsidiary objectives will be given which relate to issues which may not be central to the overall objectives but on which information will also be gathered while the study is in progress.

2.1 The idea for a study

The most creative phase of the planning of a research study is the selection of the subject area of the research and the formulation of the specific questions that will be addressed. A major motivation for most successful researchers is that they are doing something that they really enjoy doing. Their motivation may come from scientific curiosity about the causes and control of a particular disease, or about the effects of a specific intervention, or their concern may be less specific and relate to an interest in exploring different ways of improving the public health. The field researcher may be motivated by working directly with people in their communities and be stimulated by the challenges posed by working in remote or difficult situations, outside of the hierarchy that may exist, for example, in a hospital environment.

The development or refinement of a field research idea will take place in interaction with others at local, national, and possibly international levels. The research activity must not only be acceptable to the population in which it will be undertaken but also to those who will authorize it nationally and to those who will fund it. Good ideas for field research on the control of a disease which is of public health importance are likely to attract support. It may be important for investigators to make early contact with the agencies that might be sources of support for a study. These agencies may have their own agenda and have listed their priorities for the support of research. Clearly, proposed investigations that fit in with such priorities are likely to be viewed sympathetically if support is requested.

Many funding agencies encourage investigators to contact them early in the planning process when only the outline of a study has been formulated, so that the agency can advise how a proposal might be developed to fit in with their own priorities. An investigator is not obliged to follow such advice, but much work can be saved if the advice is at least considered before detailed planning of a study is undertaken. Funding agencies may publish a list of their priorities for research. For example, each of the committees that review research proposals for the UNDP/World Bank/WHO Special Programme for Research and Training in Tropical Diseases (TDR) has drawn up a research plan for their target disease which details the investigations they are anxious to support with high priority. Outline protocols may have been developed for some of these studies, which particular investigators would have to tailor for use in the situation in which they will work.

Field research that is likely to be given the highest priority, both nationally and internationally, is that directed at the control of diseases which are of greatest public health importance. Thus, an important preliminary to the development of a research proposal on a specific disease or condition may be a more general survey in the local community to determine the relative importance of the disease of interest as one of the major health problems, both medically and as perceived by the local population.

A good justification for some studies may be that they attempt to replicate observations that have been made in other geographical locations. The progress of science (and of public health) is dependent upon the replication of experiments (trials) in different settings to determine whether the findings from a study may have arisen through some kind of bias, or may apply only in special circumstances, or may be generally applicable. Replication of trials of BCG vaccination against tuberculosis and leprosy, for example, have shown substantial variations in the efficacy of that vaccine against both diseases in different parts of the world.

'Confirmatory' (or otherwise!) studies are very important for the assessment of the public health usefulness of an intervention.

2.2 Purpose

The statement of the purpose of a research project should describe the main questions to be addressed by the research without going into detail (which will be done in the specific objectives). It should give a reader a clear idea of the nature of the research that will be undertaken. The purpose of a leprosy vaccine trial might be 'to assess the protective efficacy against leprosy induced by a mixture of BCG and armadillo-derived killed *Mycobacterium leprae* bacilli among the contacts of leprosy patients in Venezuela'. For a study of the use of the drug ivermectin against onchocerciasis the purpose might be 'to assess the impact of mass treatment with ivermectin on the transmission of onchocerciasis and to measure any side effects in those treated with the drug'. For a trial of a new vaccine against the blood-stages of the malaria parasite the purpose may be 'to measure the effect of a *Plasmodium falciparum* asexual blood-stage vaccine in reducing morbidity and mortality due to malaria'.

The purpose should convey to the reader the type of intervention which is to be evaluated (without details of how it will be applied, dose, and so on) and the end-points against which the impact will be measured, without necessarily specifying the magnitude nor precise nature of the impact expected, or which the study will be designed to detect. It might also include a description of the ways in which the results of the trial may influence public health policy and contribute to scientific knowledge.

2.3 Specific objectives

In the specific objectives a quantitative statement should be made regarding the size of the effect of an intervention that a study is designed to detect and the precision with which the effect will be measured. Such specifications are necessary in order to calculate how large a study should be, using the methods described in Chapter 3. The nature of the intervention should be given in more detail than in the statement of purpose (for example, dose, frequency of administration) and the endpoints of the study clearly stated. They should also include a specification of the size of the study and detail the population in which, or to which, the intervention will be applied. Thus, for a trial of a leprosy vaccine, the specific objectives might include 'to conduct a randomized trial among contacts (aged 6 to 64 years) of leprosy patients comparing the incidence of leprosy among those given BCG alone with that among those given a mixture of BCG plus armadillo-derived killed *M.leprae* bacilli (6×10^8 bacilli/dose). The trial will have 90 per cent power to detect a protective effect of 70 per cent (of BCG and *M.leprae* versus BCG) at the 5 per cent level of statistical significance in the five years following vaccination'.

For the example on the trial of ivermectin against onchocerciasis the specific objectives would include a statement of the size of the impact of transmission which the trial would have a reasonable chance of detecting and the frequency with which adverse reactions of different kinds would have to occur to be detected in the study.

For the malaria vaccine, a more detailed description of the formulation of the vaccine would be required and statements included on the magnitude of the effects on disease that the trial would be expected to ascertain.

The proper specification of the specific objectives is a key to the conduct of a successful study. They should include a concise but detailed description of the intervention to be evaluated, the outcome(s) of interest, and the population in which the study will be conducted. The more specific and detailed the objectives are, the clearer it will be how to design a study to meet them. It is crucial to set the appropriate objectives and it is worth spending time to get these right.

2.4 Subsidiary objectives

In the context of many trials sub-studies will be included having subsidiary objectives, such as the comparison of various serological tests, or the analysis of genetic markers and their correlation with disease. It may be decided to add other objectives onto an intervention trial which do not relate to the main objectives. In a trial of ivermectin against onchocerciasis, for example, the impact on some other parasitic diseases might be assessed, or in a trial of a vaccine against leprosy, the effect on tuberculosis could also be studied. The introduction of an intervention may provide a special opportunity for determining particular key factors in the pathogenesis of disease, for example, trials of ivermectin, a microfilaricide, against *Wuchereria bancrofti* may provide evidence for the role of microfilaria, as compared to that of adult worms, in the pathogenesis of lymphatic filariasis disease. Decisions to add on studies of this kind should not be taken lightly as they will invariably need additional commitment of resources and may involve the study population in additional inconvenience. They may thus have a negative impact on the primary objectives and the final 'cost' for the study may be much greater than it appeared initially in monetary terms.

Once a large field study is underway successfully it is not unusual for the study organizers to be approached by other investigators who wish to graft on additional procedures to answer questions of interest to them. There may be considerable value in utilizing the same study for multiple purposes, but full consideration should be given to the extra work that this will entail, especially for key members of the research team, and to other possible harmful effects such as upsetting the rapport between the study team and the population.

3 SELECTION OF INTERVENTIONS

3.1 Characteristics required

The choice of an intervention to be subject to large-scale field evaluation will be influenced by the following criteria. The intervention should be such that it could be introduced into a national or regional disease control programme (though this criterion might not apply for 'explanatory' trials—see Chapter 1, Section 4). The dose (when applicable) should be optimal. Evidence would usually be required from short-term studies that the intervention is relatively safe and produces a convincing intermediate response. When an action has to be repeated several times (for example, vitamin supplements), there should be corresponding evidence that the interval between each action gives an effective schedule. For some interventions the concept of dose is meaningless, such as the application of a diagnostic or screening test. Corresponding relevant evidence would then be required that the test is adequate (for example, previous studies indicating sensitivity, specificity and predictive values). For continuous or repeated treatments, similar considerations apply to the duration of treatment. For example, with vitamin supplementation the duration required will depend on whether the outcome of interest is the acute effect of severe deficiency or the chronic effect of more moderate deficiency. In addition to being safe and giving promise of being efficacious, it must be acceptable to those to whom it is directed, relatively easy to deliver and, at least eventually, be of sufficiently low cost that it can be incorporated into the national disease control strategy.

3.2 Number of interventions compared

The choice of the number of different interventions to compare in a field trial is likely to be determined not only by the number of competing alternatives but also by the implications the choice has on the size of the study, which in turn is dependent on the frequency with which the outcome of interest occurs. 'Rare' outcomes require large studies (as discussed in Chapter 3). For example, in a trial of leprosy vaccines in South India it was planned that each 'arm' (one of the alternative intervention assignments) included in the study would include around 65 000 subjects in order that the study had the desired statistical power to detect effects. Clearly in this situation a decision to add another arm would have had enormous cost and logistic consequences (M. Gupte, personal communication).

If the outcome is common, however, studies to compare more than two interventions may be undertaken more readily. For example, if seroconversion following vaccination is the outcome of interest, it may be straightforward to compare multiple vaccines or vaccination strategies in a single study.

It is important to note, however, that many researchers try to build too many comparisons into a study. There is often a tendency to divide groups after the sample size has been calculated or to plan comparisons within groups, without going through the appropriate computations (as given in Chapter 3).

Comparisons within a study can always be made with much greater confidence than those between studies. Thus if drug A is found to be 50 per cent 'better' than a placebo in one trial and drug

B is found to be 50 per cent better than a placebo in another trial, it will not necessarily be possible to conclude that A and B are equally effective, as the circumstances in which the two trials were conducted will not have been identical. A further trial may be necessary for a direct comparison of A and B. If the need for this trial could have been anticipated in advance it would have been more efficient to conduct one trial involving both drugs A and B and a placebo. A trial like this may be more complex to organize and would probably have to be substantially larger than either of the '2-arm' studies.

3.3 Combined interventions

For some diseases there are several possible interventions that may reduce the disease impact on a population. For example, interventions against malaria include destruction of mosquito breeding sites, spraying of residual insecticide, personal protection measures (for example, use of bed-nets and repellents), drug prophylaxis, and drug treatment, and studies might be designed to evaluate each of these interventions individually. A malaria control programme may choose to use more than one intervention at the same time and may wish to evaluate the impact of the 'strategy' rather than the individual components of it. In such a case, the intervention trial might compare an integrated strategy incorporating several different measures applied simultaneously with a control group in which only the routine measures normally available would be applied.

In developed countries, several studies of this kind have been conducted for the prevention of heart disease. Those in the intervention group were advised to smoke less, take more exercise, eat less fat, and so on, and their subsequent cardiovascular disease rates were compared with those in a group who were not so advised. The advantage of this kind of study is that if no effect is seen then it may be reasonable to conclude that no one of the components of the intervention was effective (at least, as applied in the trial), but the disadvantage is that if an effect is demonstrated it is not possible to be sure what fraction of the overall result each of the various components of the intervention was responsible for. It is also possible when no effect is seen that a beneficial effect of one component of the intervention has been counter-balanced by a deleterious effect of another component.

3.4 Choice of comparison intervention

The best way to evaluate an intervention is to compare its effect with that of another intervention in the same population at the same time. The allocation of individuals or groups of individuals to the different interventions should be 'at random' (see Section 4.1 and Chapter 7). In general, the intervention that is the current 'best' should be used as the comparison, but the choice of the 'control' intervention is not always straightforward and may involve difficult ethical issues (Chapter 4). When no effective intervention is known the comparison must be with a group in which 'no intervention' is made; in general a placebo should be administered in order to preserve 'blinding' (Section 4.1). For example, before the development of ivermectin no effective and safe treatment for onchocerciasis existed. Thus, placebo-controlled trials of the drug were ethically acceptable, at least until the beneficial effects of ivermectin had been established. For most tropical diseases, however, some kinds of intervention exist and may already be deployed by the health services or by a control programme in the area where a trial is planned. Only in rare circumstances would it be ethical to withdraw these existing interventions for the purposes of a trial. A more difficult issue is with respect to the extent to which they should be introduced in the context of a trial. If it is known that regular prophylaxis with anti-malarial drugs reduces mortality from malaria, for example, would it be necessary to give this intervention to all those in the 'control' arm of a malaria vaccine trial, even though in normal circumstances few of them would be on prophylaxis? Indeed, would it even be ethical to withhold prophylaxis from those who would be receiving a malaria vaccine whose efficacy against mortality was unknown? The optimistic reader will seek a definitive answer to these questions in Chapter 4! Unfortunately, the search will be in vain as there are no general definitive solutions to problems such as this; each situation has to be considered on its own merits, taking full account of the circumstances in which a particular investigation is planned.

In a leprosy vaccine trial in Venezuela, the new leprosy vaccine consisted of a mixture of BCG and killed *M.leprae* bacilli. When the trial was designed a choice was made between using BCG for the control arm (the efficacy of BCG alone against leprosy in Venezuela was unknown) or using a placebo. BCG was chosen even though doing this might reduce the chance of showing a protective effect (as BCG alone may be protective). The inclusion of a placebo arm would have allowed the protective effect of BCG alone to be evaluated but the incidence of leprosy was too small for a third arm in the study. The major purpose of the trial was to evaluate whether a leprosy-specific vaccine (i.e. one which included *M.leprae* bacilli) would be more effective than a non-specific vaccine (for example, BCG). If the comparison had been with a placebo instead of BCG, any effect due to BCG could not have been distinguished from that due to the addition of *M.leprae* bacilli to the vaccine.

The use of a placebo may be very important to derive an unbiased measure of effect (see Section 4.1 and Chapter 7, Section 3), but it requires careful ethical justification. In a placebo-controlled trial of vitamin A supplementation in Ghana, the objective was to determine if a reduction of child mortality was produced by supplementation. As eye signs of vitamin A deficiency are effectively treated by vitamin A supplements, all in the trial were monitored for such signs and withdrawn from the placebo group immediately such signs were detected, even though this was likely to reduce the power of the study to detect an impact of vitamin A supplementation on mortality.

4 ALLOCATION OF INTERVENTIONS

4.1 Randomization and 'blindness'

Once a potential intervention has been shown to be safe and acceptable for use in humans and the dose schedule established, studies should be conducted to evaluate quantitatively the benefit attributable specifically to the intervention under trial compared to some other intervention, having excluded the confounding effect of other variables. The only general way rigorously to exclude the biasing effects of other factors is to base allocation decisions as to which intervention is applied to a particular individual or group on a random mechanism. Incorporation of randomization into the study is a most important design issue (see Chapter 7).

The randomized intervention trial is as close to a rigorously scientific experimental study involving human beings as it is possible to achieve ethically. The main study design features of a randomized trial include the following:

1. To avoid bias in assignment to the alternative interventions all eligible patients are assigned at random to the alternative treatment groups. This involves two steps; the first is selecting participants on the basis of the criteria for eligibility that have been established, and the second is the randomization procedures to ensure that each selected participant has an equal opportunity to receive a particular intervention procedure.

2. To avoid bias in the assessment of the endpoints the person(s) assessing the outcome measures should not know to which intervention group the participant is assigned (i.e. the assessor should be 'blind' to the intervention group).

3. To avoid bias in behaviour of the participant the participant should also be 'blind' (i.e. the intervention group assignment should not be known by the participant).

If neither the assessor nor the participant is aware of the intervention allocations, the study is said to be 'double-blind'. If only the assessors (or, more rarely, only the participants) are aware of the allocations, the study is called 'single-blind'. For situations in which there is no presently useful treatment or preventive method, a placebo of some sort must be used if double-blinding is to be assured. The 'double-blind' approach is the key to the elimination of bias in the assessment of the impact of an intervention and, wherever possible, a 'double-blind' design should be used. Sometimes it is not possible because of the nature of the intervention procedure, but even if the providers of the intervention must know the assignments an independent assessor may be kept 'blinded'. The more clearly defined and objective the outcome to be measured, the less critical it becomes to ensure blinding of the assessor. Similarly, the less likely a patient is to be influenced by knowledge of which treatment is being given, the less important is the blinding.

4.2 Unit of application

The unit to which an intervention is applied may be the individual, the family (household), or the community (environment). The unit for randomization will usually vary in parallel with this. The choice of the unit for application of the intervention depends upon the nature of the intervention, the administrative method for its .application, and the purpose for which the intervention is being applied. In statistical terms the most efficient design, in most circumstances, is to use the individual as the unit of application and this should be the design of choice unless there is good reason for household or community (group) application and randomization. There are four general reasons for applying an intervention to a group rather than by individual.

First, group allocation is appropriate when, by its nature, the intervention must be applied on a geographical area or community-wide basis, such as most environmental alterations, many vector control measures, and commonly used approaches to educational interventions.

Second, it may be logistically easier to administer the interventions to individuals in groups rather than on an individual basis. Often it is simpler administratively and/or more acceptable to the people to randomize by household or village rather than by individual. Furthermore, with individual randomization there may be risk of sharing medications within households or villages.

Third, if the purpose of applying the intervention is to reduce transmission of infection, the appropriate unit of application would be the 'transmission zone', i.e., the area in which humans, vectors, and intermediate hosts may be interacting and sharing a common pool of parasites. Factors of importance in defining such zones include the flight range of vectors and the movements of people, vectors, and intermediate hosts. To reduce interchange ('contamination') among transmission zones it may be useful to have intervening buffer zones that are not involved in the study. For many diseases the size of the transmission zones may be difficult to determine and may vary over time.

Some interventions may be applied to individuals but with the expectation that there may be an effect on transmission through applying them to a high proportion of individuals in the community. The extent of coverage required to produce such effects depends upon the epidemiological circumstances, the presence of other control measures, and the type of intervention procedure being introduced. For example, the use of a malaria vaccine to reduce the transmission of malaria in parts of Africa where the disease is 'holoendemic' may require so near to complete coverage that such a purpose would not be seriously considered. In some areas of south-east Asia, however, where control measures have greatly reduced transmission, the addition of vaccines may be sufficient to eliminate transmission.

For some types of intervention procedures, when the procedure itself provides individual benefit, such as ivermectin in the treatment of onchocerciasis, a further important issue is whether reduction of transmission provides a benefit in addition to the individual reductions of morbidity/mortality. Study designs to demonstrate this additional benefit are likely to be complex.

A fourth reason for applying interventions to a group or community as a unit would be for trials involving an intervention of already proven efficacy in individuals but for which the delivery may be more effectively carried out on a group or community basis. The trial might consist of a comparison of different delivery systems. Generally, the end-result desired in this type of study is based upon cost-effectiveness criteria. The issue under evaluation might be whether it is possible to achieve a greater amount of disease reduction for a given expenditure (or alternatively, a given amount of disease reduction for less expenditure) by use of a community-based distribution system than by the usual methods. Many types of community-based distribution systems require community participation studies. The principles involved in cost-effectiveness studies and community participation studies are beyond the scope of this manual.

When group randomization is adopted, the efficiency of the design can be improved by ensuring that the groups allocated to the different intervention arms are comparable. When there are large numbers of units to be allocated, randomization itself will ensure comparability, but usually when communities or other groups are the units to be randomized, the number of units is quite limited and randomization may leave considerable differences between the groups in the different arms. Attempts can be made in the analysis to allow for these differences, but the persuasiveness of the results may be reduced if the conclusions depend upon extensive statistical manipulation of the study results. A more efficient approach to increase the comparability of the groups in the different arms is to stratify the groups into 'blocks' having similar underlying, pre-intervention, risks of the disease outcome in question and then to randomize within each block. Stratification should be in terms of variables which are either strongly related to the risk of the outcome under study, or in terms of this risk itself. For example, in studies of malaria in which villages are to be randomized, the villages might be stratified according to their pre-study malaria prevalence or incidence rates, if such information is available, and the randomization done within strata. For studies comparing two interventions villages with similar malaria rates might be paired and one village in each pair randomly allocated to each intervention.

Often, good information on the distribution of the outcome measures will not be available in the study population. In such circumstances baseline studies to obtain the required information should be considered. Sometimes, as an alternative, surrogate measures must be used (i.e. measures which are thought to correlate closely with the outcome measures of principal interest). In the absence of detailed data on the population, geographical proximity and socio-economic level may be used as stratification characteristics. Thus, if a small geographic area is chosen as the randomization unit, the total study area would be divided into regions containing a small number of relatively homogeneous units and, within each region, an equal number of units allocated to each treatment arm. The regions may be limited in size so that the number of units within a region is simply the number of treatment arms (i.e. one unit per treatment arm in each region).

4.3 'Stepped-wedge' design

The issue of the ethics of randomization is presented in acute form in situations where previous studies, perhaps using short-term endpoints or a more intensive intervention than is feasible on a population basis, indicate that the intervention is likely to be beneficial. Withholding the intervention from those in one of the treatment arms for the duration of the trial may then be argued to be unacceptable. An approach that can be adopted in this situation is the phased introduction of the intervention on a group by group basis, until the entire target population is covered. The order in which the groups are given the intervention is randomized. This approach has been used in The Gambia to evaluate the long-term effects of vaccination against the hepatitis B virus (HBV). The study design is illustrated in Fig. 2.1. This type of design has been called a 'stepped wedge' design (The Gambia Hepatitis Study Group 1987). The power of this approach, compared to a simple allocation of groups to one or other treatment arms, is of the order of 75–80 per cent, depending on the number of groups. The same considerations apply to stratification and blocking as in the static allocation designs.

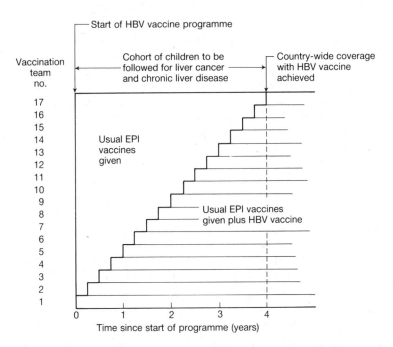

Fig. 2.1 The 'stepped wedge' study design used to evaluate the impact of hepatitis B vaccination on liver cancer rates in The Gambia (The Gambia Hepatitis Study Group 1987). Hepatitis B vaccine was introduced into the routine child vaccination programme over a period of 4 years. The order in which the different vaccination teams (there were 17 at the time of the trial was planned) began to use the vaccine was random. At the end of 4 years there was a cohort of children who had received the vaccine and a cohort who had not. These cohorts will be followed to compare the incidence rates of liver cancer and chronic liver disease.

4.4 Other approaches to allocation

The allocation of interventions to individuals based on a random mechanism is the only general approach to rigorously exclude the potential biasing effects of other factors. Reports are not uncommon in which the allocation of alternative interventions in a trial has not been randomized. A common approach is to compare the incidence or prevalence of the disease under study before and after the intervention has been applied and to attribute any difference to the effect of the intervention. This approach has little to commend it as it may be very misleading to assume that in the absence of the intervention the disease rate would have remained the same. Many diseases, and especially those of parasitic or infectious origin, vary greatly in incidence and severity from year to year and place to place, for reasons that are incompletely understood. Certainly variations in climate (for example, temperature and rainfall) can have profound effects. Some diseases show marked declines over time in some communities (for example, tuberculosis) which cannot be related to any obvious specific factor. 'Before and after' evaluations of interventions in such situations may be very misleading.

Another commonly employed approach is to apply an intervention in one community and not in another and to attribute any difference in disease rates between the two communities as being due to the intervention. This also may be very misleading for reasons similar to those outlined above.

The main reason often advanced for using a non-random allocation between intervention groups is for simplicity of design and administrative ease. Approaches like these also seem easier to explain to officials and to gain public acceptance. The rationale for randomization is difficult to communicate, even to other scientists, but the arguments in favour of randomization, as outlined above, are extremely strong, and failure to accept this approach has frequently led to studies from which erroneous conclusions have been drawn.

There are, however, situations in which allocation cannot be made on a randomized basis. There are occasions when the benefits of an intervention appear so clear that a properly randomized trial cannot be contemplated. The value of the intervention then has to be assessed by comparison of the situation before and after its introduction, or by the use of case-control studies after the intervention has been introduced (Smith 1987). Temporal comparison is clearly confounded with whatever trends in disease rates that are occurring in the population independently of the specific intervention, and with changes in the pattern of ascertainment of the outcome, a likely concomitant of the intervention introduction. Conclusions can be sharpened by comparison with time trends in disease rates in neighbouring regions where intervention has not occurred, and also by consideration of the sharpness with which changes in disease rates take place and related to the speed with which the intervention is introduced over the entire population. Knowing and recording possible confounding variables in the areas being compared may also be useful. For example, in a study in which an objective is to reduce transmission of lymphatic filariasis by treating the human population with antifilarial drugs, monitoring the vector population for changes in density and infectivity may be useful.

While acknowledging these exceptions to use of randomization as the basis of allocation, such studies cannot achieve the rigour of a randomized design and any conclusions drawn from such studies must be viewed with some caution.

5 CHOICE OF OUTCOME MEASURES

For many interventions there will be a range of outcomes that could be affected and which might be of interest to study. Nutritional supplements, for example, might effect any or all of the following:

(1) biochemical measures;
(2) short term acute consequences of deficiency;
(3) the consequences of chronic deficiency;
(4) mortality ascribed to the conditions which the intervention is intended to rectify; and
(5) total mortality.

In determining which outcome is of the greatest importance for the study, consideration must be given to:

(1) whether the outcome is of public health significance;

(2) whether the probable effect on that outcome is large enough
    to be of interest; and

(3) whether it can be accurately recorded.

Total mortality and age-specific mortality rates are of basic
public health importance, and systems can usually be set up to
ensure that they are well recorded (sometimes requiring considerable input), but they are unlikely to be sufficiently affected by
many interventions to enable effects to be detected with studies of
manageable size. Mortality from specific causes should be more
greatly affected, but may be much more difficult to ascertain
accurately. Using total mortality clearly dilutes the effect that
might be seen if specific causes were examined, since the random
variation in rates arising from the unaffected causes is included.
The choice may have to be made between setting up special
mechanisms to improve the quality of the information on cause of
death, or to allow for a dilution of the observed effect by increasing the size of the study. It should be stressed that for conditions
that are life threatening, mortality is a most important outcome to
evaluate.

Short-term outcomes are clearly attractive in that if used as the
outcome on which the design is based, then the study size will be
smaller and the duration shorter than if mortality were to be used.
The danger is that the short-term measure may in itself be of no
consequence to health and the effect of the intervention on that
outcome may not correlate well with the effect on more serious
conditions. There is, for example, little point in measuring an
antibody response to infection if it bears no relation to the risk of
disease. Conversely, however, if it is known that a short-term
outcome is highly correlated with an outcome of greater public
health consequence (and is effectively a surrogate measure of the
more important outcome) it is generally highly efficient to focus
most studies on the former outcome.

In most circumstances, the appropriate outcome for determining the duration and size of the trial would be the most serious
consequence of the specific condition at which the intervention is
aimed. For measles vaccination in technically advanced countries,
the onset of the disease would be the natural end-point, rather
than death from the disease, and certainly not total mortality. In
contrast, for countries where mortality from measles is high, death

from measles might well be the outcome of choice. If mechanisms for establishing accurate diagnosis were inadequate, total mortality might even be considered (especially as measles vaccine may reduce the risk of death attributable to diseases other than measles).

With this perspective, short-term 'intermediate' outcomes should not be discarded but included as valuable monitoring mechanisms. They provide information as to whether the programme is on target to meet its more basic goals, and if it is not on target, should help to identify what remedial action is required. When short-term outcomes are used in this way, any assumptions about the natural history of the disease should be clearly stated.

Definition of the main outcome will have consequences for the duration of the trial. Prior information should be available on the time needed for the intervention to affect the outcome. In some situations, such as the prevention of liver cancer in adult life by hepatitis B vaccination in the first year of life, the final outcome measure may not be observed for several decades. The role of intermediate outcomes then becomes important.

A final and important point to stress in this section is that it is essential that attention is given to monitoring the severity and frequency of adverse effects of an intervention. In their desire to assess the effectiveness of an intervention, investigators often do not pay sufficient attention to finding and documenting adverse effects, which may require additional effort and resources. In most situations, the future applicability of the conclusions drawn from a study will involve an assessment of the balance between positive and negative effects.

6 STUDY POPULATION

6.1 Criteria for selection of trial population

The criteria for selection of the population to be included in the trial depend primarily upon what condition the intervention is directed against and upon the purpose of the trial. In general, the population will be chosen from an area in which there is high endemicity for the condition of interest. The higher the incidence of the disease of interest, in general, the smaller the study population for the trial has to be. Sometimes, however, the purpose of the trial is to determine the efficacy under special epidemiological circumstances or in special population groups, such as pregnant women. Good community and governmental co-operation and participation are also key factors in the successful conduct of a trial. The study area should be accessible at the times surveys are to be conducted (for example, during the rainy season). Well-qualified and experienced field teams should be available or be able to be recruited. In addition, access to high-quality clinical and laboratory facilities may be necessary for the trial. If required, entomological, behavioural science, and other appropriate disciplinary expertise should be available. Planning the trial will be much simplified if baseline data are already available in an area.

If the study design involves the repeated follow-up of members of the study population over several years, as will be the case for many intervention trials, it is important to select a location for the study in which substantial migration into, or especially from, the area is unlikely to occur. Migration rates in excess of ten per cent a year are not uncommon in many rural areas and may be considerably higher in some areas and in urban or peri-urban settings. It is often not easy to ascertain migration rates during the planning of a study. A rapid survey of a sample of the proposed study population may be useful to determine if a reasonable proportion of the population have been resident in the area for several years.

6.2 Inclusion and exclusion criteria

In general, the trial population should be chosen to represent the group that will be the target for the intervention in a public health programme. Care should be taken to define the target population. To the extent feasible, those included should be the persons for whom benefit is likely to be greatest and those excluded should be the persons for whom benefit is likely to be minimal or, indeed, who may be harmed. Specific inclusion and exclusion criteria should be developed for a trial. For example, because the major morbidity and mortality associated with malaria in a holoendemic area is seen in infants and young children, these groups are likely to be the focus of a major field trial of a malaria vaccine in such an area, though adults and older children might be used in preliminary studies to test the safety of the vaccine in those who already have some immunity or may be the focus of a vaccine trial where malaria transmission is much less intense.

In early trials, of an explanatory nature, special groups at high risk or volunteers may form the study population either to maximize the potential effect, to ensure good compliance, or to facilitate the logistics. Valuable information concerning the potential of the intervention can result, but the extent to which the results may be extrapolated to the general population may be limited.

Exclusion criteria need to be carefully considered so as to eliminate subjects who may be put at greater risk by the intervention or who have underlying conditions that may interfere with the assessment. Exclusion criteria should be stated explicitly and unambiguously before the study begins. It is usual to exclude from trials those who are seriously ill, those who are very old, those who are very young, and pregnant women, unless any of these are the specific target group for the intervention. These groups are excluded either because it is considered they are unlikely to derive benefit from the intervention or because they might be considered more likely to be susceptible to possible adverse effects of the intervention. Ascertaining pregnancy is difficult, without specific testing, and in some trials it may not be feasible to detect women in the early stages of pregnancy. Sometimes all women of child-bearing age are excluded from trials if it is thought that damage may be caused by the intervention to the fetus. Against this must be balanced the potential benefit that women may receive from the intervention and it may be appropriate to include them in later trials with careful monitoring of pregnancy outcomes.

6.3 Size

Strict attention needs to be given to the required size of the study, in terms of the precision of the effect estimates and of the power to detect important differences. These aspects are discussed in detail in Chapter 3. It is important to allow for the loss of power that results from group randomization if such a design is adopted (see Chapter 3, Section 6).

For interventions that are likely to be given to large numbers of individuals if they are introduced into disease control programmes, there are strong arguments in favour of designing trials of the interventions to be large also, not only to pick up any rare side-effects, but also to obtain a relatively precise measure of their expected impact.

6.4 Compliance

Conclusions from an intervention study will be based on the comparison of the outcome measures adopted for the trial between those allocated to the alternative intervention arms of the study. Only a certain proportion of those allocated to a particular intervention will receive that intervention effectively. Effective delivery of an intervention requires both that the provider carries out the intervention procedure correctly and that the trial participants co-operate in the appropriate fashion. In field trials the provision of the intervention will usually be under the control of the investigator, but a successful trial also requires the compliance of the participants, who are not under the control of the investigator, and will depend on the understanding and co-operation of the community involved. Hence the strong emphasis in this manual on the importance of communication and feedback between the investigating team and the participating communities has a pragmatic, as well as an ethical, basis.

In most trials, however, some participants will not fully comply, and the intervention procedure either will not be carried out or it will not be done in an effective manner. For trials to determine the public health value of an intervention (pragmatic trials), some degree of non-compliance may give a more realistic measure of effectiveness than a tightly controlled study, but for explanatory studies, in which an important objective may be to determine the maximum effect possible, every effort should be made to keep compliance high and, where possible, the degree of compliance should be continually monitored, at least on a sample basis. This might be done, for example, by doing urine or blood analyses for chemoprophylaxis agents and nutritional supplements. For intervention measures that are given sequentially over time, or on a continuing ongoing basis, repeated spot samples should be taken.

A further aspect of compliance which is sometimes overlooked is that those in the 'control' arm of a trial, who are allocated to routine care may adopt the active treatment under study. For example, if those in some villages are allocated to receive an intervention and those in other villages serve as controls, those in the latter villages may go to the former villages to obtain the intervention. Monitoring for the possible occurrence of this latter form of non-compliance (sometimes called 'contamination') is of importance. Care should also be taken in the construction of the different treatment groups to minimize the opportunity for such contamination. For example, if the intervention consists of a vaccine, given by peripatetic vaccination teams, clear geographical separation of those in the different arms of this study would be one means to help prevent crossing-over.

7 IMPLEMENTATION

7.1 Community acceptance

Critical to the conduct of a successful intervention study is that the study population co-operates well during the conduct of the trial and accepts the intervention offered. They must feel a part of the trial and perceive it to be for their benefit. To ensure these aspects will require careful planning and investigation before the trial starts, including appropriate discussion with, and explanation to, community leaders and the potential participants themselves. Feedback and interaction should be continued throughout the course of the study. These aspects are discussed in several chapters and form the foci of Chapter 4 (on ethical considerations), Chapter 5 (on community involvement), and part of Chapter 10 (on qualitative research methods).

7.2 Staff recruitment and training

The dedication and commitment of the staff employed to conduct a field research project is essential. This will involve their careful selection, training, and encouragement. They must understand the importance of their role in the study and how it relates to that of others. The importance of high-quality work must be emphasized and this must be monitored throughout the study (see Section 9 and Chapters 11 and 12).

7.3 Field organization

All aspects of field procedures should be planned in advance and potential problems and solutions anticipated (for example, actions in case of staff sickness, vehicle or computer failure). The study design must reflect not only what should be done, but also what can be done given the constraints under which the study must be conducted. These aspects are considered in detail in Chapter 11 and Chapter 12. Issues relating to mapping and conducting a census of the study area are covered in Chapter 6.

8 DATA HANDLING

8.1 Data collection

A necessary part of any trial will be the collection of certain items of basic data on all participants. These will include identification information, such as name, age, sex, place of residence, and information on other factors that may influence the risk of occurrence of the outcome measures under study in the trial. Further data will be collected during the course of the trial to monitor the application of the interventions and to record information on the outcomes of interest. The conduct of a population census is described in Chapter 6 and methods to obtain information by questionnaire at the start of a trial or during its course are described in Chapter 9. Methods for obtaining data through anthropological and sociological survey methods are outlined in Chapter 10. Of crucial importance in any trial is the proper measurement of the incidence of endpoints against which the intervention is designed to protect and these aspects are discussed in Chapter 8.

8.2 Data processing

Methods of coding and computer processing of data collected in a trial are described in Chapters 9 and 13.

9 QUALITY CONTROL

In most intervention studies members of the population are invited to participate, the intervention is applied, perhaps repeatedly, and the population is kept under surveillance until the final outcomes are recorded. The quality of each step in this process must be carefully monitored. The two major reasons, which hardly need stating, are first to ensure that each operation is being performed to an acceptable standard, and second to identify areas where attention is required. A third reason is to be able to ascertain, at the end of a study which failed to show anticipated effects, the possible reasons for failure. The damage done by a misleading negative result can be serious and widespread. The following are major aspects of quality control that need attention.

9.1 The intervention

Regular monitoring of the delivery of the intervention should be an integral part of the design to ensure that there is no slippage in the quality as a trial goes on. For example, in a vaccination trial continual review would be needed of the quality of the vaccination techniques being used by field workers. The quality of the agents used in the intervention needs checking. For example, the potency of each batch of vaccine used should be assayed, together with monitoring of the maintenance of the cold chain.

Short-term endpoints may be used as monitoring assays at this stage in a trial. At the individual level, repeated surveys of physiological measures of response to the intervention will provide an overall assessment of whether an effective intervention agent has been effectively delivered. Examples would be antibody levels against a vaccine, or levels of a micronutrient in serum. Such evaluations may have to be done or be evaluated by an independent monitor for the trial, to ensure that those who will assess the main endpoints in the trial are kept blind to the identity of those in intervention and control groups.

9.2 Follow-up

For many intervention studies, the endpoints of interest may not emerge for a lengthy period after the start of the intervention. It may not be necessary to keep the entire study population under active observation, and this is often not feasible (for example, cases might be detected as they report to clinics rather than by conducting periodic surveys of the study population), but it is essential that the study is designed in such a way that losses to the study population (for example, cases who do not go to clinics) will not distort the conclusions. The follow-up rate should be monitored closely in order to identify potential problems at an early stage (for example, disgruntlement in a particular village, a fieldworker whose work quality is declining). If possible the reasons that individuals are lost to follow-up should be ascertained and this information should be analysed to assess any effect that the losses might have on the interpretation of the results of the study.

9.3 Assessment of study outcomes

Mechanisms have to be established to ensure that the quality of information on the outcomes is acceptable. This requirement may well affect the choice of outcome to be used in the main evaluation. Ongoing monitoring is required to establish that the data on outcomes are maintaining acceptable quality and that no biases are present in the way outcomes are recorded in different treatment arms. Attention needs to be paid to inter-observer variation in the assessment of the outcomes, and changes that may occur in this variation as the study progresses.

9.4 Other field and laboratory procedures

Quality control should pervade all field activities and the question as to how high quality is to be achieved and maintained should be addressed specifically for all activities. This is discussed in most of the chapters that follow.

Laboratory procedures must be subject to constant scrutiny and 'blind' coded duplicate samples should be introduced into the workload regularly to monitor performance.

In interview surveys a proportion of respondents should be re-interviewed by a second interviewer, blind to the results of the first interviewer, to check on the repeatability of the responses.

It is important that all involved in the study accept and understand the need for constant checking and re-checking. Errors are bound to occur and their detection should not result in a reprimand unless there is evidence of dishonesty or continual carelessness. Incentives or rewards to encourage high-quality work may be worthwhile.

All members of the field team are, and must be made to feel, important contributors to the research project. Feedback of results and progress should be continuous so that they can appreciate where their contribution fits into the overall project. Neglect is a great stimulus to poor quality work.

10 ANALYSIS AND REPORTING

10.1 Planning the main analyses

The main analyses that are expected to result from the trial should be developed in some detail with the use of dummy tables. Such an exercise is a great help in clarifying exactly what data are actually needed and provides a useful guide for planning the study. All specific objectives should be tied to the analyses.

10.2 Ongoing analyses

Analysing the results of a trial as data accumulate is an important way of monitoring the satisfactory progress of a study. Administrative analyses of the numbers of participants recruited each day or week and of the data collected by different field workers are important for quality control. A running tally should be kept of the numbers of subjects experiencing the different endpoints of interest to verify that the estimates of incidence rates used to plan the size of the trial were appropriate. Ideally, the investigators will be blind with respect to which interventions have been allocated to which participants, but differences in these respects between the different interventions might be analysed by a data monitoring committee (as discussed in the next section). Other aspects of ongoing analyses are reviewed in Chapter 13.

Interim reports based on ongoing analyses during the course of a trial may be required by national authorities and by the funding agency supporting the conduct of the study. These may be required to check that the original proposal is being adhered to.

10.3 Data monitoring committee

For large trials it is advisable for the investigators to set up an independent data monitoring committee. Such a committee may serve several functions.

The most important function might be to hold the randomization code for the study and to monitor the results of the trial as they accumulate. If there is evidence of a substantial risk of adverse reactions associated with any of the interventions under study, the committee would have the power to stop further recruitment. Similarly, if evidence accumulates that one intervention is substantially better than the others (or one is substantially worse), the committee would recommend that the study be ended. The advantage of these functions being undertaken by an independent committee is that it means that the investigators are kept blind to the randomization codes, which is an important way of ensuring unbiased assessment of the study endpoints. The circumstances in which a study will be prematurely ended should be carefully considered when the study is being designed and the data monitoring committee should be party to such discussions. It will not be possible to predict all possible situations that may cause a decision to be taken to end a study, but this should be done to the extent possible. In particular, there should be consideration as to how large a difference may be apparent between the interventions with respect to their impact on specific endpoints, before it is decided to end the study. In some circumstances it may be important to go on beyond the point where statistical significance is reached. These issues are discussed in Chapter 3, and there are also ethical considerations which are discussed in Chapter 4.

The committee might also set up independent quality control checks on study procedures and, for example, may arrange to review the diagnoses of all cases of the diseases of interest arising in the study (which should be done, of course, 'blind' to knowledge of the randomization codes).

In some trials the data monitoring committee may consist of one person, sometimes called the 'clinical monitor'.

10.4 Analysis methods

The analysis of a large field trial may be a complex undertaking and may well require the services of a professional statistician. It is not feasible in a manual of this kind to detail all of the analysis methods that it might be appropriate to employ in different trials. In Chapter 14 an outline is given of the main methods of analysis that are likely to be employed. It is included as it summarizes relevant methods that are not covered as comprehensively in most basic epidemiological texts or books on medical statistics.

10.5 Reporting results

Once a field trial has been completed and the results analysed it is essential that the results, and their implications, are made available to the scientific community, to those who participated in the study and to those responsible for designing and implementing regional and national disease control strategies. Some remarks on these aspects are made in Chapter 16.

REFERENCES

Smith, P. G. (1987). Evaluating interventions against tropical diseases. *International Journal of Epidemiology*, **16**, 159–66.
The Gambia Hepatitis Study Group (1987). The Gambia hepatitis intervention study. *Cancer Research* **47**, 5782–87.

3
Study size

1 INTRODUCTION

One of the most important factors to consider in the design of an intervention trial is the choice of an appropriate study size. Studies that are too small may fail to detect important effects on the outcomes of interest, or may estimate those effects too imprecisely. Studies that are larger than necessary are a waste of resources, and may even lead to a loss in accuracy, as it is often more difficult to maintain data quality and high coverage rates in a large study than in a smaller one.

In this chapter the choice of an appropriate study size is considered. In Section 2 there is a discussion of the criteria used to make this choice. In Sections 3 and 4 procedures are given for calculating study size requirements in the simplest case where two groups of equal size are to be compared. More complex designs are considered in Section 5. Special methods are necessary when the interventions are allocated to groups rather than individuals, and these are described in Section 6. Following this, two other factors that may influence the choice of study size are discussed; first, the need to allow for interim analyses of the results (Section 7.1), and second, the effects of losses to follow-up (Section 7.2). The chapter ends with a discussion of the consequences of the widespread practice of conducting intervention trials that are too small. The principal formulae given in the chapter are summarized in Table 3.4 for reference purposes.

The procedures described in this chapter should be regarded only as providing a rough estimate of the required study size, as they are often based on only approximate estimates of expected disease rates, subjective decisions about the size of effects that it would be important to detect, and the use of approximate formulae. However, a rough estimate of the necessary size of a study is generally all that is needed for planning purposes. Breslow and Day (1987) give a more comprehensive review of methods for the determination of study size requirements, but the methods given in this chapter should be adequate for most purposes. There are computer programs available that perform sample size calculations. In particular, this facility is available in the package 'Epi Info' (see Chapter 13, Section 2.1), though it does not cover the full range of possibilities considered in this chapter.

Readers who are not familiar with methods for the statistical analysis of trial data, and in particular with the concepts of confidence intervals and significance tests, may find it helpful to read Chapter 14 Section 2 before embarking on this chapter, which is placed here because of the importance of considering study size requirements at the design stage of a study.

A principal objective of most intervention trials is to *estimate the effect* of the intervention on the outcome or outcomes of interest. Any such estimate is subject to error, and this error has two main components, bias and sampling error. Possible sources of *bias* and ways of avoiding them are discussed in other chapters. The second component, *sampling error*, arises because the study data come from only a *sample* of the population. This second component of error is the focus of the chapter. Sampling error is reduced when the study size is increased, whereas bias generally is not.

2 CRITERIA FOR DETERMINING STUDY SIZE

2.1 Precision of effect measures

To select the appropriate sample size it is necessary to decide how much sampling error in the estimate of the effect of the intervention is acceptable, and to select the sample size to achieve this precision. When the data are analysed, the amount of sampling error is represented by the width of the *confidence interval* around the estimate of effect. The narrower the confidence interval, the greater the *precision* of the estimate, and the less the probable amount of sampling error. When designing a study, it is necessary, therefore, to decide the width of an acceptable confidence interval. Having made this decision, the method to select the required study size is given in Section 3.

2.2 Power of study

An alternative approach is to choose a study size which gives adequate *power* to detect an effect of a given magnitude. The focus is then on the result of the *significance test* which will be conducted at the end of the study. The significance test assesses the evidence against the *null hypothesis*, which states that there is no difference between the interventions under comparison. A *significant* result indicates that the data conflict with the null hypothesis, and that there are grounds for rejecting the hypothesis that there is no difference in the effects of the interventions under study on the outcomes of interest.

Because of the variations resulting from sampling error, it is never possible to be certain of obtaining a significant result at the end of a study, even if there is a real difference. It is necessary to consider the *probability* of obtaining a statistically significant result in a trial, and this probability is called the *power* of the study. Thus a power of 80 per cent to detect a difference of a specified size means that if the study were to be conducted repeatedly, a statistically significant result would be obtained four times out of five if the true difference was really of the specified size.

The power of a study depends on:

1. The value of the true difference between the study groups; in other words, the true effect of the intervention. The greater the effect, the higher the power to detect the effect as statistically significant for a study of a given size.

2. The study size. The larger the study size, the higher the power.

3. The probability level at which a difference will be regarded as 'statistically significant'.

The power also depends on whether a one-sided or two-sided significance test is to be performed (see Chapter 14, Section 2.3), and on the underlying variability of the data. How the power may be calculated for given values of these parameters is explained in Section 4.

When designing a study, the objective is to ensure that the study size is large enough to give high power *if the true effect of the intervention is large enough to be of practical importance.*

2.3 Choice of criterion

The choice of which of the above two criteria (precision or power) should be used in any particular instance depends on the objectives of the study. If it is known unambiguously that the intervention has some effect, it makes little sense to test the null hypothesis, and the objective may be to estimate the magnitude of the effect, and to do this with acceptable precision.

In studies of new interventions, it is often not known whether there will be any impact at all on the outcomes of interest. In these circumstances it may be sufficient to ensure that there will be a good chance of obtaining a significant result if there is indeed an effect of some specified magnitude. It should be emphasized, however, that if this course is adopted, the estimates obtained may be very imprecise. To illustrate this, suppose it is planned to compare two groups with respect to the mean of some variable, and suppose the true difference between the groups is D. If the study size is chosen to give 90 per cent power (of obtaining a significant difference with $p < 0.05$ on a two-sided test) if the difference is D, the 95 per cent confidence interval on D is expected to extend roughly from $0.4D$ to $1.6D$. This is a wide range and implies that the estimate of the effect of intervention will be very imprecise. In many situations it may be more appropriate to choose the sample size by setting the width of the confidence interval, rather than to rely on power calculations.

2.4 Studies with multiple outcomes

The discussion above related to factors influencing the choice of the study size with respect to a particular outcome measure. In most studies several different outcomes are measured. For example, in a study of the efficacy of insecticide-treated mosquito-nets on childhood malaria, there may be interest in the effect of the intervention on deaths, deaths attributable to malaria, episodes of clinical malaria over a period of time, spleen sizes at the end of the malaria season, packed cell volumes at the end of the season, and possibly many other variables.

In order to decide on the study size, the investigator should first focus attention on a few key outcomes, for which it is important that the study should be able to provide adequate results. The methods of this chapter can then be used to calculate the required study size for each of these key outcomes. Ideally, the outcome that results in the largest study size would be used to determine the size as then, for other outcomes, it would be known that better than the required precision or power would be achieved.

It is often found, however, that one or more of the outcomes would require a study too large for the resources that are likely to be available. For example, detecting changes in mortality often requires very large studies. In these circumstances it may be decided to design the study to be able to detect an impact on morbidity, and accept that it is unlikely to be able to conclude anything useful about the effect on mortality. It is important to point out, however, that if a trial shows that an intervention has an impact on morbidity it may be regarded as unethical to undertake a further larger trial to assess the impact on mortality. For this reason it is generally advisable to ensure that trials are conducted at an early stage in which the outcome of greatest public health importance is the endpoint around which the study is planned. This issue is discussed further in Chapter 4.

Sometimes, different study sizes may be used for different outcomes. For example, it might be possible to design a study in such a way that a large sample of participants are monitored for mortality, say by annual surveys, and only a proportion of these are monitored for morbidity, say by weekly visits.

2.5 Practical constraints

In practice, statistical considerations are not the only factors that need to be taken into account in planning the size of an investigation. Resources in terms of staff, vehicles, laboratory capacity, time or money may limit the potential size of a study, and it is often necessary to compromise between the results of the study-size computations and what can be managed with the available resources. Trying to do a study that is beyond the capacity of the available resources is likely to be unfruitful, as data quality is likely to suffer and the results may be subject to serious bias, or the study may even collapse completely, thus wasting the effort and money that has already been put into it. If the calculations indicate that a study of manageable size will yield power and/or precision that is unacceptably low, it is probably better not to conduct the study at all.

A useful approach to examine the trade-off between study size (and thus cost) and power is to construct *power curves* for one or two of the key outcome variables. Power curves show how the power varies with the study size for different values of the effect measure. Figure 3.1 shows power curves for malaria deaths in the mosquito-net study discussed in Section 2.4, assuming that equal numbers of children are to be allocated to the intervention and control groups and statistical significance is to be based on a two-sided test at the 5 per cent level. R represents the relative rate of malaria death in the intervention group compared to the control group, so that $R = 0.3$ represents a reduction in the death rate of 70 per cent. The assumptions used to construct these curves are described in Section 4.1. The curves indicate that if 1000 children

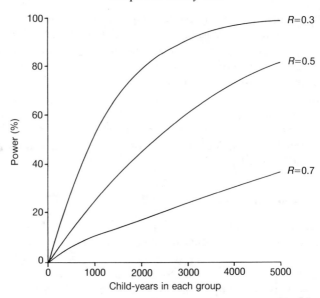

Fig. 3.1 Power curves for a trial of the effect of mosquito-nets on malaria deaths. (Malaria death rate in control group assumed to be 10/1000/yr. R = relative rate in the intervention group. Assumes equal size groups, 2-sided test, and significance at $p < 0.05$.)

were followed for one year in each group (making 2000 children in all), there would be about a 1 in 2 chance of obtaining a significant result (power = 50 per cent), even if the reduction in the death rate was as high as 70 per cent. A study four times as large as this would have a good chance of detecting a reduction in the death rate of 50 per cent or more, but would be inadequate to detect a more modest effect (say, 30 per cent reduction in the death rate).

3 SIZE TO GIVE ADEQUATE PRECISION

3.1 Introduction

This section describes how the study size is determined if the aim is to obtain an estimate of the effect of an intervention with a specified level of precision. The simplest case is considered, in which just two groups are to be compared (for example, an intervention compared with a control group, or the comparison of two interventions), and where the two groups are to be of approximately equal size. More complex designs are discussed in Section 5. The methodology varies according to the type of effect measure and the comparison of incidence rates, proportions, and means are considered in the sections that follow.

3.2 Comparison of incidence rates

Suppose a comparison of two groups is required with respect to the rate of occurrence of some defined event over the study period. Suppose the true incidence rates are r_1 and r_2 in groups 1 and 2 respectively, where each rate represents the number of events per person-year of observation. The rate ratio, R (sometimes called, incorrectly, the *relative risk*) of the incidence rate in group 1 compared to the incidence rate in group 2, is given by $R = r_1/r_2$ (see Chapter 14, Section 5 for methods of analysis for the comparison of rates). If the total follow-up time for those in each group is y years (for example, y persons are each followed for 1 year, or $y/2$ are each followed for 2 years), each group is said to experience y person-years-at-risk. The expected numbers of events in the two groups will be $e_1 = yr_1$ and $e_2 = yr_2$ respectively. When the results are analysed, the approximate 95 per cent confidence interval for R is expected to extend from R/f to Rf where

$$f = \exp\{1.96 \sqrt{[(1/e_1) + (1/e_2)]}\}. \tag{3.1}$$

This is commonly called the *error factor*.

To decide on the necessary size of the study, make a rough guess as to the likely value of R, select the precision that is required by specifying a value for f, the error factor, and calculate

$$e_2 = (1.96/\log_e f)^2 [(R + 1)/R], \tag{3.2}$$

where $\log_e f$ is the *natural logarithm* of f. The study size is then fixed so that the expected number of events in group 2 during the study period is equal to the calculated value e_2. The expected number of events in group 1 will be Re_2.

It should be noted that the above methods are only appropriate in the situation where each individual can experience only one event during the study period, or where the number of individuals experiencing multiple events is very small. If most individuals experience at least one event, and many experience two or more, it is preferable to define a *quantitative* outcome for each individual representing the number of events experienced during the study period, and to use the methods described in Section 3.4.

Example: In the mosquito-net trial, suppose the study groups are to consist of children aged 0–4 years, and that the death rate associated with malaria in the study area for that age group is estimated to be roughly 10 per 1000 child-years. If group 1 is the intervention group (treated bed-nets) and group 2 is the control group (no protection), R represents the ratio of the intervention and control death rates. Suppose R is expected to be about 0.4, corresponding to a reduction in the death rate of 60 per cent. Suppose also that f is selected to be equal to 1.25, so that the 95 per cent confidence interval for R is expected to extend from 0.4/ 1.25 = 0.32 to 0.4 × 1.25 = 0.50. In other words, it is desired to estimate the protective efficacy to within about 10 per cent of the true value (i.e. 50–68 per cent around the estimated efficacy of 60 per cent).

Then: $e_2 = [1.96/\log_e(1.25)]^2 (1.4/0.4) = 270$.

To expect 270 deaths in the control group, it would be necessary to observe an estimated 27 000 child-years [= 270/(10/1000)]. This could be achieved by following 54 000 children for 6 months, or 27 000 children for one year, or 13 500 for two years, and so on. The magnitude of the required study size (27 000 child-years of observation *in each group*) illustrates that when rare events are being studied very large samples are needed to obtain a precise estimate of the impact of an intervention.

3.3 Comparison of proportions

In this section outcomes are considered that are *binary* (yes or no) variables. This includes cumulative incidence or *risk*, for example, the proportion of children experiencing at least one episode of clinical malaria during the follow-up period. It also includes examination of the *prevalence* of some characteristic; for example, the presence of a palpable spleen in a survey conducted at the end of the study.

Suppose the true proportions in groups 1 and 2 are p_1 and p_2 respectively, giving a risk ratio (sometimes called the relative risk) of $R = p_1/p_2$. The approximate 95 per cent confidence interval for

R extends from R/f to Rf where, in this case, the factor f is given by:

$$f = \exp(1.96 \sqrt{\{[(1 - p_1)/(np_1)] + [(1 - p_2)/(np_2)]\}}) \quad (3.3)$$

where n is the number of children in each group. The required value of f is chosen and rough estimates are made of the values of p_2 and R to enable the number required in each group, n, to be calculated as:

$$n = (1.96/\log_e f)^2 \{[(R + 1)/(Rp_2)] - 2\}. \quad (3.4)$$

Example: In the mosquito-net trial, one of the outcomes of interest is the prevalence of splenomegaly (the spleen rate) at the end of the study. Prior data from the study area suggest that in the control group a spleen rate of approximately 40 per cent would be expected. Suppose the intervention is expected to roughly halve the spleen rate, so that $R = 0.5$, and an estimate of R is wanted to within about 0.15. This suggests setting f to about 1.3 [because then the upper 95 per cent confidence limit on R is $Rf = 0.5 \times 1.3 = 0.65$ which is 0.15 above R ($= 0.5$)], and thus $n = (1.96/\log_e 1.3)^2 \{[1.5/(0.5 \times 0.4)] - 2\} = 307$, so that around 300 children would need to be studied in each group.

3.4 Comparison of means

Quantitative outcomes may be analysed by comparing the means of the relevant variable in the intervention and control groups. This could be the mean of the values recorded at a cross-sectional survey, for example, the mean weight of study children at the end of the survey. Alternatively, it could be the mean of the changes recorded between baseline and follow-up surveys, for example, the mean change in weight (or weight velocity; i.e. the change in weight divided by the time between the two measurements) among the study children.

Suppose the true means in groups 1 and 2 are μ_1 and μ_2. These would generally be compared in terms of the difference in the means, $D = \mu_1 - \mu_2$. The 95 per cent confidence interval for D is given by $D \pm f$, where

$$f = 1.96 \sqrt{[(\sigma_1^2 + \sigma_2^2)/n]} \quad (3.5)$$

where σ_1 and σ_2 are the standard deviations of the outcome variable in the two groups. An acceptable value of f is chosen, values of σ_1 and σ_2 are selected, and the required number in each group is calculated as:

$$n = (1.96/f)^2 \, (\sigma_1{}^2 + \sigma_2{}^2). \tag{3.6}$$

An estimate of the standard deviation of the outcome variable is often available from other studies. It is usually reasonable to assume that the standard deviation will be roughly similar in the two study groups. If no other estimate is available, a rough approximation can be obtained by taking one-quarter of the likely range of the variable.

Example: In the mosquito-net trial, another outcome of interest is the packed cell volume (PCV) measured in blood samples taken from the children at the end of the study. From previous data, the mean PCV in the control group is expected to be about 33.0 with a standard deviation of about 5.0 (the normal range is about 33 ± 10 and it has been assumed that the normal range covers 4 standard deviations). An increase in mean PCV in the intervention group is expected of between 2.0 and 3.0, and it is required to estimate the difference D between the two groups to within about 0.5, so that $f = 0.5$. Assuming that the standard deviation is about 5.0 in both groups:

$$n = (1.96/0.5)^2 \, (5.0^2 + 5.0^2) = 768.$$

4   SIZE TO GIVE ADEQUATE POWER

4.1 Introduction

The alternative approach is now considered of selecting the study size to achieve a specified *power*. In order to do this the following must be specified:

1. How large a difference, D, between the two groups there would have to be in order to have a good chance of obtaining a significant result, and thus concluding that there is a real difference. D is the *true* difference between the two groups, not the estimated difference as measured in the study. Very small differences are generally of no public health importance, and it would not be of concern if they were not detected in the study. The

general principle, in most cases, is to choose D to be the *minimum difference* which would be regarded as being of public health relevance, and which it would therefore be important to detect in a study. Note that 'detecting' D means that a significant difference is obtained, indicating that there is some difference between the two groups. This does not mean that the difference is estimated precisely. To ensure a precise estimate is obtained, the approach of Section 3 should be used.

2. Having specified D, the investigators must decide how confident they wish to be of obtaining a significant result if this were the true difference between the groups. In other words, the *power* is set for this value of D. Note that if the difference between the groups is actually larger than D, the power of the study will be larger than the value set. The required power is specified in the calculations by choosing the corresponding value of z_2, as shown in Table 3.1. Commonly chosen values for the power are 80, 90 and 95 per cent, the corresponding values of z_2 being 0.84, 1.28, and 1.64. It would generally be regarded as unsatisfactory to proceed with a study with a power of less than 70 per cent for the main outcome.

3. The significance level must also be specified for the comparison of the two groups under study. This is entered into the calculations in terms of the parameter z_1. The most common choice for

Table 3.1. Relationship between z_2 and % power (Numbers in the body of table show power corresponding to each value of z_2)

z_2	First decimal place of z_2									
	0.0	0.1	0.2	0.3	0.4	0.5	0.6	0.7	0.8	0.9
−3.0	0.1	0.1	0.1	0.0	0.0	0.0	0.0	0.0	0.0	0.0
−2.0	2.3	1.8	1.4	1.1	0.8	0.6	0.5	0.3	0.3	0.2
−1.0	15.9	13.6	11.5	9.7	8.1	6.7	5.5	4.5	3.6	2.9
−0.0	50.0	46.0	42.1	38.2	34.5	30.9	27.4	24.2	21.2	18.4
+0.0	50.0	54.0	57.9	61.8	65.5	69.1	72.6	75.8	78.8	81.6
+1.0	84.1	86.4	88.5	90.3	91.9	93.3	94.5	95.5	96.4	97.1
+2.0	97.7	98.2	98.6	98.9	99.2	99.4	99.5	99.7	99.7	99.8
+3.0	99.9	99.9	99.9	100.0	100.0	100.0	100.0	100.0	100.0	100.0

(Note: for example $z_2 = -0.07$ corresponds to a power of 24.2 per cent)

the required p value is 0.05, corresponding to a z_1 of 1.96. Alternative values might be 0.01 or 0.001, corresponding to z_1 values of 2.58 or 3.29, respectively. It is assumed throughout this chapter that *two-sided* significance tests are to be used (see Chapter 14, Section 2.3). A significance level of 0.05 is assumed in the numerical examples unless otherwise stated.

4. In addition, certain additional information must be specified, which varies according to the type of measure being examined. This may be a rough estimate of the rates or proportions that are expected, or an estimate of the standard deviation for a quantitative variable. Note that if these quantities were known exactly, no study would be needed! Only rough estimates are required.

Having specified these values, the formulae or tables given below can be used to calculate the required study size. It is often useful, however, to proceed in the opposite direction; that is, to explore the power that would be achieved for a range of possible study sizes, and for a range of possible values for the true difference D. This enables the construction of *power curves* as illustrated in Fig. 3.1. Formulae for this approach are also given below.

4.2 Comparison of incidence rates

For a specified difference $D = r_1 - r_2$ and values of z_1 and z_2 representing the required significance level and power as explained in Section 4.1, the required study size is given by

$$y = [(z_1 + z_2)^2 \, (r_1 + r_2)]/(r_1 - r_2)^2 \qquad (3.7)$$

A rough estimate of the average of the two rates is therefore required [i.e. $(r_1 + r_2)/2$]. y gives the required person-years of observation in each group. For 90 per cent power and significance at $p < 0.05$, this simplifies to

$$y = [10.5(r_1 + r_2)]/(r_1 - r_2)^2. \qquad (3.8)$$

An alternative but equivalent formula gives the number of events required in group 2 in terms of the relative risk R for which the specified power is required.

$$e_2 = [(z_1 + z_2)^2 \, (1 + R)]/(1 - R)^2 \qquad (3.9)$$

This formula was used to construct Table 3.2, which shows the

Table 3.2. Sample size requirements for comparison of rates. (Numbers in the body of the table are expected number of events required in Group 2 to give specified power if relative rate in Group 1 is R)

Relative Rate, R*	Expected events in Group 2 to give†		
	80% power	90% power	95% power
0.1	10.6	14.3	17.6
0.2	14.7	19.7	24.3
0.3	20.8	27.9	34.4
0.4	30.5	40.8	50.4
0.5	47.0	63.0	77.8
0.6	78.4	105.0	129.6
0.7	148.1	198.3	244.8
0.8	352.8	472.4	583.2
0.9	1489.6	1994.5	2462.4
1.1	1646.4	2204.5	2721.6
1.2	431.2	577.4	712.8
1.4	117.6	157.5	194.4
1.6	56.6	75.8	93.6
1.8	34.3	45.9	56.7
2.0	23.5	31.5	38.9
2.5	12.2	16.3	20.2
3.0	7.8	10.5	13.0
5.0	2.9	3.9	4.9
10.0	1.1	1.4	1.8

* R = Ratio of incidence rate in Group 1 to incidence rate in Group 2.
† Using a two-sided significance test with $p < 0.05$. The two groups are assumed to be of equal size.

number of events needed in group 1 to detect a relative risk of R with 80, 90 or 95 per cent power.

To calculate the power for a given study size, compute:

$$z_2 = \{\sqrt{[n/(r_1 + r_2)]}\}(|r_1 - r_2|) - z_1 \qquad (3.10)$$

where $|r_1 - r_2|$ is the absolute value of the difference between the two rates. Refer the resulting value of z_2 to Table 3.1 to determine the power of the study.

Example: Assume once again in the mosquito-net trial that the death rate from malaria in the control group is 10/1000 child-years, so that $r_2 = 0.010$. 80 per cent power is wanted to detect a significant effect if the true rate in children with bed-nets is reduced by 70 per cent to $r_1 = 0.003$. The number of child-years of observation required in each group is given by:

$$y = [(1.96 + 0.84)^2 (0.003 + 0.010)] / (-0.007)^2 = 2080.$$

The power curves shown in Fig. 3.1 were constructed using the same assumption concerning the death rate in controls. For example, with $y = 2000$, and a relative risk of $R = 0.7$ (corresponding to a death rate of 7 per 1000 child-years in the intervention group)

$$z_2 = \{\sqrt{[2000 / (0.007 + 0.010)]}\}(|0.007 - 0.010|) - 1.96 = -0.93$$

giving a power of 18 per cent (see Table 3.1).

4.3 Comparison of proportions

The study size required in each group to detect a specified difference $D = p_1 - p_2$ with power specified by z_2 and significance level specified by z_1 is given by:

$$n = [(z_1 + z_2)^2 2\bar{p}(1 - \bar{p})] / (p_1 - p_2)^2 \qquad (3.11)$$

where $\bar{p}$ is the average of p_1 and p_2. For 90 per cent power and significance at $p < 0.05$ this simplifies to:

$$n = [21\bar{p}(1 - \bar{p})] / (p_1 - p_2)^2. \qquad (3.12)$$

Table 3.3 shows the required study size for a range of values of p_1 and p_2 for 80, 90 or 95 per cent power.

To calculate the power of a study of specified size, calculate

$$z_2 = (\sqrt{\{n / [2\bar{p}(1 - \bar{p})]\}})(|p_1 - p_2|) - z_1 \qquad (3.13)$$

and refer the value of z_2 to Table 3.1.

Example: Assume that the spleen rate in the control group of the mosquito-net trial is around 40 per cent. To have high power (say 95 per cent) of detecting a significant effect if the intervention reduces the spleen rate to 30 per cent (i.e. $\bar{p} = 0.35$) the number of children required in each group is given by:

$$n = [(1.96 + 1.64)^2 (2 \times 0.35 \times 0.65)] / (0.3 - 0.4)^2 = 590.$$

4.4 Comparison of means

The study size required in each group to detect a specified

Table 3.3. Sample size requirements for comparison of proportions (Shown in the body of the table are the sample sizes required in each group to give the specified power*)

Smaller prop. p_1	Difference $D = p_2 - p_1$											
	0.05	0.10	0.15	0.20	0.25	0.30	0.35	0.40	0.45	0.50	0.55	0.60
0.05	435	141	76	50	36	28	22	18	15	13	11	10
	583	189	102	67	48	37	30	25	21	18	15	13
	719	233	126	83	60	46	37	30	26	22	19	16
0.10	686	200	101	63	44	33	26	21	17	14	12	10
	919	268	135	84	59	44	34	28	23	19	16	14
	1134	330	166	104	72	54	42	34	28	24	20	17
0.15	906	251	122	74	50	37	28	22	18	15	13	11
	1212	336	163	98	67	49	38	30	24	20	17	14
	1497	415	201	122	83	60	46	37	30	25	21	18
0.20	1094	294	139	82	55	40	30	24	19	16	13	11
	1464	394	186	110	74	53	40	31	25	21	17	15
	1808	486	230	136	91	66	50	39	31	26	21	18
0.25	1250	329	153	89	59	42	31	24	19	16	13	11
	1674	441	205	119	79	56	42	32	26	21	17	14
	2067	544	253	147	97	69	52	40	32	26	21	18
0.30	1376	357	163	94	61	43	32	24	19	16	13	10
	1842	478	219	126	82	58	43	33	26	21	17	14
	2274	590	270	156	101	71	53	40	32	26	21	17

Table 3.3. (*continued*)

Smaller prop. p_1	Difference $D = p_2 - p_1$											
	0.05	0.10	0.15	0.20	0.25	0.30	0.35	0.40	0.45	0.50	0.55	0.60
0.35	1470	376	170	97	63	44	32	24	19	15	12	10
	1968	504	228	130	84	58	43	32	25	20	16	13
	2430	622	282	160	103	72	53	40	31	25	20	16
0.40	1533	388	174	98	63	43	31	24	18	14	11	
	2052	520	233	131	84	58	42	31	24	19	15	
	2534	642	287	162	103	71	52	39	30	24	19	
0.45	1564	392	174	97	61	42	30	22	17	13		
	2094	525	233	130	82	56	40	30	23	18		
	2586	648	287	160	101	69	50	37	28	22		
0.50	1564	388	170	94	59	40	28	21	15			
	2094	520	228	126	79	53	38	28	21			
	2586	642	282	156	97	66	46	34	26			
0.55	1533	376	163	89	55	37	26	18				
	2052	504	219	119	74	49	34	25				
	2534	622	270	147	91	60	42	30				

0.60	1470 / 1968 / 2430	357 / 478 / 590	153 / 205 / 253	82 / 110 / 136	50 / 67 / 83	33 / 44 / 54	22 / 30 / 37
0.65	1376 / 1842 / 2274	329 / 441 / 544	139 / 186 / 230	73 / 98 / 121	44 / 59 / 72	28 / 37 / 46	
0.70	1250 / 1674 / 2067	294 / 394 / 486	122 / 163 / 201	63 / 84 / 104	36 / 48 / 60		
0.75	1094 / 1464 / 1808	251 / 336 / 415	101 / 135 / 166	50 / 67 / 83			
0.80	906 / 1212 / 1497	200 / 268 / 330	76 / 102 / 126				
0.85	686 / 919 / 1134	141 / 189 / 233					
0.90	435 / 583 / 719						

* Upper figure: power = 80 per cent; Middle figure: power = 90 per cent; Lower figure: power = 95 per cent. Using a two-sided significance test with $p < 0.05$. The two groups are assumed to be of equal size.

difference $D = \mu_1 - \mu_2$ with power specified by z_2 and significance level specified by z_1 is given by:

$$n = [(z_1 + z_2)^2 \, (\sigma_1^2 + \sigma_2^2)] / (\mu_1 - \mu_2)^2, \qquad (3.14)$$

where σ_1 and σ_2 are the standard deviations of the outcome variable in groups 1 and 2 respectively. For 90 per cent power and significance at $p < 0.05$ this simplifies to:

$$n = 10.5(\sigma_1^2 + \sigma_2^2) / (\mu_1 - \mu_2)^2. \qquad (3.15)$$

To calculate the power of a study of specified size, calculate

$$z_2 = \{\sqrt{[n / (\sigma_1^2 + \sigma_2^2)]}\}(|\mu_1 - \mu_2|) - z_1 \qquad (3.16)$$

and refer the value of z_2 to Table 3.1.

Example: In the mosquito-net trial, the mean PCV in the control group at the end of the study is expected to be 33.0 with a standard deviation of 5.0. To have 90 per cent power of detecting a significant effect if the intervention increases the mean PCV by 1.5, the number of children required in each group is given by:

$$n = [(1.96 + 1.28)^2 \, (5.0^2 + 5.0^2)] / (1.5)^2 = 233.$$

Suppose it turns out that only 150 children are available for study in each group. The power in these circumstances is given by:

$$z_2 = \{\sqrt{[150 / (5.0^2 + 5.0^2)]}\}(|\,1.5\,|) - 1.96 = 0.64$$

corresponding to a power of about 74 per cent.

A summary of the various formulae that have been given above for calculating the study size requirements for the comparison of two groups of equal size is given in Table 3.4.

5 MORE COMPLEX DESIGNS

5.1 Two groups of unequal size

Sections 3 and 4 considered the simplest situation, where the two groups to be compared are of equal size. Sometimes, there may be reasons for wishing to allocate more individuals to one group than to the other. For example, if an experimental drug is very expensive, it may be desired to minimize the number of patients allocated to the drug, and so the trial may be arranged so that there are two or three patients given the old drug for every patient given the new drug. In order to maintain the same power as in the equal allocation scheme, a larger total study size will be needed, but the number given the new drug will be smaller.

Let the size of the smaller of the two groups be n_1, and suppose the ratio of the two sample sizes to be k, so that there will be kn_1 individuals in the other group $(k > 1)$. Then, to achieve approximately the same power and precision as in a study with an equal number n in each group, n_1 should be chosen as:

$$n_1 = n(k + 1)/(2k). \qquad (3.17)$$

Examples are shown in Table 3.5 for various values of k. Notice that the number allocated to the smaller group can never be reduced below half the number required with equal groups. Little is gained by increasing k beyond 3 or 4, since beyond this point, even a substantial increase in n_2 achieves only a small reduction in n_1.

5.2 Comparison of more than two groups

Field trials comparing two groups (for example, intervention and control, or treatment A and treatment B) are by far the most common. However, in some trials three or more groups may be compared. For example, in a trial of a new vaccine, there may be four trial groups receiving different doses of the vaccine. It is unusual for field trials to have more than four groups because of logistical difficulties, or often because of study size limitations.

It is suggested that in designing a trial with three or more groups, the investigator should decide which pair-wise comparisons between groups are of central interest. The methods of Sections 3 and 4 can then be used to decide on the study size required in each group.

6 INTERVENTIONS ALLOCATED TO GROUPS

The methods described in Sections 3 to 5 all assume that *individuals* are to be the *units of allocation*. In other words, the study

Table 3.4. Summary of formulae for calculating study size requirements for comparison of two groups of equal size.

Type of outcome	Formula	Notation	Section in text
A: Choosing study size to achieve adequate precision			
Rates:	$e_2 = (1.96/\log_e f)^2 (R+1)/R$	e_2 = Expected events in group 2 R = Rate in group 1/Rate in group 2 Gives 95 per cent CI from R/f to Rf	3.2
Proportions:	$n = (1.96/\log_e f)^2 [(R+1)/(Rp_2) - 2]$	n = Number in each group R = Prop. in group 1/Prop. in group 2 p_2 = Prop. in group 2 Gives 95 per cent CI from R/f to Rf	3.3

Means:

$$n = (1.96/f)^2(\sigma_1^2 + \sigma_2^2)$$ 3.4

n = Number in each group
σ_i = SD in group i
D = Mean in group 1 – Mean in group 2
Gives 95 per cent CI of $D \pm f$

B: Choosing study size to achieve adequate power

Rates:

$$y = (z_1 + z_2)^2(r_1 + r_2)/(r_1 - r_2)^2$$ 4.2

y = Person-years in each group
r_i = Rate in group i

Proportions:

$$n = (z_1 + z_2)^2 2\bar{p}(1 - \bar{p})/(p_1 - p_2)^2$$ 4.3

n = Number in each group
p_i = Proportion in group i
$\bar{p}$ = Average of p_1 and p_2

Means:

$$n = (z_1 + z_2)^2(\sigma_1^2 + \sigma_2^2)/(\mu_1 - \mu_2)^2$$ 4.4

n = Number in each group
σ_i = SD in group i
μ_i = Mean in group i

$z_1 = 1.96$ for significance at $p < 0.05$

Power	80%	90%	95%
z_2	0.84	1.28	1.64

Table 3.5.   Study sizes necessary to achieve approximately the same power in a trial with two groups, one of which contains k times as many individuals as the other

k	n_1	n_2	$n_1 + n_2$
1	n	n	$2n$
2	$0.75n$	$1.5n$	$2.25n$
3	$0.67n$	$2.0n$	$2.67n$
4	$0.62n$	$2.5n$	$3.12n$
5	$0.60n$	$3.0n$	$3.60n$
10	$0.55n$	$5.5n$	$6.05n$
100	$0.50n$	$50.0n$	$50.50n$

groups will be constructed by making a complete list of the individuals available for study, and randomly selecting which individuals are to be allocated to each study group. As explained in Chapters 1 and 2, however, many field trials are not organized in this way. Instead, *groups of individuals* are allocated to the interventions under study. These groups are called *communities* in this section, because in practice they often correspond to villages, hamlets, or defined sectors of an urban area.

If interventions are allocated to communities in this way, the community should also be used as the unit of analysis, even though assessments of outcome are made on individuals in the communities (see Chapter 14, Section 7). For example, suppose the mosquito-net trial is to be conducted as follows. A number of villages (say 20) are to be randomly divided into two equal-sized groups. In the 10 villages in the first group, the entire population of each village will be given mosquito-nets, while the second group of 10 villages will serve as controls. The analysis of the impact of mosquito-nets on the incidence of clinical malaria would be made by calculating the (age-adjusted) incidence rate in each village, and comparing the 10 rates for the intervention villages with the 10 rates for the control villages. This would be achieved by treating the (adjusted) rate as the quantitative outcome measured for each village, and comparing these using the unpaired *t*-test (Chapter 14, Section 4.2) or the non-parametric rank sum test (Chapter 14, Section 7.2). If analysing proportions rather than incidence rates, the principle is the same: the (age-adjusted) proportion would be treated as the quantitative outcome for each community.

When allocation is by community, the study size formulae (3.7) and (3.11) have to be adjusted to allow for intrinsic variation between communities. Suppose first that incidence rates in the two groups are to be compared. The required number of communities, c, is given by:

$$c = 1 + (z_1 + z_2)^2[(r_1 + r_2)/y + k^2(r_1^2 + r_2^2)]/(r_1 - r_2)^2 \quad (3.18)$$

In this formula, y is the person-years of observation in each community, while r_1 and r_2 are the average rates in the intervention and control communities respectively. The intrinsic variation between communities is measured by k, the *coefficient of variation* of the (true) incidence rates among the communities in each group, and is defined as the standard deviation of the rates divided by the average rate. The value of k is assumed similar in the intervention and control

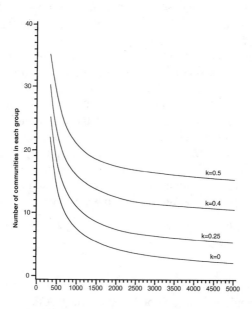

Fig. 3.2 Number of communities required in each group in a trial of the effect of mosquito nets against clinical malaria, according to the number of child-weeks of observation in each community and the extent of variation in rates of clinical malaria between communities (k is the coefficient of variation of the incidence rates—see text). The average incidence rate of clinical malaria in the absence of the intervention is assumed to be 10 per 1000 weeks of observation and the trial is required to have 90 per cent power to detect a 50 per cent reduction in the incidence of malaria at the $p < 0.05$ level of statistical significance.

groups, so that the *relative variability* remains the same following intervention.

If proportions are to be compared, the required number of communities is given by:

$$c = 1 + (z_1 + z_2)^2[2p(1-p)/n + k^2(p_1^2 + p_2^2)]/(p_1-p_2)^2 \quad (3.19)$$

In this formula, n is the study size in each community, p_1 and p_2 are the average proportions in the intervention and control groups, respectively, p is the average of p_1 and p_2, and k is the coefficient of variation of the (true) proportions among the communities in each group.

An estimate of k will sometimes be available from previous data on the same communities or from a pilot study. If no data are available, it may be necessary to make an arbitrary but plausible assumption about the value of k. For example, $k = 0.25$ implies that the true rates in each group vary roughly between $r_i \pm 2kr_i$, that is between $0.5r_i$ and $1.5r_i$. In general, k is unlikely to exceed 0.5.

Example: Suppose the mosquito-net trial is to be conducted by allocating the intervention at the village level, as described above. The incidence rate of clinical malaria among children before intervention is 10 per 1000 child-weeks of observation, and the study is to be designed to give 90 per cent power if the intervention reduces the incidence rate by 50 per cent. There are about 50 eligible children per village, and it is intended to continue follow-up for one year, so that y is approximately 2500 child-weeks. No information is available on between-village variation in incidence rates. Taking $k = 0.25$, the number of villages required per group is given by:

$$\begin{aligned}c &= 1 + (1.96 + 1.28)^2[(0.01 + 0.005)/2500 + 0.25^2(0.01^2 + 0.005^2)]/ \\ &\quad (0.01 - 0.005)^2 \\ &= 6.8\end{aligned}$$

so that roughly seven villages would be needed in each group. Note that this would give a total of 17 500 child-weeks of observation in each group, compared with 6300 child-weeks if it were possible to randomize individual children to receive mosquito-nets. Figure 3.2 shows the number of villages required in each group depending on the child-weeks of observation per village and the value of k.

Are any general results available regarding the effect of group allocation on the total study size needed? If there is no heterogeneity between communities in the outcome of interest, in the sense that the variation between the community-specific rates or means is no more

than would be expected to occur by chance due to sampling variations, the total study size will be approximately the *same* as if the
interventions were allocated to individuals. For most outcomes,
however, there will be real differences between communities, and in
these circumstances the required study size will be *greater* than with
individual allocation. The ratio of the required study sizes with
community and individual allocation is sometimes called the *design
effect*. Unfortunately, no single value for the design effect can be
assumed, as its value depends on the variability of the outcome of
interest between communities, and on the sizes of the communities,
and so it is recommended that the required sample size is estimated
explicitly as explained above.

Note that even if the calculations suggest that less than four communities are required in each group, it is preferable to have at least
four in each group, if possible. With so few units of observation, the
use of non-parametric procedures such as the rank sum test is generally preferred for the analysis, and a sample size of at least four in
each group is needed to have any chance of obtaining a significant
result when this test is used.

It may be possible to reduce the required number of communities
by adopting a matched design, as described in Chapter 2. For example, this can be done by using the baseline study to arrange the communities into pairs in which the rates of the outcome in interest are
similar, and randomly selecting one member of each pair to receive
the intervention. However, it is difficult to quantify the effect of this
approach on the number of communities required. To do this, information is required on the variability of the treatment effect between
communities, and on the extent to which the baseline data are predictive of the rates that would be observed during the follow-up period in
the absence of intervention, and this information is rarely available.
With a paired design, at least six communities are required in each
group in order to be able to obtain a significant difference using a non-
parametric statistical test.

7 OTHER FACTORS INFLUENCING CHOICE OF STUDY SIZE

7.1 Allowance for interim analyses

It is sometimes desirable to incorporate interim analyses into the study
plan, involving review of the results at (say) six-monthly or

annual intervals. If an interim analysis indicates that there is already strong evidence of the superiority of one of the interventions under study, the trial can be terminated in order that participants are no longer subjected to a regime which is known to be inferior. The incorporation of interim analyses may be particularly valuable if the trial is planned to continue for several years, with the gradual accumulation of cases of the outcome of interest, or if individuals or communities are entered into the trial sequentially.

There are also disadvantages in carrying out interim analyses, however. If the trial is terminated early, because the intervention appears to be beneficial, there may be no opportunity of detecting any long-term side-effects or other adverse consequences of the intervention. Also, although a significant effect of the intervention may be demonstrated, the precision of the estimates of effect may be too low to be of much value.

If, after careful consideration, it is decided that interim analyses are to be conducted, these need to be planned for in the study design, for two reasons. First, if such analyses are done, it is necessary to employ a more stringent significance level for each analysis to maintain the same overall level of significance. Second, to maintain the same power and precision as in a study without interim analyses, a greater maximum study size is needed, although the expected study size will be reduced, because of the possibility of early termination if there is a substantial effect.

Details of the implications of interim analyses are given by Geller and Pocock (1987). As a rough guide, the following approach is suggested. It is rarely advantageous to plan for more than three or four interim analyses. It is recommended, therefore, that for studies planned to continue for 2–4 years, the study plan should include two interim analyses (plus the final analysis). To compensate for this, the maximum study size (i.e. the maximum person-years of observation if the study proceeds to completion) should be increased by about 15 per cent. A stringent significance level of $p < 0.01$ should be used at each interim analysis to decide whether or not the trial should be terminated. This means that if the trial proceeds to completion, a significance level of $p < 0.04$ can be used for the final analysis, only a little more stringent than the overall significance level of $p < 0.05$.

7.2 Allowance for losses

Losses to follow-up occur in most longitudinal studies. Individuals may be lost because they move away from the study area, because they die from some cause unrelated to the outcome of interest, because they refuse to continue with the study, because they are away from home at the time of a follow-up survey, or for some other reason.

Losses like these are of concern for two reasons. First, they are a possible source of *bias*, as the individuals who are lost often differ in important respects from those who remain in the study. Second, they reduce the size of the sample available for analysis, and this decreases the power or precision of the study.

For these reasons it is important to make every attempt to reduce the number of losses to a minimum. However, it is rarely possible to avoid losses completely. The extent of the problem will vary according to circumstances but, as a rough guide, in a longitudinal study of a rural community with two-years of follow-up, losses of at least 20 per cent might be expected.

The reduced power or precision resulting from losses may be avoided by increasing the initial sample size in order to compensate for the expected number of losses. For example, if sample size calculations suggest that 240 subjects are required, and a 20 per cent loss rate is expected, the sample size should be increased to 300 (because 80 per cent of 300 gives 240).

8   THE CONSEQUENCES OF STUDIES THAT ARE TOO SMALL

The methods outlined in this chapter for selecting an adequate sample size have been available for many years, but it is probably not an exaggeration to say that the majority of intervention trials are much too small. Although there is an increasing awareness of the need to take a large enough sample, this chapter is concluded by discussing the consequences of choosing a sample size that is too small.

Suppose first that the intervention under study has little or no effect on the outcome of interest. The difference observed in a study is likely, therefore, to be non-significant. However, the width of the confidence interval for the effect measure (for example, the relative risk) will depend on the sample size. If the sample is small, the confidence interval will be very wide, and so even though it will probably include the null value (a zero difference between the groups, or a relative risk of 1), it will extend to include large values of the effect measure. In other words, the study will have failed to establish that the intervention has no appreciable effect. For example, in the mosquito-net trial, suppose only 50 children were included in each group, and suppose the observed spleen rates in the two groups were identical at 40 per cent, giving an estimated relative risk of $R = 1$. The approximate 95 per cent confidence interval for R would extend from 0.62–1.62 (see Section 3.3). Now a relative risk of 0.62 would imply a very substantial effect, for example a reduction in the spleen rate from 40 per cent to 25 per cent, and a small trial would be unable to exclude such an effect. If the sample size in each group were increased to 500, the 95 per cent confidence interval would extend only from 0.86–1.16, a much narrower interval.

Suppose that the intervention does have an appreciable effect. A study that is too small will have low power; i.e. it will have little chance of giving a statistically significant difference. In other words there is little chance of being able to demonstrate that the intervention has an effect. In the example, if the true effect of the intervention is to reduce the spleen rate from 40 per cent to 25 per cent, a sample size of 50 in each group would give a power of only 36 per cent. 205 children would be needed in each group to give a 90 per cent power (see Table 3.3). Even if a significant difference is found, the confidence interval on the effect will still be very wide, so there will be uncertainty at the end of the study whether the effect of the intervention is small and unimportant, or very large and of major importance.

The conduct of trials that are too small has consequences extending beyond the results of the specific trial. There is considerable evidence that studies showing large effects are more likely to be published than those showing little or no effect. Suppose a number of small trials of a specific intervention are conducted. Because of the large sampling error implied by small sample sizes, a few of these trials will produce estimates of the effect of the intervention that are much larger than the true effect. These trials are more likely to be published, and the result is that the findings in the literature are likely to overestimate considerably the true effects of interventions. This *publication bias* is much smaller for larger trials, because an adequate sample size means that such trials will give results that are much closer to the true effect and, in addition, a large trial showing little or no effect is more likely to be published than a small trial with a similar difference.

REFERENCES

Breslow, N. E. and Day N. E. (1987). *Statistical methods in cancer research. The design and analysis of cohort studies*, vol. II, pp. 272–314. International Agency for Research on Cancer, Lyon.

Geller, N. L. and Pocock, S. J. (1987). Interim analyses in randomized clinical trials: ramifications and guidelines for practitioners. *Biometrics*, **43**, 213–23.

4
Ethical considerations

1 INTRODUCTION

Ethical considerations are fundamental to the design of any research investigation involving human subjects. In most countries such research is not allowed unless the study protocol has satisfied a formal ethical review committee. All major grant-giving agencies require such review and may have an ethics committee of their own which must also approve the study plan and procedures. For both idealistic and pragmatic reasons it is important, therefore, that the ethical aspects of a study are considered from its inception and, for that reason, this chapter is placed early in the manual.

A basic assumption in this chapter is that it is difficult, and indeed dangerous, to lay down ethical rules that apply to all studies in all places. It is important that each study be judged in the context of the circumstances in which it will be conducted. A study that might be judged unethical in one place might be considered ethical in another, and both of these might be the 'right' decisions.

Most ethical issues arise from conflicts between competing sets of values. For example, the medical practitioner is dedicated to the provision of the best medical care for an individual who is his or her patient. However, this dedication may be in direct conflict with the public health goal of achieving maximum health benefits in a community with the limited resources available. Consuming large amounts of resources on one patient may deprive others in the community from benefit. The appropriate balance between benefit for the individual and benefit for the community of individuals depends very much on the particular situation. The conflict is most obvious in situations of poverty and deprivation; just those conditions in which tropical diseases flourish. Those conducting field trials of interventions against tropical diseases are likely, therefore, to be faced with especially difficult ethical dilemmas. Resolution of such dilemmas often depends upon where the investigators place their horizon of responsibility. On the one hand, if they consider that their responsibility is confined to the trial participants, as tends to be the case in many clinical trials, then studies to resolve some of the most important public health issues might be viewed as unethical. For example, to assess the likely public health impact of an intervention it may be desirable to continue a trial beyond the point when it is established that one intervention is superior to another in order to obtain a better estimate of the magnitude of the beneficial effect. On the other hand, if the horizon of responsibility is extended to the entire population to which the intervention might some time be applied, as it is anticipated will be the case for many of the readers of this manual, then the failure to conduct such trials would be unethical. For example, it may be unethical to stop a trial when one intervention is shown to be superior to another while there is still a wide confidence interval on the estimate of the magnitude of the beneficial effect. This issue is discussed further in Section 4.2.

After briefly outlining generally accepted ethical principles concerning research on human subjects, in Section 2, this chapter focuses upon those issues that are of particular concern in the conduct of field research in developing countries (Section 3), with special attention to issues related to field trials (Section 4). In the final section there is a discussion of the various levels at which ethical review takes place with respect to a particular investigation.

2 ACCEPTED ETHICAL PRINCIPLES CONCERNING RESEARCH ON HUMAN SUBJECTS

The ethical principles that are involved in medical research involving humans are well described in the 'Declaration of Helsinki, 1975'. They are reproduced and have been further elaborated, with special reference to developing countries, in the 'Proposed International Guidelines for Biomedical Research Involving Human Subjects' (CIOMS 1982). The main principles, with some comments concerning their relationship to field research in developing countries, include the following:

2.1 Scientific merit

To be ethical, research must have scientific merit. The methods of the research should be appropriate to the aims of an investigation, and results from any relevant previous or ongoing research should be taken into account in its design. The investigator is obliged to design and conduct the research investigation in such a way that the results from the study are likely to provide answers to the questions being addressed. This includes attention to the appropriate size and duration of the study as well as to other aspects of its design. Furthermore, for research concerning interventions, achievement of the objectives must be linked, directly or indirectly, to some kind of action that is expected to lead to improved health.

2.2 Equitable selection of subjects

The potential benefits of research and the potential harm should be distributed equitably among communities and among individuals within communities. The economically and socially deprived are often at the highest risk of disease. There is, on the one hand, an imperative to ensure that the appropriate research is conducted in such groups and, on the other hand, an imperative to ensure that they are not exploited in research that will mainly benefit the more wealthy and privileged. For example, it would generally be deemed unacceptable to conduct a trial of a very expensive treatment in a deprived group unless it was expected that the cost of the treatment was likely to be reduced in the immediate future to a level that could be afforded by the community or that, even if there was no reduction in cost, the treatment would be made accessible to those in the community in which the trial was conducted should it be found to be efficaceous. Such treatment should not be restricted solely to those who had participated in the trial, but should also be provided to those in similar circumstances.

2.3 Informed consent

It has become an established principle that 'informed consent' must be obtained from all participants in a medical research investigation on human subjects. Special problems arise with respect to field trials in developing countries, however, in obtaining assurance that all individuals involved understand as fully as possible the nature of the study, the reasons it is being undertaken, and the possible benefit to them and their community as well as any possible harm they might suffer.

The use of a consent form that participants must sign in the presence of a witness is required to satisfy some ethics committees and grant-giving bodies, but it may offer little guarantee of protection to the subject, especially in communities where many are not literate. Such written forms do formalize the consent procedure, however, and they force an investigator to document the nature of the explanation about the investigation that will be given to study subjects. It is *always* the investigator's responsibility to ensure that subjects are fully informed of the potential risks and benefits of participation in a study.

Special provisions must be made for potential participants who are not competent to provide informed consent, such as children. A child requires an advocate who is legally and morally responsible for decisions taken on his or her behalf. Even when the advocate provides consent, the subject should have the right to refuse; but in practice it may be difficult, for example, for a child to exercise that right. In general, research procedures should not be conducted on children unless they have already been demonstrated to be safe in adults and, if appropriate, efficacious in adults also.

The information provided to obtain informed consent in a trial would be expected to include the following (after Cowan 1982):

1. A statement that the activity involves an experiment.

2. An explanation of the scope, aims, and purpose of the research.

3. A description of any reasonably forseeable harm and the possible level of risk.

4. A description of likely or expected benefits.

5. A disclosure of appropriate alternate procedures, courses of treatment, or preventive strategies that might be advantageous; this might be expected to include an explanation about medical treatment and its availability for the condition under study.

6. A statement that subjects will be notified of new information developing in the course of research that might affect their participation.

7. A statement about how confidentiality will be maintained.

8. An offer to answer questions.

9. An explanation about medical treatment and care for research-related injury.

10. A statement that participation is voluntary and refusal to participate will involve no penalty and that the subject can withdraw consent at any time.

The check-list above was drawn up in the context of trials in developed countries, but the same principles apply for trials in developing countries. In the latter, however, it may be necessary to go to some lengths to give the required explanations in ways that will be comprehensible in the context of the local attitudes and beliefs in the communities in which the trial will be undertaken.

2.4 Confidentiality

The confidentiality of all information collected in a research investigation must be maintained and only released to others with the explicit consent of all those concerned. The proportion of individuals who agree to participate in a study, especially one in which sensitive information is being collected (for example, whether or not an individual is infected with the human immunodeficiency virus), may be increased if careful explanations are given as to how confidentiality will be maintained and who within the study team will have access to such information. For example, in some studies it may be appropriate to identify individuals on record forms by a code number only, with the list linking names to the codes being kept separately in a secure place.

2.5 Coercion

In general, there are fewer legal and institutional safeguards to protect the rights of individuals in developing countries than there are in most developed countries. When research workers are employed by, or identified with, the State authorities, or with those who provide medical care, there is a danger that they might be tempted to exploit this position, with greater or lesser degrees of subtlety, to coerce subjects to participate in a study. Coercion and deception, even when rationalized as being for the 'greater good', are unacceptable. Full and open explanations of all study procedures may be time consuming, but this is the only acceptable approach.

3 FIELD TRIALS IN DEVELOPING COUNTRIES

In general, it is easier to persuade those who are sick than those who are well to participate in a medical research investigation. Field trials often involve those in the latter category (for example, trials of preventive measures) and, unlike most clinical trials, take place in a community rather than in a clinic or hospital. The task of obtaining consent for the conduct of a study in such a setting involves some special issues.

3.1 Obtaining communal consent

In some communities in many developing countries, decisions about participation in a particular project may be taken at a communal rather than a household or an individual level. Thus, permission to conduct a research project may be obtained through trusted and respected community leaders, rather than through individual community members or through the heads of households. Though such procedures may seem strange and would be unacceptable in many 'western' cultures, they are part of the cultural norm in other societies. Furthermore, it has been suggested that 'where individual members of a community do not have the necessary awareness of the implications of participation in an experiment to give adequately informed consent directly to the investigators, it is desirable that the decision whether or not to participate should be elicited through the intermediary of a trusted community leader' (CIOMS 1982).

In a clinical trial the investigator may be able to take considerable time to explain the nature of a study to each participant, as usually the total number of subjects in a study is small. Field trials of some interventions (for example, vaccines) may be large, sometimes involving thousands or tens of thousands of participants, and it may not be feasible to explain the trial in detail to all participants. In such circumstances different methods of obtaining informed consent may be appropriate. It is important, however, that those from whom 'communal consent' is sought are able to represent properly the participants and to protect their interests.

The initial approach to a community is likely to be best made to those recognized as leaders in the community. Generally, field trials are likely to be carried out by, or in direct co-operation with, the Ministry of Health and local health authorities and, in such circumstances, it will usually be appropriate for discussions with community leaders to be initiated by such authorities. The extent of such discussions, and precisely who within a community should be involved, depends on the nature of the intervention that is to be studied. Most communities are heterogeneous and sometimes there are factions within a community that have their own leaders whose co-operation must be sought. Those who are considered as the official leaders may not be recognized by the people, and others must be brought into discussions. Public notices and public meetings may also be useful.

It must be emphasized that obtaining communal consent for a study does not relieve investigators of their responsibility to explain the study procedures and the potential risks and benefits to those individuals who might participate, and those individuals must also be informed and be aware that they are free to refuse to participate or to withdraw from the investigation at any time without penalty of any kind.

3.2 Potential benefit and the risk of harm

The simple Hippocratic caveat to do no harm is not a satisfactory guide to ethical decisions concerning trials of interventions. The introduction of a new intervention requires the demonstration of benefit. Furthermore, since almost any intervention procedure involves some risk of harm, albeit often small, it is necessary to assess in intervention trials the balance of benefits against risks. In general, ethical review committees are disinclined to approve studies in which healthy persons will be exposed to more than very small risks in the context of a research investigation. Thus, it may be unacceptable to carry out a trial using a vaccine associated with serious side effects even if it offers protection against a disease which is more serious than the side-effects. For example, if two persons die as a result of vaccination for every ten persons who are saved from dying, it is unlikely that such a product would be used, even though the 'public health' balance appears to be in favour of the vaccine. More weight is given to harm that results from a deliberate medical intervention than is given to the harm done by the 'natural' disease against which the intervention protects. Furthermore, legal concerns of litigation may sometimes be given greater weight than would seem appropriate from a strictly public health viewpoint.

A proposed research investigation should be viewed within the context of the overall problems facing the community in which it is to be conducted. The community should have a reasonable expectation of benefiting from the research in both the short- and the long-term. The effects of the conduct of a field trial in a community may be immediate and evident or may be quite subtle. Even the mere presence of the research workers in a community will have side effects (for example, increased cash flow, availability of transport to other centres), and the impact of such effects should be considered in planning the research. The possibility of long-term harm must be considered even if there are short-term benefits. For example, if a greatly improved standard of health care is provided to a community during the course of a trial, there may be major problems created if this facility must be withdrawn from the community at the completion of the trial. During a trial it may be necessary to strengthen the local health care services in order to obtain information about the endpoints of interest in the study. When this is done, it is important to implement the strengthening in such a way that the effects will persist beyond the end of the study. This may involve the incorporation of some study procedures into the routine services (for example, training, improved record keeping). In general, the provision of health care for a community is the responsibility of the national or local health services and the research should not usurp nor undermine existing services. It is essential that the organizers of a field trial develop and maintain a close liaison with those responsible for the normal provision of health care.

3.3 Incentives

In some circumstances it may be reasonable to provide direct incentives as an encouragement to participation in a research project. If this is done, it must be recognized that there may be a fine dividing line between compensating individuals for time and income lost as a result of participation in the study and 'bribing' subjects to take part. In many circumstances it would be considered reasonable to give sweets or candy to children (or some more 'beneficial' reward!) after a blood sample has been taken, or to repay bus or taxi fares to participants who travel to a research centre, or to give simple medications for minor ailments, but monetary payments to encourage individuals to participate in a trial that are greater than the wages they forego or the expenses they incurred may be viewed as a form of coercion. It is difficult to lay down any absolute rules as to what is acceptable and it is necessary to review each situation on its merits in the local context.

3.4 Feedback of results

At the completion of an investigation there is a responsibility to inform the community of the results of the study in such a way that its members can understand the implications of the findings. Indeed, such feedback should be ongoing as the research progresses. Not only is it inherently reasonable that participants should be kept informed of the progress of the research, but if this is done it is also likely to encourage their continued participation. The procedures to ensure this feedback takes place should be planned from the start of an investigation.

There is also a responsibility to feedback the results of the research to the relevant local or national health services or disease control programmes, so that these groups can assess the implications of the findings for their own activities. These aspects are also discussed in Chapter 16.

3.5 Anonymity of communities

The same rights of confidentiality should apply to communities as to individuals. The members of a community in which a study has been conducted should have the right to see documents before publication and it may be appropriate to keep the identity of the community anonymous, particularly if sensitive areas of behaviour are discussed, such as hygienic practices. Sometimes it is not possible to disguise a particular location and in some circumstances it may be important that the community be identified to aid interpretation of the study results. Indeed, communities are sometimes proud to be associated with a particular research programme and the name of the community or place may be used as the title of the project [for example, the Garki malaria project (Molineaux and Gramiccia 1980)].

4 CONSIDERATIONS SPECIALLY RELEVANT TO INTERVENTION TRIALS

Trials of an intervention should be undertaken only when there is uncertainty about the balance of potential benefit and potential harm with respect to the intervention. The assessment of the extent of such uncertainty will be a critical factor in deciding whether or not it is justifiable to conduct a trial. If one trial provides good evidence of a beneficial effect, further trials of the same agent or procedure, even under very different epidemiological circumstances, will be more difficult to justify than if the first trial had not been conducted. Only if there are good reasons to believe that the results might be different under these different circumstances would further trials be indicated and, indeed, a case could be made that it would be unethical not to conduct a further trial in such circumstances.

In communities which are poor and deprived and whose inhabitants may be at substantial risk of premature death and serious disease from many causes, the balance between the potential benefits of an intervention and the risk of harm may be different from that which might apply in a more privileged community. For example, a higher level of vaccine-related adverse effects might be acceptable in a trial of a vaccine against a disease that was responsible for many deaths in a community than would be acceptable in a study in a community in which the disease was of smaller public health significance.

4.1 Choice of 'control' interventions

A generally accepted principle in the design of intervention trials is that any 'new' intervention should be compared with the intervention that is regarded as the 'best' currently available intervention at the time the trial starts. Comparison with a placebo is acceptable only if there is no convincing evidence that any intervention is effective. This principle must be interpreted, however, according to the circumstances prevailing in the proposed area for the trial and it may be important to take into account the comparative cost of different interventions. If an effective intervention is known, but its cost is beyond that which would make it feasible to introduce it into the local health care system, then it may well be acceptable to exclude it from consideration as a possible comparison intervention in a trial. In some circumstances it may be acceptable to try a new intervention that might be, at best, equivalent to an existing intervention or may be inferior to it, if, for example, it is cheaper or simpler to apply, or more stable, or associated with fewer adverse reactions, or is more acceptable to the community than the existing intervention. In such circumstances, the purpose of the trial might be to show that the efficacy of the intervention was 'equally good or not much worse than' the existing intervention.

4.2 Duration of a trial

In field trials it may be necessary to establish the efficacy of the intervention not only in the population as a whole but also in special sub-groups. This may involve the measurement of efficacy in persons of certain ages or for persons with underlying or associated conditions such as malnutrition. It will also be necessary to determine the duration of efficacy and to have a reasonably precise estimate of the degree of efficacy (as discussed in Chapter 3, Section 3).

It may be argued, therefore, that the appropriate point at which to stop a trial should be when sufficient evidence has been collected to support, or reject, the introduction of the intervention by the health services generally, rather than at the point when the difference in response in intervention and control groups is first established. For many interventions it is important to establish both the degree and the duration of protection. Thus a trial might be continued beyond the point at which protection is first established to determine if there is long lasting protection. For example, it may be established in the first few years of a vaccine trial against leprosy that the vaccine is protective but, to be of public health value, it may be necessary to demonstrate that long-lasting protection is achieved. This may necessitate continuing the trial for a decade or more with the maintenance for this period of an unvaccinated group, or of a group whose members had received an inferior vaccine. In some circumstances this will be considered acceptable, but in others it will not. Again, each situation must be considered on its own merits and much depends on how far the investigators extend their horizon of responsibility.

4.3 Multiple endpoints

Often the most important endpoint in a trial may not be observed until a considerable time after the intervention has been applied. There may be intermediate endpoints against which the intervention is also assessed. For example, a vaccine may produce a good antibody response long before any protection against disease is established. Demonstration of efficacy against such an intermediate point might be considered grounds for ending a trial if it was considered reasonable to assume that the effect observed on the intermediate endpoint would necessarily carry over to the more distant endpoint, even though efficacy against that endpoint had not been formally demonstrated. What 'it is reasonable to assume' is often a matter of considerable debate, and the ethics of continuing a trial once protection against intermediate endpoints has been established must be argued in the particular circumstances surrounding a trial. Immunological measures which are thought to correlate with protection against clinical disease may not so do. For example, in the one trial in which this aspect was examined the protection that BCG conferred against tuberculosis did not correlate well with the induction by the vaccine of sensitivity to a tuberculin skin test (Hart *et al.* 1967), even though it was possible to put forward plausible immunological arguments for believing that such a correlation should exist.

An example of the ethical difficulties that may arise is provided by proposed trials of malaria vaccines. Early treatment with appropriate antimalarials is normally curative for falciparum malaria and in a trial it would be unethical to withhold such treatment from those with clinical malaria. Yet the main purpose of such a vaccine is the prevention of death from malaria, not of infection, nor minor clinical illness. Indeed, it is conceivable that there may not be a good correlation between the protection of a vaccine against the last two endpoints and the protection against the first endpoint. The dilemma is that in most of Africa where malaria continues to kill hundreds of thousands of children annually, medical services are not adequate to provide the level of curative care that would be provided in a trial nor are they likely to be so in the immediate future. To what extent should the participants in a trial be provided with a level of treatment for malaria that is beyond that which they would receive if the trial was not conducted? There is no simple answer to this question, but one strategy that some would consider ethical might be to ensure that early studies were very large, so large that it would be impossible to treat adequately all cases of malaria outside of any existing system of medical care.

There are very strong reasons for conducting early trials of a new intervention to assess the impact of the intervention against the endpoints which are of greatest public health importance, rather than starting with trials against intermediate endpoints, if by studying intermediate endpoints further trials against more important endpoints may be compromised. Sometimes the body of knowledge from other trials or studies may be sufficient to enable the investigator to be very confident that if effects are demonstrated against intermediate endpoints then impacts on more important endpoints will necessarily follow, but in many circumstances, it may be hazardous to make such assumptions.

There are strong reasons for conducting very large trials of interventions that are likely to be used on large numbers of people in the future if the interventions are effective; much larger than would initially seem necessary to achieve only a statistically significant difference in outcome. The results of very large trials, if the trials have been adequately managed, can be much more convincing and are more likely to lead to the implementation of the intervention in disease control programmes than are the results of small trials.

Again, part of the dilemma relates to where the investigator places his or her horizon of responsibility. If the view is taken that the investigator, by taking on the responsibility of a field study, also takes on responsibility to provide full medical care of the subjects under study, then, for example, a study of a malaria vaccine with prevention of death as the endpoint could not be undertaken. If the view is taken that the horizon of responsibility extends to all those who are at risk of dying from malaria, including those who would not be included in the trial but who may benefit eventually from the vaccine, then a trial might be conducted with death as an endpoint.

5 LEVELS OF REVIEW

Most research investigations must go through several levels of review to assess their acceptability (see WHO 1989). The number of levels will depend on the nature of the research, national regulations, and from which agencies support for the research is being sought.

All ethical review bodies will require that each individual participant in a study is provided with sufficient information on potential risks and benefits to enable them to make an informed decision on whether or not to participate. Illiteracy and differing cultural concepts of health and disease do not alter the basic requirements for informed consent. If, as has been discussed above, informed consent has been achieved by virtue of a communal decision, the research worker and the ethics committee must assure themselves that there is no coercion on individuals to participate. The principles that assent must be given rather than assumed, and that all potential participants have the right of refusal, must be regarded as the minimal safeguards.

As well as being acceptable to individual participants a trial may be reviewed at a community level through either a formal or an informal review committee. In addition there may be local and national ethical and scientific review bodies to satisfy. If funding for a study is sought from an international agency there may be a further level of ethical review. For example, research proposals submitted to the WHO are reviewed by the WHO Secretariat Committee for Research Involving Human Subjects. This ethics committee will only review proposals that have first been through national and, if appropriate, local ethics committee review.

REFERENCES

Council for International Organizations of Medical Sciences (1982). *Proposed international guidelines for biomedical research involving human subjects*. CIOMS, Geneva.

Cowan, D. H. (1982). Research on the therapy of cancer. In: *Human subjects research: a handbook for institutional review boards*. (ed. Greenwald, R. A., Ryan, M. K., and Mulvhill, J. E.) pp. 151–67. Plenum Press, New York.

Hart, P. D., Sutherland, I., and Thomas, J. (1967). The immunity conferred by effective BCG and vole bacillus vaccines in relation to individual variations in induced tuberculin sensitivity and to technical variations in the vaccine. *Tubercle*, **48**, 201–10.

Molineaux, L. and Gramiccia, G. (1980). *The Garki project. Research on the epidemiology and control of malaria in the Sudan savannah of West Africa*. World Health Organization, Geneva.

World Health Organization (1989). *Manual of epidemiology for district health management. Appendix I. Ethical guidelines for epidemiological investigations*. (ed. Vaughan, J. P. and Morrow, R. H.). World Health Organization, Geneva.

5
Community involvement

1 INTRODUCTION

The active co-operation of those in the communities in which an intervention trial will be conducted is essential for the successful execution of most trials. A trial may involve some or all of the members of a single community or may include those in a few or many different communities. For the conduct of a trial a good rapport must be established and maintained between the investigators and those in the study communities, the nature of which will be determined largely by the kind of intervention and the study procedures to be employed. The participation necessary by those in the trial may be relatively passive, such as accepting vaccination and the subsequent disease monitoring procedures, or it may have to be intense if the intervention involves, for example, substantial behavioural change.

Some interventions may not appear to need much community participation. For example, the larvicidal spraying of rivers from aircraft, by which means the Onchocerciasis Control Programme is endeavouring to reduce morbidity from onchocerciasis in West Africa by control of the simulium fly which is the vector of the infection, requires little participation from villagers in the sprayed areas. The evaluation of the Programme, however, requires that affected communities are surveyed on a regular basis. These surveys involve taking skin snips from all those in the sampled communities and such investigations can only be conducted successfully, on a sustained basis, if the members of the communities understand and accept the importance of the evaluation and co-operate with the field teams.

In this chapter approaches and methods are outlined that may be adopted to gain community acceptance of, and participation in, a community intervention trial, or any similar kind of epidemiological study.

2 PRELIMINARY INVESTIGATIONS IN THE STUDY COMMUNITY

An informal approach should be made to appropriate representatives of potential study communities at an early stage in the planning of an investigation in order to ascertain if the questions that the proposed study is designed to address are considered to be relevant and important in the communities concerned. Co-operation is likely to be greatest if community members are involved in the identification of the health problems for study and these problems are considered to be of major importance locally. Local perceptions of problems may differ considerably from those of the investigator. For example, in some areas where infection with *Schistosoma haematobium* is endemic, blood in the urine is regarded as a normal part of a child's development and the absence of this may be regarded as abnormal (which in such communities it may indeed be!). In such circumstances, health education may be an essential component of the preliminary stages of an intervention trial against this disease.

The research team will need to investigate how the proposed study will be viewed in the communities in which it will be sited. Such investigations are particularly important, and may be more difficult, for investigators who are not native to the country or region of the country where the study is to be conducted. The unwary investigator may jeopardize the possibility of conducting a study if these preliminary investigations are not made tactfully with careful regard to possible local sensitivities. It is generally not sufficient just to write a letter to village leaders informing them of the study and the planned procedures. A visit to them is essential. It is important to identify those with local knowledge and expertise who might advise or help with these investigations. Social scientists often have the kind of training that facilitates such enquiries and if such a person is not already a part of the team, it may be useful to recruit such help.

3 SEEKING FORMAL APPROVAL

3.1 National and regional administrations

Due regard must be paid to the local and national social, political, and administrative structures and procedures. It is important to determine in which order the various preliminary contacts should be made. For example, the district administration may be offended if those in the villages are approached before clearance has been obtained from the district administrator and from the district medical officer. Similarly, it may be important to gain support for the study from relevant persons or groups in the national administration (including a national research council and an ethics committee) before making any approaches at regional or district levels. In some countries there is a political organization that operates in parallel with the civil administration and this may be as, if not more, important with regard to obtaining clearances for a study. In some places it may be important also to consult non-governmental organizations and religious groups, without whose co-operation it may be difficult to proceed.

3.2 Community leaders

Discreet local enquires should be made to determine who in a community should be approached first when a consultation is opened. If other investigators have conducted research in an area they may be able to advise on this. Otherwise the district medical officer or local administrators or political representatives may be consulted. The initial contact in a community is likely to be with the formal and informal leaders but, at an early stage, it will be important to meet with those from the population who may better represent the group or groups on which the intervention study will be focused. For example, if the intervention is against a childhood disease it may be important to consult with a group of mothers (for example, women's associations, traditional birth attendants) who carry influence in the community. Enquiries to investigate social and political aspects of the structure of the community may be necessary to identify the appropriate individuals or groups.

A good rapport is only established if the investigator observes local customs. It is often important that the person, or persons, who enter into the consultation process are of the appropriate gender and age. In many rural societies age is associated with authority and it may be best to choose an older member of the research team to speak to village elders. In West African villages, leaders will often expect a gift from a visitor. Those with local knowledge should be consulted as to what would constitute an appropriate gift. If the members of the research team do not speak the appropriate language an interpreter should be found who has an understanding of local customs and who will be accepted by the community concerned.

At the first meeting with community leaders it is usually best to avoid detailed discussions. The concepts of the study can be introduced and a later meeting arranged. These later meetings require thorough preparation, and advice should be sought from those with knowledge of the area as to how best to communicate the aims and objectives of the study in ways that will be comprehensible locally.

The investigators will usually be ill-advised to try to impose a predetermined and rigid study design on a community. It is better to try to adapt the design according to the wishes and needs of those representing the community. The investigator may not wish to modify the objectives of the study in a radical way but if changes in the study design or procedures proposed by the community can be accommodated, without compromising the objectives substantially, a more successful study is likely to result.

An objective of meetings with community leaders is to obtain their explicit approval of the study once the relevant objectives and procedures have been presented and discussed and, if necessary, modified. The persons involved in these meetings should be present when the study is started in the community so that they can see that the procedures described are being adhered to and, if necessary, they may reassure community members regarding the study. Indeed, if village leaders are seen to be the first to enter a study, this may increase the confidence of others to participate.

3.3 Health care providers

Consideration should be given as to how the trial might interfere with the local health care system. Health care providers must be involved in the planning of the trial in order to discuss the ways in which it may affect their services and to what extent the activities of the study will affect their work load and, in particular, how the trial might help them to improve their own services and will integrate with their activities. The population may well turn to local health care workers for advice and opinions regarding the trial, and it is essential, therefore, that these workers understand the reasons for the trial and do not feel threatened or challenged by the study. The conduct of a trial may introduce improved standards of diagnosis and treatment in the community. The health care workers must be made part of this rather than feel threatened by it.

Informal health care providers within the community should be not excluded from such considerations. Local healers and traditional birth attendants often have considerable influence in a community and co-operation, rather than confrontation, with them is likely to be the most productive strategy. Ideally, a trial will have an educative function and will leave behind an improved health care system for the community.

3.4 Potential participants

After approval to proceed has been obtained from community leaders, it is necessary to consult those who will be the participants in the study. In the first instance this may involve the community leaders communicating their discussions with the investigators back to the members of the community. As a result of this the leaders may come back with further questions and suggestions regarding the study. In some circumstances this may be all that is required before the start of the study, and explanations of the study to participants may be made as they are enrolled into the study. Sometimes, however, it is useful to organize a public meeting, or series of meetings if several communities are involved, to which everyone in the community is invited. At such meetings the objectives and methods of study proposed should be described and individuals should be told what is asked of them and what benefits they may receive as a consequence of the study and to what risks they may be exposed through participation. Any questions they have should be solicited and complete and honest answers given.

4 THE INFORMATION TO CONVEY

In the meetings with the community leaders and in any public meetings the information given about the trial should be presented in such a way that it can be understood by the audience, taking account of their educational background and their beliefs regarding the causes of illness and effective interventions. The information given should contain all of the relevant details of the trial and deception, including by the withholding of information, should be avoided. It should be remembered that in deprived communities the uneducated may nevertheless be highly intelligent. The voluntary nature of studies should be emphasized to community leaders. Once a leader is supportive of a study, he or she may tend to be coercive towards reluctant or unwilling members of the community, seeing their authority questioned by failure to participate. Leaders must understand that anyone is free to refuse to enter or to withdraw from a study.

Visual aids tailored to the particular socio-cultural context may be useful to convey some aspects of a study. For example, in studies of hepatitis B vaccination in Senegal a 'flannel-graph' was developed, consisting of a picture of a person to which could be attached pieces of red felt cut in circles (the virus) or yellow circles (the vaccine) or yellow markers (antibodies). This was considered to have made a substantial contribution to local understanding and acceptance of the studies (J. Chotard, personal communication). Such innovative methods should be field tested, however, and they may require considerable development time and expertise before being suitable for use.

Any prior image the community have of the research team, and that of the organization that it represents, will colour initial consultations. The investigator will have to be prepared to answer criticisms of other activities of its parent organization (for example, the Ministry of Health, the University or the control programme) and, indeed, of any other research activities in the community even if he or she is not a part of these. If the research is not being conducted by the government, it may be important to emphasize this if it is thought this will increase the participation rates. Individuals will need reassurance that information collected for the purposes of the study will not be used for other purposes, for example, to compile tax lists. Assurance should be given regarding the confidentiality of any information collected and the community should be told who will have access to the study records and what will be done with them when the study is finished.

Individuals, as well as community leaders, must be told that participation in the study is voluntary and those who refuse will not be discriminated against in any way. This may be particularly important if the research team is identified with the government.

The concept of 'research' may be difficult to communicate in some communities. In particular, it may be difficult to explain randomized studies and those which include control groups whose members receive no intervention or who are given a placebo treatment, and in which assessment is 'blinded' so that the investigators do not know who has received which intervention. In many countries there are national or local lotteries and it may be possible to use the principle of these to convey concepts of randomization.

In trials in which only some in a community will be included in the study, the co-operation and collaboration of those excluded may be as important for the success of the study as of those included. Individuals will want to know why only some are included. Explanations regarding sample size and statistical power will not satisfy many unless considerable efforts are made to explain the reasons in language that has local relevance. Reassurance that everyone will be offered the intervention if it is found to be effective may help.

If biological specimens are required detailed discussions may be necessary to ascertain the best way of organising their collection. Finger-prick blood sampling may be preferred to venepuncture, especially for children. The frequency of blood sampling from each individual should be agreed and may represent a compromise between scientific requirements and individual tolerance. If specimens of urine or faeces are to be collected there should be discussion as to how this might be best organized. Certain containers may be too similar in shape to cultural motifs and transparent containers for specimens may not be acceptable. Examples of possible containers might be presented to the participants and the most acceptable one chosen.

5 ENSURING SUSTAINED INVOLVEMENT

To maintain the co-operation of those in a study there must be a dialogue between the research team and the community throughout the course of the study. This can be done by holding regular meetings with the community leaders to discuss the problems perceived by the investigators and those experienced by the participants, or by making a time available for such meetings if they are requested. This is especially important for studies that continue for several years as the perception of the trial by participants may change over time and initial enthusiasm may wane unless suitably reinforced. As the study progresses results should be conveyed back to those in the community. A common reason for refusing to provide a second blood sample is that no information was provided regarding the result of tests on the first sample. In some circumstances this problem may be solved by performing some of the laboratory tests on site. Methods are available which allow haemoglobins, malaria smears, and other tests to be evaluated in the field. For example, two thick blood smears might be taken for assessment of malaria infections. One might be stained immediately and read in the field and the other kept for more careful staining and reading in the laboratory. With such a system most individuals can be given their results and treated immediately, only a small proportion might have low levels of parasitaemia that may require additional follow-up (D. Brandling-Bennett, personal communication).

It is also important to keep the local health workers informed of the progress of the study and of the results as they accumulate and at the end of the study. One way of doing this is by sending a regular newsletter to all the health staff. In a large trial of hepatitis B vaccination in The Gambia this was found to be particularly effective when it becomes a two-way process with letters published from workers in the newsletter (A. J. Hall, personal communication).

Some surveys will involve community members in substantial inconvenience. If the survey procedures are time consuming it may be important to discuss what time of day, or even what time of year, is most convenient for a survey. It may be appropriate to consider compensating individuals, in the form of money or food, for time lost from farming or other activities. In some cultures it is considered appropriate to compensate in such a way if a blood sample is taken. Such compensation must be viewed carefully from an ethical standpoint, however, and it is generally discouraged. This issue is discussed further in Chapter 4, Section 3.3.

One specific form of compensation that the community might expect is improved health care, especially for the disease(s) under study. Some of the issues relating to this are discussed in Chapter 4, Section 3.2. In some studies it will be possible to involve local health workers directly in the conduct of a trial. This may provide a means of strengthening the local health services both during the trial and after it has finished (by the training and encouragement provided during the trial and by the collection of relevant health and population information in the study).

At the completion of the study the final results of the study should be communicated to the participants and the implications for the community should be discussed with them. Such feedback is essential not only from an ethical point of view (Chapter 4, Section 3.4) but will also pave the way both for co-operation in future research activities and, more importantly, for sustained health-seeking behaviour on the part of the community members.

6
Censuses and mapping

1 INTRODUCTION

In most intervention trials it will be necessary to compile a register of individuals included in the trial. The register should include sufficient identification information on each person to enable participants to be followed over time with minimal possibility of confusing one individual with another. To assemble a suitable group for inclusion in a trial it may be necessary to enumerate (i.e. count and identify) all the members of a geographically or otherwise defined population, or a specific subgroup of it (for example, children aged less than 5 years). Such a population enumeration may serve as a sampling frame to select a representative group, or may be used to assess how representative the study group is of the whole population, if some individuals refuse to participate or are not included in the trial for other reasons.

Identification and follow-up of the members of a population, and selecting a sample of them, may be facilitated if a map is drawn of the area, marking individual homes and prominent topographical features. Mapping may also be valuable in studying the epidemiology of a disease; for example, to determine if cases of a disease tend to occur near water courses or in some other non-random fashion geographically.

Mapping and enumeration of a population are not always necessary, but often such information collected at the start of a trial may be vital to its successful conduct. For example, in a leprosy vaccine trial in Venezuela, the trial group was defined as the household and other close contacts of prevalent leprosy cases. The prevalent cases were distributed over a very wide area, in which most of the population were not included in the trial. It was necessary to enumerate the household and other contacts of prevalent cases, but it would have been inappropriate to enumerate the entire population or to map the locations of all households, other than was necessary to be able to find the contacts during the course of the trial. Conversely, in a malaria chemoprophylaxis study in The Gambia, an attempt was made to include all children in a defined area and detailed mapping and enumeration were undertaken to facilitate the conduct of the study.

In this chapter guidelines are given on mapping and on ways of compiling a population register to facilitate long-term follow-up in a trial.

2 USES OF MAPS AND CENSUSES IN INTERVENTION STUDIES

A map of an area and a population enumeration provide:

1. A sampling frame for the selection of those to be included in a trial from the target population.

2. Denominators for the computation of morbidity and mortality rates.
3. Baseline population characteristics, which may affect the impact of an intervention and which can also be monitored for changes during the study.
4. A means of studying geographical variations in disease rates.

Age, sex, and place of residence affect the risk of most tropical diseases and information on these, and other factors that may influence exposure or susceptibility to disease, or which may influence the outcome of an infection, should be recorded carefully at the start of a trial.

3 PREPARATIONS FOR A CENSUS

3.1 Planning

Early in the planning a census of an area it is useful to find out what information already exists about the population, either in national censuses or from local surveys that may have been conducted. In some populations local administrative offices maintain up-to-date lists of tax payers that may give a good indication of the size of a population (or may not in situations in which significant numbers of people avoid registering for tax collection!). Lists of voters or of residents may also be available through local administrative offices. Special health surveys or other surveys may also have been conducted previously. Gathering this information will entail visits to the study area, to government statistical offices, and possibly to universities or other institutions from which special surveys may have been organized.

Some data are usually available from national censuses, conducted periodically in most countries. National or regional census data may be used in the planning of a trial to select a suitable area (for example, a group of contiguous villages whose population is likely to be of adequate size to meet the objectives of the trial). Often, the information in a census may be out of date, however, or may be inaccurate and may be of limited value for planning. From a national census it may be possible to obtain data for an area regarding the distribution of the population with respect to age, sex, ethnic group, household size, and population density. Estimates of mortality, fertility, and migration rates may also be available. The last may be especially useful to estimate potential losses to follow-up in a longitudinal study.

For detailed planning and conduct of a trial, a special enumeration will usually be necessary. The population may be enumerated at the same time as the intervention is being applied or as a separate exercise in advance of the intervention. There are advantages and disadvantages associated with either approach and the decision regarding which to use will depend on the circumstances under which the trial is being conducted. The initial census may be the first formal contact that ordinary members of a population have with a study, though it will have been preceded by liaison of the trial organizers with local officials and local leaders (discussed in Chapters 4 and 5). The enumeration exercise may be used, therefore, as an opportunity to explain the aims, objectives, and procedures to be employed in the trial. An interval might be left between this discussion and the actual application of the intervention so that potential trial participants may have time to consider whether or nor they wish to take part in the study. The basic principles of enumeration are similar, however, whether it is conducted before or at the same time as the intervention. In this chapter it is assumed to take place prior to the intervention.

It is important to allocate adequate time for enumeration and mapping, but it will usually be desirable to conduct these tasks fairly rapidly to minimize problems associated with migration, including from one house to another house in the study area, during the course of the census. There may be an optimum time to conduct the census. In areas where there is significant seasonal migration the census might be planned for a time when most of the people are at their normal residence. Trading seasons are times when people temporarily migrate and censuses conducted during this time may suffer from omissions. It may be important to avoid the rainy season when areas may be inaccessible or when people may spend most of the day away from their homes working in their fields. It may be best to avoid market days. In urban areas weekends may be the best time for surveys. The time of day may also be important. In some areas it has been found best to conduct a census after dark, when people have returned from work.

It may be tempting to try to collect as much information as possible on the study population during the initial census, such as information on socio-economic characteristics, education, and fertility histories. In the interests of speed, however, it may be preferable to collect such information in a separate round of interviews after the initial census, possibly when the intervention is being applied or at a later date. Once it has been entered into a microcomputer, data from the census may be used for printing questionnaires, lists of children, and so on, which will aid subsequent surveys (see, for example, Imo State Evaluation Team 1989).

In a recent census in the People's Republic of China villagers were told to report to a central point at a set time. Participation rates were very high. In most populations, however, this method is likely to be less successful, unless ways can be found of motivating the population to attend, and a house-to-house census is more common. The 'assembly method' may be the only one suitable for nomadic populations. In densely populated villages, and with only a few items of data being collected, a fieldworker going from house to house might be expected to complete census schedules for about 200 people in a day. In less densely populated areas or with a longer census schedule, 50 persons a day might be a more reasonable target.

It is important to plan in detail how the collected information will be recorded and processed and how it will be utilized during the conduct of the study and in subsequent analyses.

It will usually be important to seek the active collaboration of the local health services in the planning and execution of a census, utilizing the special local knowledge of the staff. This will also enable these workers to get to know their area better and they may wish to use the information collected for the benefit of the population while the trial is in progress and after it has finished. Indeed, if local health workers are not involved in the planning they may be antagonistic to the study and may transmit these feelings to the study population (Chapter 5, Section 3.3).

3.2 Pre-testing techniques

The design and testing of questionnaires is discussed in Chapter 9. This process will involve several steps, from initial drafting to testing under field conditions on, say, between 50 and 200 households. At each step, improvements in the wording of questions and to the composition and layout of the forms should be sought. Field testing will provide an opportunity to train staff and may assist in the identification of those suitable to become supervisors for the main enumeration.

3.3 Recruitment and training of field staff

Guidelines for the recruitment of staff are given in Chapter 11. Census clerks and supervisors should be selected from those who are meticulous in their attention to detail and who have clear hand-writing. Secondary school leavers are often suitable candidates. It may be desirable to choose census clerks who are from the study area. If several language groups are resident in the area clerks might be chosen from the different language groups. Training in census techniques is a good way of introducing staff to field investigations. Training will be greatly facilitated if a manual is prepared that includes information on the specific techniques and questionnaires to be used during the trial. Field staff should be able to refer to this manual regarding specific queries on the completion of question-naires and for details of protocols used in estimating dates of birth, and so on. Training should emphasize that the manual is the 'Bible' for the study and the clerks should fully understand its contents and be trained in its use. It would be naive to assume, however, that field workers will refer to the manual routinely unless such behaviour is thoroughly indoctrinated during training sessions and reinforced by supervision during the fieldwork.

Fieldwork is likely to be of highest quality if those conducting it understand the objectives of the study, the uses to which the information they will collect will be put, and the purposes of the procedures they will perform. Formal 'classroom-like' sessions might be organized where instruction is given and discussions are held without the distractions that are likely to be around during 'on-site' training in villages, though the latter will be important at a later stage of the training.

The instruction given to the survey clerks should include discus-sion of the following items:

1. A statement regarding working conditions, including information on normal working hours, holidays, working at

weekends, details of overnight/fieldwork allowances and the circumstances under which these will be paid. It may be advisable to exaggerate a little on how difficult working conditions and how long working hours will be. Care should be taken in making statements about payments as they are often misinterpreted by fieldworkers (often to their advantage!).

2. How to organize their day-to-day activities.

3. How to organize their time to avoid unnecessary travelling and the importance of punctuality and systematic working.

4. How to introduce themselves to household members and to describe the study. The importance of politeness and their personal appearance.

5. Neatness and clarity in the completion of forms.

6. The need for completeness and accuracy. Staff must be continually reminded that information they record should be checked and double-checked for omissions and inconsistencies.

7. The need to follow set protocols and to avoid introducing personal variations. This will include set ways to ask questions, for example, asking 'when were you born?' may lead to a different assessment of age than asking 'what is your age?'.

8. How to avoid bias and leading questions.

9. Detailed discussion of all items in the questionnaire.

10. What to do about visiting again when participants are absent.

Following instructional sessions, field staff should practice interviewing and coding questionnaires themselves. Initially this can be done by having staff interview each other in the classroom. Combinations could include trainee acting as interviewer, trainee acting as respondent, trainee acting as observer, and trainer acting as observer. Such role-playing is very useful for all members of the census team. Trainees should then move to communities not included in the study to test out all the field procedures under supervision. The practice sessions in the non-study communities should begin with interviewers working in pairs. It may be useful to tape-record interview sessions to check that interviewers are using the correct wording and that their approaches to the villagers are correct. The recordings can be used for feedback in the training programme to highlight problems.

3.4 Mapping

A census can be conducted without a map being drawn and it may
not be necessary to map an area in order to be able to trace
inhabitants during the course of a study. For many studies, however, and especially large ones, maps will be very useful for
planning and conducting a survey and for following-up the trial
participants. Departments of Lands and Surveys, or their equiva-
lents, may provide information on official maps and it may even be
possible to get copies of maps which are out of print through
specialist sources. For example, Stanford's (12 Long Acre, London WC2) is a specialist map agency in London which holds large
stocks of maps for many different countries. Other maps may be
available from special sources, such as the Army, Agriculture
Departments, Tourist Offices, and the Central Statistics Office
(where maps might be held that were specially drawn for a
national census). It may be possible to obtain aerial or satellite
photographs of an area or to have these specially commissioned,
but this is likely to be expensive.

Even if maps are obtained, the information recorded may be
incomplete or inaccurate and it should be checked in the field.
Names of villages may have changed or they may be known by
different names locally, and villages may have disappeared or
arisen if the maps are not recent. Checks, and alterations as
necessary, should be made on the positions of roads and tracks,
health centres, health posts, dispensaries, markets, churches,
mosques, boreholes and other locally important features.

A map of the whole study area may be too small for each house
in each village to be marked. Existing maps might be enlarged
(which can be done using a photocopier) and the enlargements
used for the mapping of houses, or it may be necessary to redraw
maps. Separate maps should be drawn for each village (or small
area) showing the locations of all houses and prominent land-
marks. The accuracy with which these need to be drawn and the
detail they should include depends upon how they will be used.
For example, if detailed studies are to be made of the transmission
of a disease within a community it may be important to have
accurate measures of the distances between all houses, which may
involve measuring or pacing out distances between dwellings.
Alternatively, if the map is only being made to enable houses to be

found on a subsequent occasion, a rough sketch map will be adequate, especially if it is possible to mark identification numbers on houses also. An example of a village map used in a study of schistosomiasis is given in Fig. 6.1. (WHO Workshop 1980).

Detailed maps are easiest to construct if aerial photographs can be obtained, even if they are not recent, and suitable tracings made. The tracings can be updated as the survey teams go from house-to-house. In the absence of aerial photographs mapping may be undertaken using compass, theodolite, (and tape measure if great accuracy is required) to relate the position of each house to the others in an area. For most purposes, good maps can be constructed by carefully pacing out distances between houses and using a compass to locate directions. All maps should show the north line and the scale (even if this is only approximate).

An accurate way of mapping the position of houses, roads, etc. has been developed using satellite technology. Compact, hand-held global positioning systems (GPS) use signals from at least three of the more than 20 commercial satellites orbiting the earth to estimate the longitude and latitude of the hand-held device. Most GPS receivers have a facility for storing up to 100 data recordings, which can be down-loaded into desk-top computers at the end of each day's field work. The hardware is robust and can withstand temperatures up to 60°C and 95 per cent condensing humidity. The accuracy of the positioning depends upon the number of satellites from which a signal can be received and the strength of their signals. Most manufacturers maintain that the accuracy of the commercial systems are within 25 metres. The cost of the simplest GPS is around $700. Commonly used systems are produced by Trimble Navigation Europe Ltd (Trimble House, Meridian Office Park, Osborn Way, Hook, Hampshire RG27 9HX, UK) and Garmin International (9875 Widmer Road, Lenexa, Kansas 66215, USA).

There is an increasing amount of software available for the analysis and presentation of geographical data collected using GPS (for example, MapInfo, IDRISSI, EpiMap, POPMAP). This provides the opportunity, for example, to experiment with different sampling unit sizes and to present disease data spatially. Snow *et al.* (1993) provide an example of how GPS data can be used for descriptive purposes in epidemiological studies. However, the approach has yet to be fully exploited in intervention trials.

It is good practice to assign a code number to each house on a

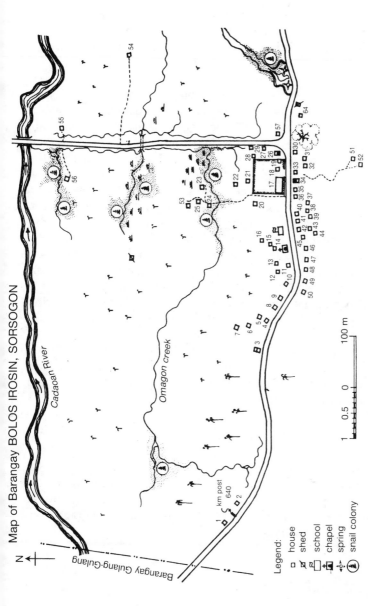

Fig. 6.1 Example of a map of a village. Map of a village in which schistosomiasis was studied in the Philippines (WHO Workshop 1980). (The map was kindly provided by K. Mott and drawn for the workshop by I. T. Cruz.)

map. This may consist of a letter or number to indicate the village code and a number to indicate the house within a village (for example, B374). If it is locally acceptable, it is useful to paint this number on the house or to affix a board with the number on it (numbers painted on mud walls may be washed off in the rains). This helps to ensure that each house is only mapped once and also the number might be used subsequently in the identification numbers for individuals in a house. For example the head of the household might be assigned the code B374/01, his wife B374/02, and so on.

It may be preferable to use a numerical rather than an alphabetical code for villages (for example, 02 instead of B) as it is slower for data entry clerks to type a mixture of alphabetic and numerical information into a computer than it is to type numerical information alone. Against this must be balanced a slightly more cumbersome identification system.

To use the house number in this way the numbering system should be designed to take account of the local family structures and their living arrangements. For example, in studies in Africa the same number might be assigned to all houses that comprise a 'compound' and individuals in the compound might be given additional numbers. This is of special relevance when a census is conducted as it may be important to design the numbering system such that related individuals, or those who normally live together, share a common number. This is not always straightforward to do and is discussed further in Section 4.2.

4 ENUMERATION

A census of the population may be conducted after or at the same time as mapping. The census will involve the collection of information on the composition of each household and demographic, and possibly other, data on each member.

4.1 Organization

A combination of speed and accuracy is required in the conduct of a census. It is useful to draw a flow chart of the data collection and processing operations. A simple example of such a chart is given in Fig. 6.2.

The field manual should include a check list of equipment that the census clerks will need to take with them each day (for example, pencils, paper, erasers, census schedules, village maps, and other necessary equipment) and they must be trained to check the list on a daily basis, as much time may be wasted otherwise through unnecessary trips back to the study base to retrieve forgotten items.

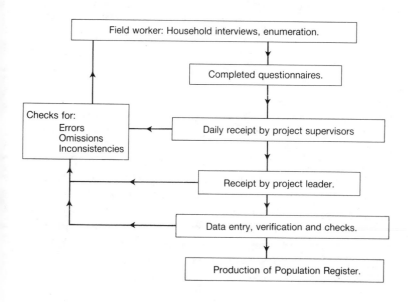

Fig. 6.2 Flow chart of census data collection.

4.2 Definition of dwelling units

The definition of a village and of a household (or compound) within a village will vary depending on the location of the trial. Villages generally share the same leaders although the inhabitants may be dispersed over a wide area. A compound in West Africa is a cluster of households fenced or partitioned off from other compounds and may have features such as a well or latrine which all the households of a particular compound share. A household might be distinguished as a nuclear or extended family structure whose members share the same kitchen (the 'cooking-pot' definition of a household). A definition of a household should be decided before mapping and enumeration begin. Households can be spread over several buildings or several households may share the same building. There are not uniquely correct ways of defining households, or compounds, or dwellings, but in any particular study it is important that clear definitions are constructed for all of the different terms to be used in describing people's living arrangements. Only if this is done will confusion be avoided in the mapping and enumeration of the study population. New investigators in an area would be well advised to find out what systems others have used who have worked in the same area, and whether or not these worked satisfactorily.

4.3 *De facto* and *de jure* populations

Before conducting a census it is necessary to decide who will be registered as a member of the population. The two simplest options are the so-called *de facto* and *de jure* populations. The *de jure* population comprises the 'normal residents' and includes individuals who usually live in a particular village but who may be absent during the enumeration. The *de facto* population consists of those who slept in the village the night before the census. In national censuses it is usual to enumerate the *de facto* population but for the purpose of most intervention trials the *de jure* population is the most appropriate. In some African cultures the definition of household membership may be difficult to specify. Some individuals may live in one household but spend a significant amount of time in another household in the study area. These individuals are likely to be enumerated twice unless care is taken to assess the true 'normal' domicile of each person. During the course of the enumeration residential status can be recorded as 'absent' or 'present'. This will give some indication of the degree of temporary migration. Similarly, field workers will have to distinguish between 'temporary' visitors and those who will remain for a long time. It may be difficult to obtain such information reliably as respondents may inform a field worker that a temporary visitor is 'permanent' if it is thought that some benefit may derive from this. The definition of who is a normal resident will depend upon the objectives of the trial. It is important to decide upon a period of time that a person should have been in or out of a community to be considered as having migrated in or out. In general, a clear and full definition is required as to who should be considered as a resident, especially in long-term studies which may involve multiple census updates. The definitions should be included in the field manual.

4.4 Ensuring completeness

As houses may be empty at the time the interviewer calls or some residents may be away, the fieldworker will have to rely upon proxy reporting in some instances. If a house is empty, arrangements should be made to call back at a time when someone is likely to be there. Only as a last resort should someone from another house be asked to provide details of the missing residents and in such instances it is best to check the information using some independent source, such as another neighbour.

Information about the composition of the household is best elicited if there is a standard order in which information is sought on individuals (discussed in Section 4.5). It is not necessary that the information on all members of a household should be given by a single respondent, nor that the interviews are held privately, unless sensitive information is being collected. Respondents might be encouraged to consult others in the compound to provide information. It is useful to specify in advance who would be regarded as an acceptable informant in a household. For example, for information on young children, the list in order of preference might be first the mother, second an adult female relative living in the household, and third the father.

If possible, interviewers should walk around the household and ask who sleeps in each of the beds, and ask also where those who appear not to have a bed sleep. This method is not foolproof, however, as in some societies children (and sometimes adults also) may sleep in different beds from night to night.

Whether or not a respondent is willing to co-operate in the study may depend on the initial impression a field worker makes and on the respondent's understanding of the reasons for the census. Co-operation may be poor if the study subjects suspect that the information collected may be used to their disadvantage. The field workers must introduce themselves properly to the respondents, explain the purpose of the study and assure them that any information given will be regarded as confidential. It may be necessary to reassure them specifically that the information will not be made available to the local administration for compiling lists of tax payers. If those in a household refuse to participate the field supervisor and the project leader should be informed and the situation investigated as soon as possible. An initial refusal should not be taken as final. Individuals may not collaborate merely because they have not properly understood the objectives of the survey or have not appreciated the potential benefits to them. If more than a small proportion of individuals refuse to participate, the effects can be serious, as not only may this introduce bias into the trial, but it may discourage others from participating. Discussions should be held with village leaders if it appears that such problems are developing in order to ascertain the reasons and to seek suitable remedies.

At the end of each day interview schedules should be carefully checked by the fieldworkers and by a supervisor for errors or omissions so that these may be corrected on the following day before moving on to another area. Plans should be made to visit again any household that could not be enumerated because of the absence of reliable informants or because the house was empty.

4.5 Numbering individuals

Part of the purpose of a census is to allocate a unique identification number to each member of the population. This number will usually remain assigned to the individual for the duration of the trial and only in very exceptional circumstances will it be changed, since it may be used to link information on an individual from

different sources (for example, interviewing, clinical examinations, and laboratory studies). There are several different ways
which are commonly used to allocate identification numbers. As
an example of one such system, suppose in village B the first
compound is numbered 01. Within compound 01 the first household is numbered 01 and the household head is given the number
01 within the household. Thus, this individual has the unique
identifying number B010101. [Note that such a numbering system
assumes there are fewer than 100 compounds in every village,
fewer than 100 households in every compound and fewer than 100
persons in every household, and that there are fewer than 27
villages in the study (see also Chapter 13, Section 4.2).]

Alternatively, numbers might be allocated in a simple continuous sequence to each member of the trial population, with no
attempt to build codes for village or household into the number.
An advantage of this system is that forms can be pre-numbered
before they are taken to the field and the number allocated to an
individual is simply that on the form that is filled in for them. If a
system such as this is used it may be worthwhile to supplement the
number with a check digit or character to aid the detection of
transcription errors. An example of such a check-digit system that
was used in a vaccine trial in Venezuela is given in Box 6.1. and an
example of a different system used by the Centers for Disease
Control in the United States (W. Meade Morgan, personal communication) is given in Box 6.2.

In addition to, or instead of, the check-digit system the practice
in some trials has been to record always, for data-linkage purposes,
both an individual's identification number and the first, say, five
letters of their name. Checks are made that both of these items
match before any linkage procedures are undertaken. In the case
of discrepancies the relevant items may be listed out so that
attempts can be made to trace the source of, and correct, any error.

4.6 Household or individual forms or cards?

After mapping the study area and assigning numbers or codes to
villages, compounds, and households, survey forms or cards can be
marked with household identification numbers. Whether all members of a household should be recorded on one form or whether
separate forms or cards should be made up for each individual will

Box 6.1. Algorithm for assigning check letter to six-digit code
number

The algorithm given below has been designed to assign a check
character to guard against the commonest kind of transcription
error; i.e. reversing the order of two adjacent digits. For example,
common transcription errors would be to write 2374 as 3274, 2734,
or 2347, by reversing the order of two consecutive digits. The
algorithm below ensures that each of the four possibilities is
assigned a different check letter.

Suppose the trial number consists of 6 digits, represented by
abcdef (for example, for the number 2374: $a = 0$, $b = 0$, $c = 2$, $d = 3$,
$e = 7$, and $f = 4$).

Step 1: Add and subtract the consecutive digits of the number as
below:

$$+a \; -b \; +c \; -d \; +e \; -f$$

Thus,   2374 gives $+0 \; -0 \; +2 \; -3 \; +7 \; -4 = +2$
3274 gives $+0 \; -0 \; +3 \; -2 \; +7 \; -4 = +4$
2734 gives $+0 \; -0 \; +2 \; -7 \; +3 \; -4 = -6$
2347 gives $+0 \; -0 \; +2 \; -3 \; +4 \; -7 = -4$
492673 gives $+4 \; -9 \; +2 \; -6 \; +7 \; -3 = -5$

Step 2: Add 30 to the result.

Step 3: Divide by 20 and use the *remainder* to assign the check letter
according to the table below:

Remainder:	1	2	3	4	5	6	7	8	9	10	11	12	13	14	15	16	17	18	19	0
Check letter:	A	B	C	D	E	F	G	H	J	K	L	M	N	P	R	T	V	W	X	Y

Thus, for the examples above:

Number	Step 1	Step 2	Step 3*	Final code
2374	+2	32	12	2374M
3274	+4	34	14	3274P
2734	−6	24	4	2734D
2347	−4	26	6	2347F
492673	−5	25	5	492673E

* Remainder, after dividing the number in Step 2 by 20

Thus, if a code number is written as 3274M it could be detected as an error (as the check character associated with 3274 should be 'P'). When such an error is found it may be possible to trace it back and ascertain the correct code number (for example, if a number has been poorly transcribed or entered wrongly into the computer). If the correct code cannot be ascertained reliably it will usually be appropriate to discard the information associated with the incorrect code as it cannot be linked back to the correct individual.

The method works equally well for numbers consisting of less than or more than 6 digits. The only modification that may be necessary is to change the number which is added in Step 2 to ensure that the final number is always positive.

The algorithm used can be put into a simple computer program so that the checking procedure can be done automatically once the data are entered into a computer.

Note: In the assignment of the check letters the following have been avoided:

I because of possible confusion with 1
O because of possible confusion with 0
Q because of possible confusion with O
S because of possible confusion with 5
U because of possible confusion with V
Z because of possible confusion with 2

Box 6.2. Alternative method of assigning check digit to six-digit number

Suppose the trial number consists of a six-digit number and it is desired to add a one-digit check number that will guard against transcription errors (such as reversing the order of two digits or recording one digit incorrectly). The number will take the form:

	d1	d2	d3	d4	d5	d6	c
(Prime:	11	7	5	3	2	1)	

The first 6 prime numbers are shown below the digits of the trial number. The check digit c is calculated by multiplying each digit by

Box 6.2 (*continued*)

the corresponding prime, summing the results and the *last* digit of
the result is taken as the check digit. Thus, for example, we have:

Trial number		Trial number *with check digit*
467913	$4 \times 11 + 6 \times 7 + 7 \times 5 + 9 \times 3 + 1 \times 2 + 3 \times 1 = 153$	4679133
476913	$4 \times 11 + 7 \times 7 + 6 \times 5 + 9 \times 3 + 1 \times 2 + 3 \times 1 = 155$	4769135
567913	$5 \times 11 + 6 \times 7 + 7 \times 5 + 9 \times 3 + 1 \times 2 + 3 \times 1 = 164$	5679134

(W. Meade Morgan, personal communication)

depend on the way in which the survey is organized and on the
design of the data processing system. If the information collected
is to be transferred into a microcomputer soon after collection,
household forms may be the best way of recording information as
separate forms can be produced for each individual, if required,
using the computer. If a computer is not to be used, however, it
may be best to make a separate card for each individual as these
are then easy to transfer (say, between storage boxes) if an individual changes houses during the study, which will be a common
occurrence in some areas, or if different individuals in a household
are followed-up at different times. Sometimes both a household
form and individual forms will be required, the former to collect
basic demographic information on all members of a household and
the latter to record more detailed information on some, or all,
members of the household.

   If the census is being conducted at the same time that other
procedures are being undertaken on the study subjects it may be
best to use individual cards instead of, or in addition to, household
forms, as otherwise it may be necessary to wait until a complete
household has been registered before other procedures can start.
If household sizes are large this may lead to significant delays for
those following the census clerks, especially at the start of each
day.

Figure 6.3 is an example of a simple household form to collect basic demographic information.

General issues related to the production and coding of questionnaires and forms are considered in Chapters 9 and 13.

4.7 Coding relationships

Interviewers should be instructed regarding the order in which individual household members should be registered, as a systematic approach is less likely to lead to omissions. In studies in Africa it would be usual to begin recording with the household head, followed by his first wife, and all her children living in the household; his second wife and her children; and so on. Next might be any brothers of the household head, each followed by their wives and children, as for the head. Unrelated individuals such as lodgers and servants might be recorded last. Relationships between different household members may be coded so that, in so far as possible, everyone is linked to one or two others in the household in a simple way using as close a relationship as is possible. Codes for brother, sister, mother, and so on, should only be used when wife, son, or daughter cannot be used to describe a relationship. To the extent possible, terms such as granddaughter, grandson, grandmother, grandfather, niece, nephew, uncle, aunt, and cousin should be avoided. An example of a coding system for relationships that was used in a vaccine trial in Uganda (Smith *et al*. 1976) is given in Box 6.3. Two alternatives to this procedure may be better in some circumstances; either everyone is related to the household head or detailed records are made of the name of each individual's mother and father (even if they are dead or do not live in the household).

In some societies it may be very difficult to ascertain the precise relationship between individuals. For example, no apparent distinction may be made between the children of a man and his brother, each might refer to them as his children. So long as this is appreciated it may cause little confusion, but it may be very important if, say, genetic studies are being conducted.

4.8 Names and addresses

The most important way of identifying an individual will be

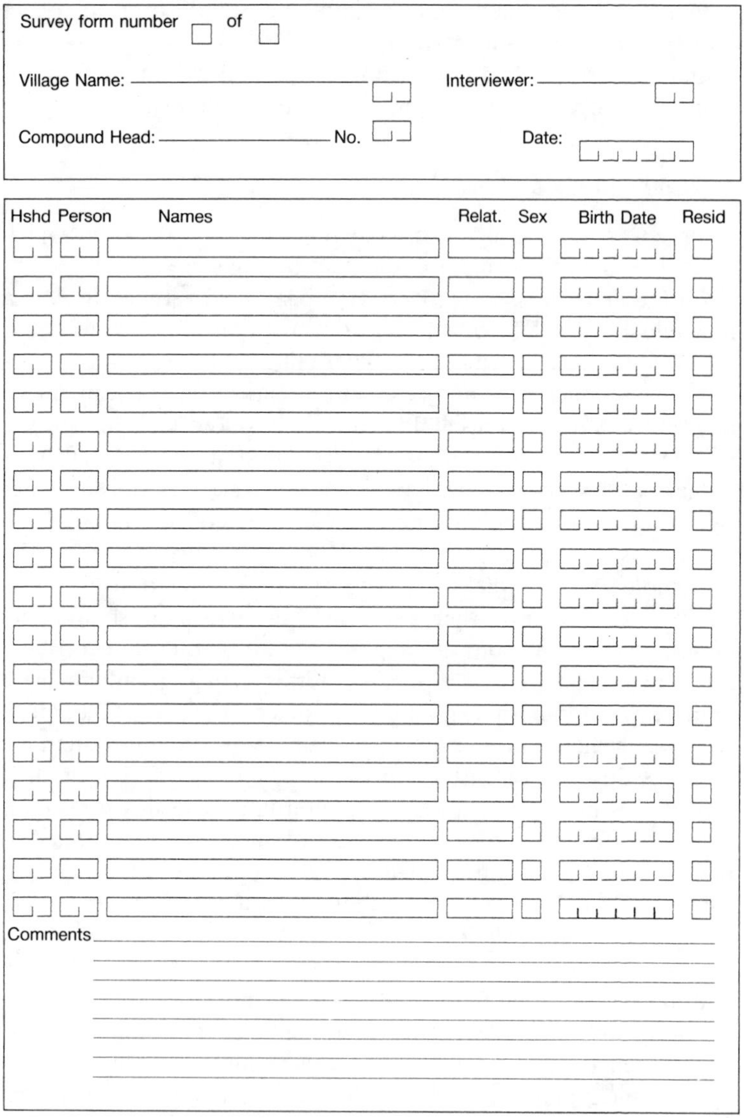

Survey form number ☐ of ☐		
Village Name: ——————— ⌐⌐	Interviewer: ——————— ⌐⌐	
Compound Head: ——————— No. ⌐⌐	Date: ⌐_____⌐	

Hshd	Person	Names	Relat.	Sex	Birth Date	Resid
⌐⌐	⌐⌐			☐	⌐_____⌐	☐
⌐⌐	⌐⌐			☐	⌐_____⌐	☐
⌐⌐	⌐⌐			☐	⌐_____⌐	☐
⌐⌐	⌐⌐			☐	⌐_____⌐	☐
⌐⌐	⌐⌐			☐	⌐_____⌐	☐
⌐⌐	⌐⌐			☐	⌐_____⌐	☐
⌐⌐	⌐⌐			☐	⌐_____⌐	☐
⌐⌐	⌐⌐			☐	⌐_____⌐	☐
⌐⌐	⌐⌐			☐	⌐_____⌐	☐
⌐⌐	⌐⌐			☐	⌐_____⌐	☐
⌐⌐	⌐⌐			☐	⌐_____⌐	☐
⌐⌐	⌐⌐			☐	⌐_____⌐	☐
⌐⌐	⌐⌐			☐	⌐_____⌐	☐
⌐⌐	⌐⌐			☐	⌐_____⌐	☐
⌐⌐	⌐⌐			☐	⌐_____⌐	☐
⌐⌐	⌐⌐			☐	⌐_____⌐	☐
⌐⌐	⌐⌐			☐	⌐_____⌐	☐
⌐⌐	⌐⌐			☐	⌐_____⌐	☐
⌐⌐	⌐⌐			☐	|_|_|_|_|_|	☐

Comments ———————————————————
————————————————————————
————————————————————————
————————————————————————
————————————————————————
————————————————————————

Fig. 6.3 A census schedule.

Box 6.3. Example of instructions for coding relationships
(Smith *et al.* 1976)

Coding of relationships

In this column write down the relationship of the individual to the other persons in the household. Since each person will be entered against a person number (the second item in the columns), the relationship can conveniently be expressed by reference to these numbers; for example 'Wife of 1' or 'Son of 1 and 2'.

The following abbreviations may be used:

Head of household	H	Grandson	GS
Wife	W	Granddaughter	GD
Son	S	Grandfather	GF
Daughter	D	Grandmother	GM
Mother	M	Other blood relative	R
Father	F	Unrelated	X
Brother	BR		
Sister	SR		

Example: A household consists of the head, his two wives and five children (three by his first wife and two by his second), his mother, and an unrelated visitor and her child. These would be coded:

Person no.	Person	Code
01	Head	H
02	Wife 1	W1
03	Child 1 (M)	S1,2
04	Child 2 (F)	D1,2
05	Child 3 (M)	S1,2
06	Wife 2	W1
07	Child 1 (F)	D1,6
08	Child 2 (M)	S1,6
09	Mother	M1
10	Visitor	X
11	Child 1 (M)	S10

through his or her names and these must be recorded with special care. Interviewers must be instructed how to spell names given by illiterate individuals. It is important to try to record all of the names of a person, including nicknames, as it is not uncommon in some cultures for individuals, and especially children, to employ different names in different situations. In Madagascar, for example, adults may change their name, officially, up to three times (A. Degremont, personal communication). The most frequently used names should be recorded first. In some areas confusion may arise as many people have the same names, especially in cultures in which the first born males or females are always given a set name, or in which they are always named after their grandmother or grandfather. In many West African societies very young children are not named until sometime after birth and until this time they may have to be recorded as 'unnamed'. In some cultures, young infants are not thought to be part of society and careful questioning may be necessary to elicit information about their existance.

In addition to the names, the complete addresses of study participants should be recorded. In some instances, this will be just the name of a village, but if there is some system of sub-units within a village, then this also should be recorded. Often it will be useful to record the name of the local chief or elder who has some responsibility in the area in which a participant resides, though it should be remembered that this person may change during the course of a study.

4.9 Ages

In some societies it takes a few seconds to elicit an individual's age or date of birth through a simple question, but in others these are very difficult to obtain as individuals do not know their age and it has no special significance to them.

The emphasis placed upon collecting accurate information on ages or dates of birth will depend upon the objectives of the trial. Accurate dates of birth may not be necessary for all age groups, and those in age groups not pertinent to the trial may not have age recorded at all. In some trials accurate estimates of dates of birth may be needed for all age groups. It is generally better to record date-of-birth rather than age last birthday, as the latter may lead to confusion because it changes during the course of a trial. During the census, field staff can convert ages to dates-of-birth using transcription tables (relating ages to years of birth) which should be included in their manual. Protocols and methods of estimating dates of birth, such as those described in this section, should be an integral part of the census clerks training and form part of their field manual. Many countries in the tropics do not have reliable civil registration of births, but various other sources of information may be available. For children, health cards and the mother's antenatal card may be a good source of information. Health cards generally have a date of birth written on them which is reasonably accurate. For children who are not taken to a health centre immediately after birth they may be less accurate. Mothers can be questioned as to how big the child was when taken to the health centre. Antenatal cards should have dates of delivery or, if not, when the mother was seen and the estimated gestational age. In the absence of any documentation, various other methods of estimating dates of birth of a child have to be employed.

Primary teeth of children can be counted and age estimated from the presence or absence of molars, premolars, and so on (see McGregor *et al*. 1968). This can be a laborious process, however. For those in the age range 6–24 months, age in months can be estimated crudely as 6 more than the number of erupted teeth. Developmental characteristics, such as the ability of the child to place the right arm over the head to touch the left ear (5 year olds), the ability to sit upright unaided, walking, talking, and so on, can all be used to estimate the developmental age and hence date of birth for very young children.

Older children are more difficult to age by means of physical and developmental characteristics due to variations in growth patterns. Age may be inferred from their grade in school, or the grade they would be in if they went to school. However, some educational systems retain pupils in lower grades if they are thought unsuitable for higher grades, or a child may start school only when the parents can afford it.

If the fieldworker can accurately age one child the 'index child' method can be used. The mother is asked about her other children in relation to this child. For example, the fieldworker might ask questions such as: 'before Ebrima, did you deliver a live birth?; is the child here?; for how long did you breast feed the child?; how many rainy seasons did you wait before becoming pregnant again?'. With such information on the birth interval, the preceding child's date of birth may be estimated. Similarly, procedures can be used for the following child's date of birth and all her other children.

To estimate the month of birth, calendars can be constructed. The calendar will list the months of rains, dry season, and so on. For example, a mother might be asked if her child was born in the rains, and if so at the beginning, middle or end of the rains? At set times of the year members of the village will be planting, sowing, weeding, ploughing, or harvesting different crops. An example of part of a monthly event calendar that was used in a study in Ghana is given in Table 6.1 (D. Ross, personal communication). Having estimated the ages of all in a household the fieldworker should then look at all the family together to assess if the ages are reasonable, bearing in mind any infant or childhood deaths, still-births or abortions. Children whose dates of birth are known to be well-estimated can be used in other households as index children. Children grow-up and play together and mothers care for each other when pregnant and such information can be used to ascertain the ages of other children within the same compound or village.

The age of adult females can be estimated in several ways. Age at menarche varies between populations but may be a reasonable marker to use in the estimation of the age of a young adult woman (though in some cultures it may be difficult to discuss). Age at marriage for women may be quite uniform in some societies. Women can be asked if they married early or late compared to their contemporaries. But it must also be elicited when marriage occurs, as in some societies the marriage process is a lengthy one and involves numerous stages before the woman goes to stay with her husband.

Given an estimated age at first marriage, birth histories can be elicited to estimate a woman's current age. Under conditions of natural fertility, on average approximately 2.5, 1.5, 1 and 1 years elapse between births, which are respectively, a live birth that was weaned, a live birth that died in infancy, a stillbirth, and an abortion. This method assumes no infertility, spouse separation, or use of contraception. In areas where these phenomena are common different assumptions have to be made.

Table 6.1. Example of part of a monthly event calendar used in Ghana Vitamin A Supplementation Trial (D. Ross, personal communication)

SEPTEMBER
Specific dates:
Farming: * Harvesting of groundnuts, cowpeas, and maize starts
          * Harvesting of sweet potatoes, peas, and wet-season rice starts
General: * Heavy rains continue (Duliu)
          * Drumming and other loud noises banned
          * Beginning of the school year

OCTOBER
Specific dates: 1–31 Rosary
Farming: * Harvesting of groundnuts, cowpeas, maize, sweet potatoes,
            pesa, and wet-season rice ends
General: * Rains slackening off
          * Season of abundant food (Womodaabu Chana)
          * Ban on drumming and other loud noises is lifted

NOVEMBER
Specific dates: 1 All Saints
                2 All Souls
Farming: * Late millet harvest
          * Construction of dry-season gardens starts
          * Coccidiosis disease (Choguru) starts in fowls
General: * Harmattan starts
          * Cutting of 'sange' and grass starts
          * Firewood collecting season starts
          * Frog hunting season starts
          * School Nov/Dec exams start

DECEMBER
Specific dates: 19   Feok Festival in Sandema
                25   Christmas Day
                26   Boxing Day
                27–29 Fao Festival in Navrongo
                31   Anniversary of the 31 December Revolution
Farming: * Dry season tomatoes and other vegetables start to become
            available
          * Collection of kapok starts
          * Harvest of ebony fruits starts
          * Gathering of millet stalks starts
          * Storing of grain
          * Animals allowed to move about freely again
General: * Harmattan continues
          * Making of bricks and repairing of houses etc. starts
          * Bush fire season starts
          * Hunting season starts
          * Many Northerners start to move South looking for farm work
          * Christmas school-holidays start

Historical event calendars are one of the most commonly used methods to estimate ages. This method is especially useful where societies have a predominantly oral tradition. Historical event calendars require much effort to develop, and before doing this it is worth finding out if they already exist in government census departments or elsewhere. If they do not a calendar can be created with the assistance of local members of staff, village teachers and village leaders. The calendar should include all the major national historical events and their dates and all outstanding local events, such as major bush fires, murders, drownings, deaths of religious and political leaders, wars, droughts, famines, and so on. If an individual can remember an event and can estimate how old he or she was (for example, just married, in school), their date of birth can be estimated. This method is time-consuming and should be piloted before use. It may be decided that it is too slow and cumbersome to be of use or there may be too few significant events for individuals that can be dated for the method to be used. An example of an event calendar that was used in a study in Ghana is given in Table 6.2 (D. Ross, personal communication). It was found, however, that this calendar needed to be supplemented by another calendar that was more locally orientated to the study area.

Other workers have found also that, to be most useful, it is necessary to construct calendars which focus on local rather than national events and which are particular to a relatively small geographical area.

The age of adult males can also be estimated using event calendars but there are fewer cross-checks such as parity to confirm the approximate date-of-birth. Occasionally, adult males may have documentation such as military service papers, voting cards, and other official papers, which may include age information.

As for children, if the age of some adults can be determined accurately that of others may be estimated in relation to those of known age by asking if any of them attended circumcision ceremonies together, grew up together, played together, or went to school together. If not, perhaps they did so with the older brothers or sisters of the index individuals, and so on. Field staff must review their census schedules to check that the age information derived is reasonable. For example, a woman born in 1935 could not have had a child in 1942; it is unlikely that a woman would be

Table 6.2. Example of part of a calendar of local events used in Ghana Vitamin A Supplementation Trial (D. Ross, personal communication)

1900 (approx)	War with Zabog people from Burkina Faso
1906	Founding of the Catholic Mission in Navrongo (Father Oscar Morin)
1908	First Kassenas enrolled for Catechism training
1913	Baptism of the first Kassenas in Navrongo
1916	First conscription of local people into the British army for the First World War
1918	Collection of mats from each household for roofing of houses for British people to stay in
1919	Bad plague of locusts
⋮	⋮
1977	Introduction of First Phase of Junior Secondary Schools
1978	1 Achaempong overthrown by Gen. Akuffo (5 July)
	2 Change of currency notes (50 cedi note added)
1979	1 J.J. Rawlings first came to power (4 June)
	2 Shooting of Col. Felli and others by firing squad
	3 Elections for the Third Republic (Hilla Liman elected)
1981	PNDC revolution (31 December)
1983	Year of drought, bush fires, caterpillars, and food shortages
1984	1 Bumper harvest
	2 Cancellation of all O and A level results throughout West Africa
1985	1 Major dust storm, when it was dark all day (13 March)
	2 25th anniversary celebrations of Navasco and Notre Dame
	3 Start of the Mamprusi/Kusasi War in Bawku
	4 Fighting between Saboro and Wusungu started (Nov–Dec)
1986	1 Good harvest
	2 Heavy rain storm which destroyed part of the Bolgatanga-Navrongo road
1987	1 Introduction of Second Phase of Junior Secondary Schools (September)
	2 Ritual murder of an old man in Navrongo
1988	1 Start of armyworm invasion (June)
	2 Ordination of 3 local men to the RC priesthood in Navrongo (23 July)
	3 The bodies of 3 Kassenas who had been killed in a road traffic accident in Nigeria were brought back (August)
	4 Very heavy rain storm and floods with many houses destroyed
	5 J.J. Rawlings visit to Sandema (15 December)
	6 Navro Fao (27–29 December)

10 years older than her husband at marriage; and birth intervals of less than 9 months are uncommon and of less than 7 months are not possible. Field staff must be trained to check for such inconsistencies.

Well-known problems with age reporting are age 'heaping' and 'shifting'. Age heaping refers to terminal digit preference, the tendency for ages to be recorded as 10, 20, 30, 40 years or 25, 35, 45 years and so on. Field staff should be made aware of this during training. However, this was emphasized to enumerators of the 1955 Guinean census and at the end of the census there were too few individuals with ages ending in 0 or 5! Such effects may be of no great consequence for adults, for whom precise age estimation is rarely necessary. Age shifting is more difficult to detect and is most common where age is a criterion of social status. Individuals may falsify their ages so that they will appear to fieldworkers to have higher 'age status'. Women who have not yet married may falsify their age downwards, as may young men who wish to avoid military draft. In Muslim communities the ages of women may be especially difficult to estimate as women may be secluded and the men may respond on their wives' behalf (Bradley *et al*. 1986).

4.10 Other identifying information

In some countries full name and date-of-birth are sufficient to identify a person. If dates-of-birth are not known the addition of parental names, place of residence, and relationships to other household members is likely to be sufficient to identify individuals at a later date. Individuals may be issued with an identity number by the state or with a social security number which they keep throughout life. For studies involving adults it may be worthwhile to take polaroid photographs of all those registered; possibly giving one to the participant to keep in a plastic wallet which includes the study number they have been allocated, and keeping one in the trial records. In some studies, involving long follow-up of large populations in which only a small proportion are expected to develop the disease outcome of interest, hand-, foot-, or finger-prints may be used to check identities. This last method was used in a large BCG trial against tuberculosis in South India (Tuberculosis Prevention Trial Madras 1979), and also in a large study to assess whether vaccination with hepatitis B vaccine shortly after birth protects against liver cancer in adult life (The Gambia Hepatitis Study Group 1987).

5 DATA PROCESSING

Most censuses involve the collection of substantial amounts of data. It is important to plan how these data will be processed before the study is started. Usually it will be desirable that the information is entered into a computer shortly after it is collected so that a large backlog of work does not accumulate. Rapid data entry and validation is especially important if the information collected at the census is to be used to produce forms for the recording of additional procedures to be performed on the study participants shortly after the census. Furthermore, once the information is in a computer, consistency checks can be conducted and errors or queries referred back to the relevant fieldworkers. Such feedback should occur as soon as possible after the information has been collected.

The computer system should be situated in, or close to, the study area if possible, so that data can be entered into it rapidly. These aspects are discussed in Chapter 13. The design of the recording system may need to allow for changes in the composition of the study population over time, due to in-and-out migration, and for movement between households within the population. It will often be desirable to seek help and guidance from a statistician or data analyst for these aspects. This should be done at the start, rather than in the middle of a study.

6 POST-ENUMERATION CHECKS AND QUALITY CONTROL

Arrangements should be made for quality control at all stages of an investigation. Interview schedules that have been completed by fieldworkers should be checked daily; first by the fieldworkers themselves and then some or all should be checked by field supervisors and the project leader. Not all errors can be detected through visual checks of forms and some may only come to light in subsequent surveys or be detected by computer programs written to check for inconsistencies and other errors. The field staff should be aware that quality checking is a continuous process throughout the study. It is important to emphasize the great importance of having a system of routine supervision and regular checks to maintain the quality of work. In addition, it is important that project leaders and principal investigators should work with the field teams periodically. This serves to maintain morale and enables problems to be detected that field staff and supervisors may have missed or considered unimportant. If it appears that the work of field staff is not being examined error rates are likely to increase. For a random sample of households the census schedule should be completed again independently to check for errors. This is not always straightforward to do as people may not appreciate having to answer the same questions twice, and it may be difficult to be sure whether any inconsistencies are a result of interviewer or respondent error. Such post-enumeration checking is specially important during the early phases of a survey as the results may highlight any ambiguities in the interpretation of responses to questions or misunderstandings regarding the techniques to be used, for example, with respect to the methods used for age estimation or that used for the definition of temporary visitors. A post-enumeration survey might be conducted in conjunction with the collection of more detailed data on some or all members of the household; for example, when collecting information on household characteristics and assessing socio-economic status. If individual field staff prove unreliable, they may need to be retrained or dismissed and a re-enumeration undertaken of the areas they surveyed.

After the census the list of the population can be checked against other sources of information on the population. For example, school attendance records can be compared to the eligible age bands in the census and the information collected can also be compared with other census data either from the Central Statistics Offices or elsewhere. Population pyramids can be drawn to see if there are any unusual features, such as age heaping or disproportionate numbers of individuals at older ages. Sex ratios can be checked in areas where there is no selective migration of males or females.

7 VITAL REGISTRATION

In some trials the enumeration of the population at the start of the study is all that is required and there is no reason to monitor the population 'continuously' for births, deaths, and migration. In other trials, however, a system of registration of vital events may be required.

After the initial census and when the intervention has started or been applied, follow-up surveys may be required to assess the effects of the intervention. For diarrhoeal episodes, weekly or twice weekly visits may be required, whereas for deaths annual or quarterly surveys may be adequate. These visits provide an opportunity to update the census by ascertaining births, deaths, address changes, and migration into or out of the study area.

Maintaining an up-to-date census in this way may be difficult. It requires good organization, especially in areas with substantial migration, such as in peri-urban slums. For example, in a study carried out in southern Brazil, one half of the families with young children changed address within two years (Barros *et al.* 1990). It may be difficult to conduct long-term follow-up studies in such populations.

A census is relatively easy to update if a computer or other listing is available which gives the names of the residents in each household at the previous survey, with appropriate spaces for updating information (for example, see Stephens *et al.* 1989). Pregnant women should be noted, so that in the next survey enquiries may be made about the child. Maps should be updated, marking any new or abandoned houses. To obtain reasonable information on births and deaths the maximum interval between surveys probably should not exceed a year, and preferably will be less.

The recording of deaths occurring in the population is usually of special interest. Information on these may be obtained by employing 'village informers' to notify the trial investigators when deaths occur. Information may also be available through hospital, church, or cemetery records. Usually it will be necessary to supplement this information with a re-survey of the population if complete ascertainment of such events is required. Deaths tend to be missed unless specific questions are asked about each individual who was registered in the last round of the fieldwork. Such questioning must be done with sensitivity and the responses may need to be interpreted in the light of any local taboos against speaking of the dead.

REFERENCES

Barros, F. C., Victora, C. G., and Vaughan, J. P. (1990). The Pelotas (Brazil) birth cohort study 1982–1987: strategies for following up 6000 children in a developing country. *Perinatal and Paediatric Epidemiology*, **4**, 267–82.

Bradley, A. K., MacFarlane, S. B. J., Moody, J. B., Gilles, H. M., and Musa, B. D. (1986). Malumfashi endemic diseases project XXI: some aspects of the collection of demographic data. *Annals of Tropical Medicine and Parasitology*, **80**, 635–40.

McGregor, I. A., Thomson. A. M., and Billewicz, W. Z. (1968). The development of primary teeth in children from a group of Gambian villages and critical examination of its use for estimating age. *British Journal of Nutrition*, **22**, 307–14.

Imo State Evaluation Team (1989). Evaluating water and sanitation projects: lessons from Imo State, Nigeria. *Health Policy and Planning*, **4**, 40–9.

Smith, P. G., Revill, W. D. L., Lukwago, E., and Rikushin, Y. P. (1976). The protective effect of BCG against mycobacterium ulcerans disease: a controlled trial in an endemic area of Uganda. *Transactions of the Royal Society of Tropical Medicine and Hygiene*, **70**, 449–57.

Snow, R.W., Armstrong Schellenberg, J.R.M., Peshu, N., Forster, D., Newton, C.R.J.C., Winstanley, P.A., Mwangi, I., Waruiru, C., Warn, P.A., Newbold, C. and Marsh, K. (1993). Periodicity and space–time clustering of severe childhood malaria on the coast of Kenya. *Transactions of the Royal Society of Tropical Medicine and Hygiene*, **87**, 386–90.

Stephens, J., Alonso, P. L., Byass, P., and Snow, R. W. (1989). Tropical epidemiology: a system for continuous demographic monitoring of a study population. *Methods of Information in Medicine*, **28**, 155–59.

The Gambia Hepatitis Study Group (1987). The Gambia Hepatitis Intervention Study. *Cancer Research*, **47**, 5782–87.

Tuberculosis Prevention Trial Madras (1979). Trial of BCG in South India for tuberculosis prevention. *Indian Journal of Medical Research*, **70**, 349–63.

WHO Workshop (1980). Quantitative aspects of the epidemiology of *Schistosoma japonicum* infection in a rural community of Luzon, Philippines. *Bulletin of the World Health Organization*, **58**, 629–38.

Additional reading

Casely, D. J. and Lury, D. A. (1987). *Data collection in developing countries*. Chapter 3. Oxford University Press.

Pison, G. (1985). *Selected papers on population: calculating age without asking for it. Method of estimating age and age distributions of the Fula Bande (Eastern Senegal)*. INED-INSEE-ORSTOM Publications.

Shryock, H. S. and Siegal, J. S. (ed.) (1976). *The materials and methods of demography*. Chapters 2, 3, 6. Academic Press. New York.

World Health Organization (1978). *Geographical reconnaissance for malaria eradication programmes*. WHO, Geneva. Document PA/264.65.

World Fertility Survey (1976). *Training manual. Basic documentation, number 4*. International Statistical Institute, Voorberg, The Netherlands.

World Fertility Survey (1975). *Supervisors instructions. Basic documentation, number 5*. International Statistical Institute, Voorberg, The Netherlands.

World Fertility Survey (1975). *Interviewers instructions. Basic documentation, number 6*. International Statistical Institute, Voorberg, The Netherlands.

World Fertility Survey (1976). *Editing and coding manual. Basic documentation, number 7*. International Statistical Institute, Voorberg, The Netherlands.

Woods, R. (1979). *Population analysis in geography*. (Chapter 2). Longman group. London.

7
Randomization and coding

1 INTRODUCTION

The importance of randomization in the design and conduct of intervention trials has been stressed in Chapter 2, Section 4.1. Only if the units to which the interventions are applied (for example, individuals, households, or communities) are randomized between the interventions under study is it possible to be confident that any differences in the outcome measures of the trial among those in the different intervention groups are due to the effects of the interventions, rather than to underlying differences between the groups.

Randomization eliminates the possibility of any subjective influence in the assignment of individuals to the different intervention groups. It is superior to any systematic method of allocation, such as alternate assignment of the different interventions to successive trial entrants, or allocation based upon date-of-birth or date of entry (with, say, one intervention being assigned to those reporting on even dates and another to those reporting on odd dates). With systematic allocation, it is possible for the investigator to know in advance the group to which a participant will be allocated and this may introduce conscious or unconscious bias into the allocation procedure. For example, such knowledge may affect the investigator's judgement as to whether or not an individual is eligible for entry. For this reason it is essential that the randomization is done (or the randomization code is opened) only *after* it has been ascertained both that an individual is eligible for entry into a trial and also that he or she is prepared to participate in the trial no matter which intervention is assigned.

In this chapter various ways are described in which interventions may be randomly assigned among trial participants. The simplest method, if there are two intervention groups, is by tossing a coin to decide the allocation for each individual. This can either be done literally or an equivalent procedure may be simulated using a table of random numbers, as described in Section 2.1. If the total number of persons in a study is small, such an assignment procedure may result in the compositions of the different intervention groups being markedly different with respect to factors that may affect the outcome measures in the trial, or markedly unequal numbers of participants may be recruited to each intervention group. Such imbalance may arise by chance as, for example, it is possible that if a coin is tossed 10 times it will come down heads, say, only twice. For trials involving several hundred participants or more, any such imbalance is likely to be small and can be taken into account in the analysis of the study. In a small trial, imbalance may make the trial more difficult to interpret and it is advisable to design the randomization procedure to ensure balance. For this purpose 'restricted' or 'blocked' randomization (Section 2.2) can be used to ensure balance in group sizes, while either stratum-matched (Section 2.3) or pair-matched (Section 2.4) designs are employed to produce balance in the composition of the groups with respect to those variables on which the matching is based.

Whenever possible, intervention studies should be both randomized and 'double-blind'; that is, neither the participants nor the investigator should know to which group each participant has been allocated. This guards against biases that may result from knowledge of the intervention affecting the way an individual is treated or monitored during the trial, or assessed at the end. 'Blinded' designs are described in Section 3, which includes a description of suitable coding systems (Section 3.1) and a discussion of circumstances in which it may be necessary to 'break' the intervention code for an individual (Section 3.2).

The techniques described below may be used whether the intervention is assigned to communities or to individuals. It is common, however, for a matched-pairs design (Section 2.4) to be employed for trials in which communities are randomized, since the number of randomization units (communities) may be small (often 20 or less).

2 RANDOMIZATION SCHEMES

2.1 Unrestricted randomization

Simple random allocation of individuals between the different intervention groups is carried out most conveniently by using a table of random numbers, such as that given in Appendix 7.1 at the end of this chapter. An arbitrary starting point is chosen in the table, for example, by placing a pencil point on a page of the random numbers, with eyes closed. Numbers are then read from the table from that point according to some predetermined sequence. For example, row-by-row across the page, or column-by-column down the page, or row-by-row within a block or column-by-column within a block, and subsequent blocks are selected from those adjacent either horizontally or vertically. Some calculators have a key which generates a 'random' number on the display (usually a decimal number between 0 and 1) and random numbers can also be generated using a microcomputer (for example, there is a specific instruction in the computer programming language BASIC to do this). Unfortunately, some of these 'random number generators' do not produce numbers that are 'sufficiently random' and there is a danger that there may be an unacceptably long run of allocations to one of the treatment groups. Although for most purposes the random numbers so generated may be used instead of random number tables, in general it is probably safer to use a table of random numbers.

If randomization is required between two groups, one-digit random numbers are selected (for example, the first digit after the decimal point on a calculator display of a random number). Odd numbers (1,3,5,7,9) might be assigned for one intervention group

(A) and even numbers (0,2,4,6,8) for the other group (B), or vice versa. For example, suppose numbers are selected row-by-row across the page starting at the top left hand corner of Appendix 7.1(d). The first ten numbers selected are 8,4,3,7,9,0,6,1,5,6. Thus, the first and second participants would be allocated to group B, the third, fourth and fifth to group A, the sixth and seventh to group B, the eighth and ninth to group A, and the tenth to group B. This is illustrated in the first section of Table 7.1. Procedures for randomizing between three or four intervention groups are also shown in the table, together with an alternative procedure for allocating to 2 groups.

Random number tables are generated in such a way that each of the digits 0 through to 9 is equally likely to occur. If equal numbers of participants are required in each intervention group, the same number of one-digit numbers should be assigned for each group, even if this means that some digits do not correspond to any group. Thus, in the case of three groups, three of the ten one-digit numbers are assigned to each group. Selection of the number zero

Table 7.1. Examples of allocation procedures for unrestricted randomization, for 2, 3, or 4 intervention groups

Number of intervention groups	Allocation procedure	Example of sequence of random members with corresponding allocation
2	A: 1,3,5,7,9 B: 0,2,4,6,8	8 4 3 7 9 0 6 1 5 6 B B A A A B B A A B
	A: 0–4 B: 5–9	8 4 3 7 9 0 6 1 5 6 B A A B B A B A B B
3	A: 1–3 B: 4–6 C: 7–9 (0 ignored)	8 4 3 7 9 0 6 1 5 6 C B A C C – B A B B
4	A: 1–2 B: 3–4 C: 5–6 D: 7–8 (9, 0 ignored)	8 4 3 7 9 0 6 1 5 6 D B B D – – C A C C

from the random number tables is ignored, and the selection proceeds to the next number.

It has been emphasized above that the allocation of an intervention to an individual should be made only after the individual has been accepted for entry into the trial. A commonly used procedure is to prepare a set of sealed and numbered envelopes containing the allocations (or possibly the actual interventions if these are drugs). The envelopes are opened in sequence as each new person is entered into the trial. Entry criteria must be checked and eligibility satisfied before an envelope is opened, in order to exclude the possibility that the decision to accept a subject into the trial is influenced by the knowledge of the group to which he or she would be allocated. For large trials the use of envelopes may be too cumbersome. Coding systems and alternative procedures appropriate for use in the case of 'double-blind' designs are discussed in Section 3.1.

If only some individuals in a community are to receive an intervention, the trial may be more acceptable if the community is involved in the randomization procedure. For example, the village head might be asked to draw slips of paper from a bucket containing the names of all those in the village eligible for entry into the trial, the names being allocated as they are drawn alternately to intervention or control groups. In this way it is apparent that the allocation is random and that no favouritism is operating. Codes can be used to indicate which intervention is to be allocated so that 'blindness' can be preserved (see Section 3.1).

2.2 Restricted randomization

Although an 'unrestricted' randomization procedure should lead to approximately equal numbers of participants in each group, this is not guaranteed. For example, there is more than a 5 per cent chance that if 20 participants are allocated to one of 2 groups at random, 6 or fewer may be allocated to one group and 14 or more to the other. A better balance may be achieved by using a 'restricted randomization' procedure, also called 'blocked randomization' or 'randomization with balance'. This procedure ensures equal numbers in each group after fixed numbers of allocations. For example, the allocation procedure might be designed in blocks of 10 such that, in every 10 allocations, 5 are to one group and 5 to the other.

The size of the blocks must be a multiple of the number of intervention groups.

In order to minimize the possibility that an allocation can be deduced from previous allocations, the block size should not be too small (in particular it should not be two) and, if possible, it should not be known to the investigator responsible for the administration of the interventions. Indeed, as far as possible, those giving the interventions should not be aware that blocking has been carried out. Another safeguard may be to use several different block sizes for allocating interventions in a trial. For example, sometimes using 8, sometimes 10, and sometimes 12.

Two different procedures for carrying out restricted randomization are described below, one appropriate for small block sizes and the other appropriate for larger block sizes, say 8 or more.

2.2.1 Small block sizes

If two interventions, say A and B, are to be allocated using a block size of, say 4, it is possible to list all the different possible combinations of the allocations that will yield two As and two Bs. This is illustrated in Table 7.2. A number is allocated to each combination and a random number is chosen to select a particular allocation.

The selection of each random number generates four allocations. For example, starting in the middle column of the first block of the second row of blocks on Appendix 7.1(a), and reading down

Table 7.2. Example of allocation rule for a block size of 4, with two intervention groups, A and B

Allocation	Corresponding random number
AABB	1
BBAA	2
ABAB	3
BABA	4
ABBA	5
BAAB	6
Ignore	codes 7,8,9,0

the column, gives the first five random numbers in the sequence as 7,1,6,1,8. Since codes 7 and 8 have no corresponding sequence in Table 7.2, the 5 numbers yield a list of twelve allocations as follows:

7	1	6	1	8
____	AABB	BAAB	AABB	____

2.2.2 Larger block sizes

Listing all possible combinations of allocations within a block becomes unmanageable as the block size increases. For example, with a block size of ten, there are 252 different possible combinations each yielding five participants in each of two intervention groups, A and B. An alternative approach is necessary, therefore. Suppose the block size is to be 12 and six allocations are to be made to group A and six to group B. Appendix 7.1 may be used to select six different two digit random numbers between 01 and 12. For example, starting at the top left of the middle block in Appendix 7.1 (b) and reading down the page gives the random numbers 67,02,79,87,34,11,52,07, 04,01, . . . If numbers are ignored that fall outside the range 01 and 12 or that duplicate a number previously selected, the sequence obtained is: 02,11,07,04,01,12.

Thus the second, eleventh, seventh, fourth, first, and twelfth participants within the block are allocated to one of the interventions, say A, and the other participants to B. The complete sequence for the block of 12 is:

Participant:	01	02	03	04	05	06	07	08	09	10	11	12
Group:	A	A	B	A	B	B	A	B	B	B	A	A

A similar procedure is used to allocate interventions in the next block (i.e. 13 to 24), and so on.

In general, it is better to choose block sizes which are not too large to reduce the risk of a long sequence of individuals being allocated to the same intervention. A maximum block size of 12 is suggested.

2.3 Stratified randomization

If the effect of an intervention may be different in different subgroups of participants, say in males and females, it may be desirable to design the allocation procedure such that the interventions are equally divided in each subgroup. This may be achieved though 'stratified' randomization. The population is stratified, for example, by sex, and the allocation of the interventions is carried out separately in each stratum.

Stratification may be based on more than one factor. For example, there may be a separate allocation of interventions in each of a number of different age–sex groups. The greater the number of strata, the more complex is the organization of the randomization and, in general, the number of strata should be kept to a minimum. Different coloured sets of envelopes, packages, or sticky labels, might be employed for each stratum.

Stratified randomization should be considered if it is known that there are large differences in disease risk between different individuals in a trial and that it is possible to place individuals in strata corresponding to different levels of risk prior to entry to the trial. The objective of stratification is to try to include in each stratum those at similar risk of disease and to randomize between interventions separately within each stratum.

2.4 Randomization with a matched-pair design

A matched-pairs design is a special case of stratified randomization in which the strata are each of size 2. Individuals (or communities) are matched into pairs, chosen to be as similar as possible for potential confounding variables, such that in the absence of any intervention they would be expected to be at similar risk of the disease under study. One member of each pair is assigned at random to one intervention group and one to the other intervention group. A random number is selected and this determines to which group the first member of a matched pair is allocated; the other member of the pair is allocated to the other group. For example, consider the random number sequence given as an example at the top of Table 7.1, namely 8,4,3,7,9,0,6,1,5,6, with odd numbers corresponding to group A and even numbers corresponding to group B. This would lead to the following distribution for the first ten matched pairs recruited: BA BA AB AB AB BA BA AB AB BA.

Similar matching procedures can be employed when there are more than two intervention groups. For example, with three groups matched triads would be employed. The randomization procedure would be based on the allocation of numbers to each of the six possible combinations of order of the three groups (ABC,ACB,BAC,BCA,CAB,CBA), in the way described in Section 2.1.

Matching is unnecessary in large trials, as it is likely that any imbalance between the intervention groups, with respect to risk factors for the occurrence of the outcomes of interest, will tend to even out. Furthermore, it is possible to adjust for any residual imbalance during the analysis of the study without important loss of statistical power.

For small trials more serious imbalance may arise which may be difficult to adjust fully for in the analysis. This is likely to be a special problem in trials in which communities are randomized, as it is unusual to be able to include large numbers of communities in such studies. Pair-wise matching of similar communities (i.e. communities in which the rates of the disease under study are likely to be similar in the absence of the interventions to be applied) before the allocation of interventions is likely to be a useful strategy in such situations.

3 BLIND DESIGNS

Whenever possible, neither the participants nor the investigators should know to which intervention group each participant belongs until after the end of the trial. Such 'double-blind' designs (both the investigator and the participants are 'blind') eliminate the possibility that knowing to which intervention an individual is allocated may affect the way the individual is treated or monitored during the trial, or the way an individual responds to the intervention, or the way an individual is assessed at the end of the trial. Sometimes, a double-blind trial is not possible and a 'single-blind' design might be used, in which the investigator knows to which group a participant belongs but the participant does not.

'Blinded' designs are especially important when those in one of the groups under comparison are given no intervention; that is, an intervention that is expected to have no effect on the outcome of interest. To maintain blindness in these circumstances, a placebo should be used, if possible, which should be as similar as possible to the intervention itself (with respect to appearance, taste, and so on). Sometimes an identical-looking placebo cannot be obtained and, in these circumstances, the investigator (and the participants) may be kept blind to which treatment is the active one. While this may be the best that can be done in some trials, it is generally undesirable. Either the participants or the investigator may form a view as to which is the active treatment (possibly erroneously) and this may affect differentially the amount of other care given to the participants or the likelihood that a participant reports apparently beneficial or harmful effects. For example, patients may express a strong preference for red rather than blue tablets, and report different effects even if both are inactive (Huskisson 1974)!

For some interventions it may be possible to preserve blindness in the initial phase of a trial, but this may be more difficult later. For example, in placebo-controlled studies of ivermectin against onchocerciasis it was found that some participants were able to guess that they had received an active drug rather than a placebo because of the effect of ivermectin on other helminth infections, such as ascaris, through the passage of worms in their stools, whereas those receiving placebo rarely experienced this effect. In placebo-controlled trials of BCG vaccination most of those who have received BCG develop a lasting scar, whereas those who have received placebo do not. The possible bias that this might induce in the assessment of whether or not a participant developed leprosy following vaccination was overcome in a trial in Uganda by covering the vaccination site with sticking plaster for all participants before each clinical examination (Brown and Stone 1966).

For some intervention trials in which the unit of randomization is the community, the use of a placebo is straightforward and is no different in principle from the situation for an individually randomized trial (for example, if a drug or a vaccine is the intervention under study). For other interventions, however, a suitable placebo may be impossible to find. For example, what would be a suitable placebo for an improved water supply and sanitation programme in a village?

If effective interventions are already known for the disease under study, it will usually be considered unethical to include a placebo-treated group in a trial, and so the comparison made must be of the currently-used therapy (or preventive measure) against the new one under test. For example, in a trial of a new measles vaccine it would be unacceptable to leave a comparison group unvaccinated (or to give a placebo) in most, if not all, circumstances. Even if effective interventions are not available, some investigators may be unwilling to allocate some of the trial participants to a placebo from which the participants can expect to receive no benefit. What is sometimes done is to use instead another intervention that would be expected to have no effect on the outcome under direct study in the trial but which may prevent or treat other diseases.

3.1 Coding systems

In some circumstances, it may be necessary to break the intervention code (Section 3.2) for an individual (say, if a severe side-effect becomes manifest) and the coding system should be designed such that, if this is necessary, the blindness of the investigator with respect to the interventions received by other trial participants should be preserved. For example, if one intervention is coded A and the other B, breaking the code for one individual effectively breaks the code for all participants (if the investigator knows who has received A and who B). The use of a single code for each intervention is, generally, a poor design. It is better to have a unique code for each participant and to have a separate list linking participant numbers with the intervention allocated, or to have only a very small number of participants sharing the same code number. For example, in a BCG trial in South India for tuberculosis prevention, ampoules (each containing several doses of vaccine) were packed in boxes of three. Each box held 3 vials containing 1 of 2 different vaccine doses or a placebo preparation. The three ampoules were randomly coded 1, 2, and 3. The vaccine received by a participant was coded in the trial records by a combination of the box number and the ampoule number (Tuberculosis Prevention Trial Madras 1979). If it had been necessary to break the vaccine code for an individual it would only have been broken for those participants who received vaccine from the same ampoule in the same box.

The randomization list should usually be prepared in advance of the trial and the codes assigned by someone other than the principal investigator. If the intervention is a drug or a vaccine, the manufacturer may agree to supervise the packaging and coding, but the allocation procedure should be overseen, and the code should be held during the trial by a disinterested party. It is also worth checking, for a random sample of the drugs or vaccines, that the codes are correct and errors have not been made in the packaging.

3.1.1 Individual allocations

Suppose 2 interventions are to be allocated between 200 individuals. A good coding scheme would be to chose 100 random numbers between 1 and 200 and allocate these codes for intervention A, say, and allocate the other 100 for intervention B (there may also be some 'blocking' within the total group of 200, say in blocks of size 10; see Section 2.2). When an intervention is allocated to the 127th patient in the trial, they might be given the drugs, if this was the intervention, say in envelope number 127, and this would be noted in their trial record. A master list of the interventions corresponding to each number would be kept in a secure place by a third-party not directly connected with the trial. If it was necessary to break the code for an individual patient the third-party could do this without revealing any of the other codes to the investigator. Only at the end of the trial would the list be released to the investigator for the analysis of the results of the trial.

3.1.2 Group allocations

If a trial involves many thousands of participants it may be too time-consuming to allocate a separate treatment code number to each participant. An alternative approach is to use a fixed, but not too small, number of codes for the different interventions. If there are N participants in the trial and C codes for the interventions, then breaking the code for one participant would break the codes for N/C in total. For example, the coding system that was used for a vaccine trial in Venezuela is given in Box 7.1. In this trial 998 different codes were used (499 for one vaccine and 499 for the other) for about 30 000 participants. Breaking the code for one individual would break it for about 30 others.

A simpler system might be required if participants had to be given the same intervention on a number of occasions. A method

Box 7.1. Assignment of check letter for three-digit vaccine code

The coding system described below was that used in a leprosy vaccine in Venezuela. Randomization was to one of two vaccines. The vaccine vials were labelled with a number between 1 and 998. 499 of these numbers were allocated at random for one vaccine, and the other 499 for the other vaccine. A check letter was added to each number so that transcription errors would stand a high chance of being detected. The code was devised such that every possible permutation of the same three digits in a number had a different check letter, as illustrated below:

```
001A   010B   100C
002D   020E   200F
 .
 .
 .
009M   090N   900P
010B—already allocated—see above
011R   101S   110T
 .
 .
123W   132X   213Y   231A   312B   321C
124D   142E   214F   241G   412H   421J
 .
 .
```

and so on.

In some countries 1's and 7's are distinguished clearly when written by the 7 having a horizontal stroke put through it. In other countries, however, this is not done and there is a danger that these numbers will be confused. In such cases it would be advisable to change the check coding system such that if a 1 is confused with a 7, or vice-versa, the check letter will enable the error to be detected. Thus the system outlined above might be modified as indicated below:

```
001A   010B   100C   007D   070E   700F
002G   020H   200J
003K    .      .
 .
 .
011R   101S   110T   017V   107X   170Y   701A   710B
077C   707D   770E
012F    .
```

that was used in a trial of ivermectin against onchocerciasis in Sierra Leone was to allocate 20 codes for ivermectin or placebo treatments (A,B,C,D, ... and so on). The drugs were taken to the field in 20 tins with the code letters on them (10 ivermectin, 10 placebo) and participants were allocated to 1 of the 20 codes at random. If a participant was allocated, say to code E, then each time they were treated the dose was taken from tin E. About 1000 patients were included in the trial so that breaking the code for one individual would have also broken it for 1000/20 = 50 others (J. Whitworth, personal communication).

With either individual or group allocations it is helpful if the intervention codes are on removable sticky labels that can be affixed to the individual's form, thus minimizing the likelihood of any recording errors. Where possible the coding system should be devised so that transcription errors in recording may be detected. How this was achieved in the leprosy vaccine trial in Venezuela is illustrated in Box 7.1.

3.2 Breaking the code

There are several circumstances in which it might be necessary to break the trial codes. First, an individual in the trial may become seriously ill and knowledge of the intervention received may be needed to decide the appropriate treatment to give. It should be noted, however, that in most situations knowledge of the intervention is unlikely to be needed to treat such illnesses.

Second, adverse reactions may appear to be occurring as a consequence of the intervention and if these are sufficiently serious or frequent it may be necessary to consider stopping the trial. In such circumstances it is best if a 'monitoring group', not directly involved in the organization of the trial, is charged with breaking the code and assessing the results (see Chapter 2, Section 10.3). This group need not reveal the codes to the investigator unless it is considered that there is sufficient evidence to recommend stopping the trial. If it is found, for example, that apparent adverse reactions are equally prevalent among those receiving a placebo and those receiving the active drug then it may be decided there are no grounds for stopping the trial or revealing the codes to the investigators.

Third, it may be unethical to prolong a trial beyond the time it is apparent that one group is faring substantially better than another.

If this is a possible concern, a 'monitoring group' might also be asked to break the code and review the trial results periodically without revealing either the results or the codes to the investigators. Only when this group is satisfied that the trial should stop should the code be broken to the investigators.

In a trial of the drug ivermectin against onchocerciasis in West Africa, a computer program was written that would allow the data to be analysed during the course of the trial according to whether individuals were receiving ivermectin or placebo. The analyses were done only by group and the treatments received by individuals were not revealed (J. Whitworth and G. Maude, personal communication).

In practice, the necessity to break the code is very rare. It is important to decide before the start of the trial the conditions under which the code will be broken, and the extent to which it will be broken. It is preferable that the decision rests with an independent disinterested party, such as a data monitoring committee, rather than with the investigators themselves.

REFERENCES

Armitage, P. and Berry, G. (1987). *Statistical methods in medical research*, (2nd edn). Blackwell, London.
Brown, J. A. K. and Stone, M. M. (1966). BCG vaccination of children against leprosy: first results of a trial in Uganda. *British Medical Journal*, **1**, 7–14.
Fisher, R. A. and Yates, F. (1974). *Statistical tables for biological, agricultural and medical research*. Longman Group UK Ltd, London (previously published by Oliver and Boyd Ltd, Edinburgh).
Huskisson, E. C. (1974). Simple analgesics for arthritis. *British Medical Journal*, **3**, 196–200.
Tuberculosis Prevention Trial Madras (1979). Trial of BCG in South India for tuberculosis prevention. *Indian Journal of Medical Research*, **70**, 349–63.

Appendix 7.1 Random numbers

(Reproduced from Table XXXIII of Fisher and Yates 1963, by permission of authors and publishers)

(a)

03	47	43	73	86	36	96	47	36	61	46	98	63	71	62	33	26	16	80	45	60	11	14	10	95
97	74	24	67	62	42	81	14	57	20	42	53	32	37	32	27	07	36	07	51	24	51	79	89	73
16	76	62	27	66	56	50	26	71	07	32	90	79	78	53	13	55	38	58	59	88	97	54	14	10
12	56	85	99	26	96	96	68	27	31	05	03	72	93	15	57	12	10	14	21	88	26	49	81	76
55	59	56	35	64	38	54	82	46	22	31	62	43	09	90	06	18	44	32	53	23	83	01	30	30
16	22	77	94	39	49	54	43	54	82	17	37	93	23	78	87	35	20	96	43	84	26	34	91	64
84	42	17	53	31	57	24	55	06	88	77	04	74	47	67	21	76	33	50	25	83	92	12	06	76
63	01	63	78	59	16	95	55	67	19	98	10	50	71	75	12	86	73	58	07	44	39	52	38	79
33	21	12	34	29	78	64	56	07	82	52	42	07	44	38	15	51	00	13	42	99	66	02	79	54
57	60	86	32	44	09	47	27	96	54	49	17	46	09	62	90	52	84	77	27	08	02	73	43	28
18	18	07	92	46	44	17	16	58	09	79	83	86	19	62	06	76	50	03	10	55	23	64	05	05
26	62	38	97	75	84	16	07	44	99	83	11	46	32	24	20	14	85	88	45	10	93	72	88	71
23	42	40	64	74	82	97	77	77	81	07	45	32	14	08	32	98	94	07	72	93	85	79	10	75
52	36	28	19	95	50	92	26	11	97	00	56	76	31	38	80	22	02	53	53	86	60	42	04	53
37	85	94	35	12	83	39	50	08	30	42	34	07	96	88	54	42	06	87	98	35	85	29	48	39
70	29	17	12	13	40	33	20	38	26	13	89	51	03	74	17	76	37	13	04	07	74	21	19	30
56	62	18	37	35	96	83	50	87	75	97	12	25	93	47	70	33	24	03	54	97	77	46	44	80
99	49	57	22	77	88	42	95	45	72	16	64	36	16	00	04	43	18	66	79	94	77	24	21	90
16	08	15	04	72	33	27	14	34	09	45	59	34	68	49	12	72	07	34	45	99	27	72	95	14
31	16	93	32	43	50	27	89	87	19	20	15	37	00	49	52	85	66	60	44	38	68	88	11	80
68	34	30	13	70	55	74	30	77	40	44	22	78	84	26	04	33	46	09	52	68	07	97	06	57
74	57	25	65	76	59	29	97	68	60	71	91	38	67	54	13	58	18	24	76	15	54	55	95	52
27	42	37	86	53	48	55	90	65	72	96	57	69	36	10	96	46	92	42	45	97	60	49	04	91
00	39	68	29	61	66	37	32	20	30	77	84	57	03	29	10	45	65	04	26	11	04	96	67	24
29	94	98	94	24	68	49	69	10	82	53	75	91	93	30	34	25	20	57	27	40	48	73	51	92

Appendix 7.1 (contd.)

(b)

16	90	82	66	59	83	62	64	11	12	67	19	00	71	74	60	47	21	29	68	02	02	37	03	31
11	27	94	75	06	06	09	19	74	66	02	94	37	34	02	76	70	90	30	86	38	45	94	30	38
35	24	10	16	20	33	32	51	26	38	79	78	45	04	91	16	92	53	56	16	02	75	50	95	98
38	23	16	86	38	42	38	97	01	50	87	75	66	81	41	40	01	74	91	62	48	51	84	08	32
31	96	25	91	47	96	44	33	49	13	34	86	82	53	91	00	52	43	48	85	27	55	26	89	62
66	67	40	67	14	64	05	71	95	86	11	05	65	09	68	76	83	20	37	90	57	16	00	11	66
14	90	84	45	11	75	73	88	05	90	52	27	41	14	86	22	98	12	22	08	07	52	74	95	80
68	05	51	18	00	33	96	02	75	19	07	60	62	93	55	59	33	82	43	90	49	37	38	44	59
20	46	78	73	90	97	51	40	14	02	04	02	33	31	08	39	54	16	49	36	47	95	93	13	30
64	19	58	97	79	15	06	15	93	20	01	90	10	75	06	40	78	78	89	62	02	67	74	17	33
05	26	93	70	60	22	35	85	15	13	92	03	51	59	77	59	56	78	06	83	52	91	05	70	74
07	97	10	88	23	09	98	42	99	64	61	71	62	99	15	06	51	29	16	93	58	05	77	09	51
68	71	86	85	85	54	87	66	47	54	73	32	08	11	12	44	95	92	63	16	29	56	24	29	48
26	99	61	65	53	58	37	78	80	70	42	10	50	67	42	32	17	55	85	74	94	44	67	16	94
14	65	52	68	75	87	59	36	22	41	26	78	63	06	55	13	08	27	01	50	15	29	39	39	43
17	53	77	58	71	71	41	61	50	72	12	41	94	96	26	44	95	27	36	99	02	96	74	30	83
90	26	59	21	19	23	52	23	33	12	96	93	02	18	39	07	02	18	36	07	25	99	32	70	23
41	23	52	55	99	31	04	49	69	96	10	47	48	45	88	13	41	43	89	20	97	17	14	49	17
60	20	50	81	69	31	99	73	68	68	35	81	33	03	76	24	30	12	48	60	18	99	10	72	34
91	25	38	05	90	94	58	28	41	36	45	37	59	03	09	90	35	57	29	12	82	62	54	65	60
34	50	57	74	37	98	80	33	00	91	09	77	93	19	82	74	94	80	04	04	45	07	31	66	49
85	22	04	39	43	73	81	53	94	79	33	62	46	86	28	08	31	54	46	31	53	94	13	38	47
09	79	13	77	48	73	82	97	22	21	05	03	27	24	83	72	89	44	05	60	35	80	39	94	88
88	75	80	18	14	22	95	75	42	49	39	32	82	22	49	02	48	07	70	37	16	04	62	67	87
90	96	23	70	00	39	00	03	06	90	55	85	78	38	36	94	37	30	69	32	90	89	00	76	33

(c)

```
53 74 23 99 67   61 32 28 69 84   94 62 67 86 24   98 33 41 19 95   47 53 53 38 09
63 38 06 86 54   99 00 65 26 94   02 82 90 23 07   79 62 67 80 60   75 91 12 81 19
35 30 58 58 46   06 72 17 10 94   25 21 31 75 96   49 28 24 00 49   55 65 79 78 07
63 43 36 82 69   65 51 18 37 88   61 38 44 12 45   32 92 85 88 65   54 34 81 85 35
98 25 37 55 26   01 91 82 81 46   74 71 12 94 97   24 02 71 37 07   03 92 18 66 75

02 63 21 17 69   71 50 80 89 56   38 15 70 11 48   43 40 45 86 98   00 83 26 91 03
64 55 22 21 82   48 22 28 06 00   61 54 13 43 91   82 78 12 23 29   06 66 24 12 27
85 07 26 13 89   01 10 07 82 04   59 63 69 36 03   69 11 15 83 80   13 29 54 19 28
58 54 16 24 15   51 54 44 82 00   62 61 65 04 69   38 18 65 18 97   85 72 13 49 21
34 85 27 84 87   61 48 64 56 26   90 18 48 13 26   37 70 15 42 57   65 65 80 39 07

03 92 18 27 46   57 99 16 96 56   30 33 72 85 22   84 64 38 56 98   99 01 30 98 64
62 95 30 27 59   37 75 41 66 48   86 97 80 61 45   23 53 04 01 63   45 76 08 64 27
08 45 93 15 22   60 21 75 46 91   98 77 27 85 42   28 88 61 08 84   69 62 03 42 73
07 08 55 18 40   45 44 75 13 90   24 94 96 61 02   57 55 66 83 15   73 42 37 11 61
01 85 89 95 66   51 10 19 34 88   15 84 97 19 75   12 76 39 43 78   64 63 91 08 25

72 84 71 14 35   19 11 58 49 26   50 11 17 17 76   86 31 57 20 18   95 60 78 46 75
88 78 28 16 84   13 52 53 94 53   75 45 69 30 96   73 89 65 70 31   99 17 43 48 76
45 17 75 65 57   28 40 11 72 12   25 12 74 75 67   60 40 60 81 19   24 62 01 61 16
96 76 28 12 54   22 01 11 94 25   71 96 16 16 88   68 64 36 74 45   19 59 50 88 92
43 31 67 72 30   24 02 94 08 63   38 32 36 66 02   69 36 38 25 39   48 03 45 15 22

50 44 66 44 21   66 06 58 05 62   68 15 54 35 02   42 35 48 96 32   14 52 41 52 48
22 66 22 15 86   26 63 75 41 99   58 42 36 72 24   58 37 52 18 51   03 37 18 39 11
96 24 40 14 51   23 22 41 88 57   95 67 47 29 83   94 40 07 06 07   18 16 36 78 86
31 73 91 61 19   60 20 72 93 48   98 57 07 23 69   65 95 39 69 58   56 80 30 19 44
78 60 73 99 84   43 89 94 36 45   56 69 47 07 41   90 22 91 07 12   78 35 34 08 72
```

Appendix 7.1 (contd.)

(d)

84	37	90	61	56	70	10	23	98	05	85	11	34	76	60	76	48	45	34	60	01	64	18	39	96
36	67	10	08	23	98	93	35	08	86	99	29	76	29	81	33	34	91	58	93	63	14	52	32	52
07	28	59	07	48	89	64	58	89	75	83	85	62	27	89	30	14	78	56	27	86	63	59	80	02
10	15	83	87	60	79	24	31	66	56	21	48	24	06	93	91	98	94	05	49	01	47	59	38	00
55	19	68	97	65	03	73	52	16	56	00	53	55	90	27	33	42	29	38	87	22	13	88	83	34
53	81	29	13	39	35	01	20	71	34	62	33	74	82	14	53	73	19	09	03	56	54	29	56	93
51	86	32	68	92	33	98	74	66	99	40	14	71	94	58	45	94	19	38	81	14	44	99	81	07
35	91	70	29	13	80	03	54	07	27	96	94	78	32	66	50	95	52	74	33	13	80	55	62	54
37	71	67	95	13	20	02	44	95	94	64	85	04	05	72	01	32	90	76	14	53	89	74	60	41
93	66	13	83	27	92	79	64	64	72	28	54	96	53	84	48	14	52	98	94	56	07	93	89	30
02	96	08	45	65	13	05	00	41	84	93	07	54	72	59	21	45	57	09	77	19	48	56	27	44
49	83	43	48	35	82	88	33	69	96	72	36	04	19	76	47	45	15	18	60	82	11	08	95	97
84	60	71	62	46	40	80	81	30	37	34	39	23	05	38	25	15	35	71	30	88	12	57	21	77
18	17	30	88	71	44	91	14	88	47	89	23	30	63	15	56	34	20	47	89	99	82	93	24	98
79	69	10	61	78	71	32	76	95	62	87	00	22	58	40	92	54	01	75	25	43	11	71	99	31
75	93	36	57	83	56	20	14	82	11	74	21	97	90	65	96	42	68	63	86	74	54	13	26	94
38	30	92	29	03	06	28	81	39	38	62	25	06	84	63	61	29	08	93	67	04	32	92	08	09
51	29	50	10	34	31	57	75	95	80	51	97	02	74	77	76	15	48	49	44	18	55	63	77	09
21	31	38	86	24	37	79	81	53	74	73	24	16	10	33	52	83	90	94	76	70	47	14	54	36
29	01	23	87	88	58	02	39	37	67	42	10	14	20	92	16	55	23	42	45	54	96	09	11	06
95	33	95	22	00	18	74	72	00	18	38	79	58	69	32	81	76	80	26	92	82	80	84	25	39
90	84	60	79	80	24	36	59	87	38	82	07	53	89	35	96	35	23	79	18	05	98	90	07	35
46	40	62	98	82	54	97	20	56	95	15	74	80	08	32	16	46	70	50	80	67	72	16	42	79
20	31	89	03	43	38	46	82	68	72	32	14	82	99	70	80	60	47	18	97	63	49	30	21	30
71	59	73	05	50	08	22	23	71	77	91	01	93	20	49	82	96	59	26	94	66	39	67	98	60

8
Outcome measures and case definition

1 INTRODUCTION

Most field trials are designed to assess the impact of one or more interventions on the incidence, prevalence, or severity of some specified diseases, or on some intermediate variables which are considered to be closely related to some or all of these measures of disease load (for example, reduction in the density of the vector of a parasite or human behavioural changes that are likely to lower the risk of disease). The measures chosen to assess the impact of the interventions are called the *outcome* measures in the trial (or may also be called the *endpoints*). Such measures should be defined at the time the trial is designed in such a way that the outcomes can be compared between those in the different groups in the trial without bias, and there should be consistency in the definitions during the course of the trial. Clear definitions are also necessary so that the measures can be replicated in other trials and meaningful comparisons made between trials, which may be conducted at different times by different investigators. Failure to pay sufficient attention to the precise definition of the outcome measures at the start of a trial may lead to confusion in interpreting the results.

As discussed in Chapter 2, Section 5 several different outcome measures may be employed in an intervention trial and it is important to decide which is of most interest as this has major design implications, particularly in terms of the study size and duration. For interventions aimed at preventing disease, the outcome measure of most interest is likely to be the difference in the incidence of the disease between groups receiving different interventions. Even though an intervention may be designed to induce immunity (for example, a vaccine) which prevents or inhibits infection, or to reduce vector density leading to reduction of transmission of infection, or to change behaviour to reduce the risk of infection, the goal is to reduce disease incidence, particularly severe disease which may lead to permanent disability or death. Similarly, for intervention strategies designed to find and treat cases of disease, the outcome measures of most interest are likely to be a reduction in disability and death. Thus, the main outcome measures for many intervention studies are likely to be based on clinical criteria.

It will often be desirable to measure also short-term or intermediate effects, such as the incidence of infection and intensity of infection, changes in immune response, vector-biting density, infectivity of vectors, knowledge, attitudes and practices, or economic productivity.

In this chapter, the different kinds of outcome measures are reviewed (Section 2) and factors influencing the selection of these are also discussed (Section 3). The importance of standardizing measurements between different observers is stressed (Section 4.1) and there is a discussion of how the results of a trial may be influenced by poor sensitivity or specificity in the outcome measures (Section 4.2). Finally, ways of avoiding bias and maintaining quality control in case ascertainment methods are reviewed (Sections 4.3 and 4.4).

2 TYPES OF OUTCOME MEASURE

2.1 Clinical diagnosis

Clinical criteria provide the basis for defining disease and will be the basis of the outcome measures of primary interest in many intervention trials. A clinical diagnosis is usually based on a medical history and physical examination and may utilize the results of laboratory tests and X-ray or similar examinations. The taking of a medical history and the conduct of a physical examination are commonly considered to be the province of the medically qualified doctor and constitute important tools for understanding and diagnosing diseases in individual patients. For field trials specific questions concerning previous illness or present symptoms and specific kinds of physical examination may be of key importance for diagnosing the disease, which may be the outcome measure in a trial. Interviewing techniques and questionnaire design are discussed in Chapter 9 and issues concerning laboratory tests of relevance to diagnosis in field trials are outlined in Chapter 12.

The extent and nature of the physical examination needed depend upon the disease in question and the objectives of the trial, but usually the observations required are limited in number and often can be more efficiently carried out by specially trained paramedical workers than by physicians. Measures of body temperature, height, weight, and blood pressure are commonly done by paramedical staff. Also, measures such as liver and spleen size, lymphedema, and even assessment of cardiac size and grading of leprosy lesions, can be performed by well-trained and supervised paramedical staff.

Carrying out physical examinations may pose particular problems for the conduct of a trial. Special arrangements that provide for privacy and adequate lighting may be required and the examination procedure itself can be time-consuming. Since the removal of some or all clothing and the touching of the participant's body by the examiner is often needed, physical examinations are virtually always highly personal and may raise sensitive issues concerning individual dignity. When privacy is required, a third person in the examination room is often important both to reassure the patient and to provide against possible charges of misconduct. In the case of children, the mother's presence should normally be requested;

for the examination of women, a nurse and appropriate family members may be needed, even when the examiner is a woman. If there are local codes of behaviour that cover such circumstances, these must be adhered to.

The quality control and variability issues discussed in Section 4 apply to physical findings. Inter-observer variability in measuring such physical findings as liver and spleen size may be of particular importance, but measuring reproducibility, which requires repeat examination by different observers on a sample of the participants, may create difficult logistical problems. It is usually easier for the patient to remain in the same place and position and to be examined by a second observer immediately after the first than it is for them to have to dress and undress again and go through the whole procedure a second time, but the logistics to ensure that a second examiner is promptly available are not readily achieved and require careful organizational planning.

2.2 Standardized criteria for defining disease

For many diseases standardized criteria for defining a 'case' have been established. The criteria may be revised periodically as improved diagnostic tests become available and there is a better understanding of the disease process. For example, such criteria have been developed and revised for the diagnosis of AIDS, diarrhoeal diseases, and acute respiratory tract infections. They do not enable all cases of disease to be classified correctly. The aim has been to devise criteria that are reproducible between investigators. This facilitates comparisons of results from different studies. The International Classification of Diseases (WHO 1977), which is revised about every ten years, provides a basis for coding all diseases (using a four-digit code) in a systematic way and it is widely used for clinical and epidemiological research. The publication does not aim to give the criteria for making the diagnoses on which the codes are based, however.

If standardized criteria for 'case definition' have not been developed for the disease under study, a suitable definition should be established before the trial starts. This is often done by constructing a case definition that is agreed by clinicians experienced in the diagnosis of the disease. For several of the tropical diseases demonstration of the parasite may be diagnostic of the infection, but defining 'disease' is much more problematic, particularly for helminth infections. If the disease is such that a definite diagnosis can be made on the basis of other criteria (for example, an antibody test), the validity of the clinical criteria can be tested among individuals whose disease status can be confirmed. In a trial it may be necessary to base diagnosis on clinical criteria if, for example, there is not convenient access to a suitable laboratory.

Often several different definitions of a 'case' are possible and it will be important to choose the one that is most relevant for the objectives of the study. For example, for interventions against malaria a spectrum of different outcomes may be considered, ranging from the detection of asymptomatic parasitaemia through clinical disease to severe malaria and death. A variety of definitions are possible for the diagnosis of 'disease' due to malaria. In an area where malaria is holoendemic many children might have malaria parasites in their blood but show no clinical symptoms of malaria. In such an area possible definitions of disease due to malaria might include:

1. History of fever without other specific symptoms or signs with or without confirmation of fever by thermometer (temperature >38°C).
2. History of fever without other specific symptoms or signs and with or without confirmation of fever by thermometer (temperature >38°C), plus malaria parasites in a blood film.
3. History of fever without other specific symptoms or signs and with or without confirmation of fever by thermometer (temperature >38°C), plus a malaria parasite count 10,000 per μl blood or greater than or equal to 2 malaria parasites per white blood cell.

A variety of other definitions are possible.

It may be decided that 'severe malaria' would be the most appropriate outcome measure for a trial. In that case the diagnostic criteria should be carefully specified, taking account of the diagnostic facilities likely to be available to the investigators in the trial. A discussion of such diagnostic criteria is given in WHO (1986). If death from malaria is chosen as an outcome measure it may be necessary to develop criteria for the diagnosis of cause of death based on a 'verbal post-mortem' (see Section 2.3).

For some diseases there may be a gradient of diagnostic certainty and it may be possible to develop criteria to classify suspected cases as definite, probable, possible, or not cases. For example, in a large leprosy study in Malawi a diagnostic algorithm was devised to classify each suspected case of leprosy into one of four groups, as shown in Fig. 8.1. Using this algorithm individuals are classified as in the 'narrow' (N) group ('definite' leprosy), the 'middle' (M) group ('probably' leprosy), the 'wide' (W) group ('possibly' leprosy) or the 'not leprosy' (O) group (Ponnighaus *et al.* 1987).

2.3 Death and verbal post-mortems

Death is often assumed to be an outcome variable for a trial that can be measured with high sensitivity and specificity. It should not be assumed, however, that deaths can be ascertained without error. Individuals may have various reasons to encourage uncertainty about the vital status of their household members (for example, tax evasion). For young infants it may be difficult to distinguish still-births from early neonatal deaths unless mothers are questioned closely to establish whether the baby showed any sign of life, such as movement of limbs or crying. Infants whose birth and death occurs between two survey rounds may not be reported. In many cultures there is a reluctance to report deaths, and individuals who are said to be temporarily away may, in fact, have died.

Deaths may be best identified by some kind of continuous surveillance of the study population. For example, local informers might be recruited who live in the community and whose task is to report any deaths soon after they occur. Information on deaths may also be ascertained through regular complete surveys of the population, with careful enquiries being made regarding the vital status of anyone who does not present at a survey round. Special attention should be paid to households for which all members are absent because the death of an adult may lead to dissolution or migration of households. Enquiries should be made to neighbours in such circumstances. Recall periods of three to six months, and possibly as long as a year, are sufficiently short to obtain reliable information on deaths. The two approaches, surveillance and repeated surveys, may be used together and the results cross-checked. If the two systems for ascertaining deaths can be considered to be independent the discrepancies between the two can be

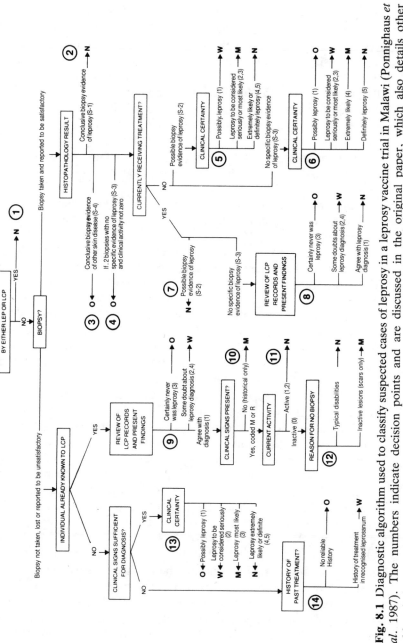

Fig. 8.1 Diagnostic algorithm used to classify suspected cases of leprosy in a leprosy vaccine trial in Malawi (Ponnighaus *et al.* 1987). The numbers indicate decision points and are discussed in the original paper, which also details other abbreviations used. Suspected cases of leprosy are classified into one of four groups: 'narrow' (N: definite), 'middle' (M: probable), 'wide' (W: possible), 'not leprosy' (O).

used to estimate the proportion of deaths likely to have been missed by both systems (Chandrasekar and Deming 1949).

Childhood mortality levels and trends in large populations may also be estimated indirectly using demographic techniques. Estimates of child mortality rates may be made from information on the proportions of children surviving who were born to mothers of specified ages. Similarly, adult mortality can be estimated from survey questions on orphanhood and widowhood. However, these estimates refer to the past (typically to periods at least two years prior to the survey) and are only useful as evaluation measures in trials of long duration (United Nations 1983; Hill and David 1988; Hill and Aguirre 1990; David *et al.* 1990).

While it is relevant to measure overall mortality rates for the evaluation of many interventions, and indeed this may be the most important measure of the overall public health impact, an intervention is likely to effect different causes of death differentially. For example, BCG vaccination might be expected to reduce mortality from tuberculosis, but to have no appreciable effect on other causes of death. In a trial of BCG vaccination it would be highly desirable to ascertain the causes of death of those in the trial groups as well as the total numbers of deaths. This is not a straightforward task. Even in developed countries with highly sophisticated death registration and certification systems, there is often uncertainty as to the correctness of the cause of death recorded on a death certificate, especially when the death has occurred outside of a hospital. In developing countries the reliability of death certificate information is even more suspect. In many developing countries only a small proportion of deaths take place in hospital and have a cause of death assigned by a doctor at the time of death and, even then, due to lack of diagnostic facilities in many hospitals in developing countries, diagnoses are often not reliable. It may be necessary to assign the probable cause of death on the basis of a 'verbal post-mortem', obtained by interviewing someone close to the deceased person (for example, the mother of a dead child) soon after the death (but probably not for a week or two after the death, during which time the mother is likely to be very distressed) to obtain a history of the symptoms and signs of the final illness. Specially trained lay reporters may be used to record the symptoms and signs and a clinician familiar with the patterns of mortality in the study area might then be able to use the information collected to assign a probable cause of death. Verbal post-mortems have been used to ascertain deaths from malaria and other causes in studies conducted in The Gambia (Greenwood *et al.* 1987).

A verbal post-mortem may be conducted by first asking the respondent to describe in their own words the circumstances of the death. The investigator then reads through a list of symptoms and for each ascertains if it occurred and for how long it was present. The symptom list should not be long (say, not exceeding 15 items) and should not include rare conditions (unless they are the subject of study). The list should be adapted for local disease patterns and the questions should be asked in a culturally acceptable and comprehensible manner. Usually the questions will seek information on fever, diarrhoea, vomiting, abdominal pain, cough, breathlessness, and chest pain. Information on any contact with the health services around the time of death should also be noted as hospital and clinic records may be available that will assist diagnosis.

An example of such a verbal post-mortem questionnaire that has been used in studies of child mortality in The Gambia is given in Appendix 8.1 at the end of this chapter (A. de Francisco, B. Greenwood, and P. Alonso, personal communication). An addendum to this, used for neonatal deaths, is given in Appendix 8.2.

The experience in The Gambia has been that examination of the completed questionnaires by a medical officer has enabled probable causes of death to be assigned to a high proportion of deaths among children and there has been reasonable consistency between different medical officers in the diagnoses derived. It is difficult to validate verbal post-mortem techniques but attempts to do this have given encouraging results (Alonso *et al.* 1987). There is less experience with this method for ascertaining causes of death among adults.

2.4 Behavioural changes

Interventions may be directed at altering knowledge and attitudes in order to change some specific behaviour thought to increase the risk of disease. Changes in knowledge or attitude can be assessed with reasonable reliability using questionnaires or appropriate interview methods, but observational studies may be required to determine if behavioural changes have actually occurred. For example, in a study to investigate the effectiveness of a health education campaign to promote use of latrines, it may be relatively straightforward to assess after the campaign whether individuals have a better knowledge of why using latrines is desirable, but observational studies, before and after the campaign, may be necessary to ascertain whether or not the frequency of use of latrines had changed. Further studies may then be needed to determine whether the changed behaviour has led to a reduction in disease.

2.5 Transmission reduction

The purpose of interventions based on vector control or environmental alteration is to reduce or to interrupt transmission of the infectious agent. A detailed discussion of the many possible intermediate outcome measures for these interventions is beyond the scope of this manual. Generally, the first priority is to determine whether the intervention has accomplished the immediate changes intended. For example, in trials in which insecticides are applied to reduce vector populations in order to reduce the transmission of some infectious agent, the first step would be to determine the impact of the intervention on the vector population. If the vector population is little affected it may be reasonable to conclude that any impact on human disease is unlikely. However, if there is a reduction in vector population it may be hazardous to conclude that the disease load will also fall. Thereafter, a study to determine the impact on disease may be required. Similarly, if interventions are being evaluated that may reduce indoor air pollution as a measure against respiratory disease, it may be best to focus initial studies on the assessment of changes in pollution levels, before assessing the impact on respiratory diseases. Usually, it will be more efficient to carry out trials to monitor the impact on disease only after there is evidence of an effect on the vector or on the agent against which the intervention is directed.

In order to assess a change in transmission any or all of several different outcomes may be used:

(1) a change in incidence of disease;

(2) a change in disease severity levels;

(3) a change in prevalence of disease;

(4) a change in density of infection (particularly for helminths);

(5) a change in the intensity of the infective agent in the vector.

The impact on these different outcomes will occur at different times. For example, in the Onchocerciasis Control Programme, the first evidence that the intensive larviciding of *Simulium damnosum* (black fly) breeding sites was having an effect was a dramatic drop in fly-biting rates in the intervention area. Over the next several years there was a steady fall in the intensity of micro-filarial infections among those living in the endemic area, but only after some years was it possible to detect evidence of a fall in the prevalence of infection, and later still was it possible to demon-strate an impact on blindness rates which is the major adverse health consequence of onchocerciasis.

2.6 Adverse reactions

The detection of adverse effects of an intervention may be an important part of a study. The problems of measuring such effects are similar to those of measuring other outcome variables but an important difference is that their nature may be ill-defined at the start of the study. Thus, adverse effects may be missed because neither participants nor the trial staff anticipate the particular effects produced. Participants may correctly or erroneously attri-bute all sorts of ailments, such as a painful knee or a headache, to the intervention. In general, it will only be possible to determine if the alleged effects are attributable to the intervention if the trial includes a suitable comparison group, possibly untreated.

It is important for the trial organisers to anticipate possible adverse effects of an intervention. Clues to these may come from earlier studies on animals or from experience with interventions of a similar kind. A decision will have to be made whether to seek information on such effects 'actively' or 'passively'. If each partici-pant is asked if they suffered any adverse effects of treatment, a wide range of different complaints may be volunteered, many of which may be relatively minor and of no great significance. None the less, if the trial includes a suitable comparison group, it may be of interest to compare the incidences of such effects. Alternatively, it may be decided not to ask about adverse effects specifically, but to record any that are volunteered by the participants, either when they are seen after the intervention or through them seeking medical attention at a local clinic. Fewer effects will be recorded in this way and those detected are likely to be for more serious conditions.

The intensity of the monitoring system for adverse effects will depend upon how much experience there has been with the intervention in the study area prior to the trial. A relatively 'new' intervention may demand close monitoring. For example, when it was planned to introduce ivermectin on a widespread basis for the treatment of onchocerciasis, a series of community trials involving many thousands of subjects was set up whose main objective was to assess the safety of the drug when given on a mass basis in affected communities (WHO 1989).

3 FACTORS INFLUENCING CHOICE OF OUTCOME MEASURES

In some trials the only outcome measure of interest is the change in the all-cause mortality rate attributable to an intervention, whereas in others a variety of different outcome measures may be employed, including changes in, for example, the incidence of both infection and disease due to a specific agent, the prevalence and intensity of infection, knowledge, attitudes and practices, economic productivity, and the density of disease vector populations.

The choice of the outcome measures in a specific trial may be constrained by economic, logistic, or ethical considerations. Often such constraints will make it necessary to focus evaluation of the impact of an intervention on variables intermediate to the outcomes of most interest. For example, if the intervention is a health education programme designed to persuade individuals to have fewer sexual partners in order to reduce the risk of HIV infection, it may be decided to measure the impact of the programme on behaviour rather than on changes in HIV incidence. Even if the latter was done, it would still be highly desirable to include measures of behaviour change to aid interpretation of the results. In studies on vaccines, the prime interest is often in the reduction of mortality or severe morbidity due to a specific disease, but in practice what is often done is to assess the impact of vaccination on infection rates or on mild disease and to assume that any protection observed will carry over to the more serious consequences. Otherwise a study of much greater size would be necessary to measure the outcomes of prime interest. For example, in trials of measles vaccines it is common to take cases of measles rather than deaths from measles as the main outcome variable. Often there are ethical constraints in observing the outcome of most interest in the context of a controlled field trial, especially when effective treatments are potentially available for the condition of interest.

Discussed below are some of the factors that may influence the choice of the outcome variables to be used in a specific field trial.

3.1 Relevance

Interventions are generally designed to reduce disease or to promote health in some way (i.e. to make people 'feel better'). The outcome measures chosen should reflect these objectives as fully as possible, but when intermediate variables are used rather than those of main interest, great care must be taken to choose variables of direct relevance to the main outcome. This is not always straightforward. For example, it may be decided to assess the impact of a vaccine by measuring the proportion of individuals who develop antibodies following vaccination against the agent that causes the disease of interest. This may be reasonable if it is known that there is a high correlation between the development of antibodies and protection from clinical disease. For many diseases, however, this relationship has not been established, and it would not be warranted to base conclusions regarding protection against disease simply on antibody determinations.

A health education intervention may be designed to change behaviour to reduce disease risk. Asking individuals if they have changed their behaviour may give a measure of impact that correlates poorly with changes in the risk of disease. Are individuals responding truthfully? Are they doing what they say they do? Even if behaviour changes, is this associated with a lowering in the incidence of disease?

The outcome variable measured should be as close as possible to the outcome of main interest. While this may seem a very obvious suggestion it may have major impact on the design of a study. For example, if the prevention of death is of prime interest, then whenever possible this should be made the endpoint of the trial.

The consequence might be to increase the size of the trial from hundreds to thousands of individuals. Not all investigators will be in a position to make such a jump, but it is important that some do, as otherwise there may never be an adequate test of whether the intermediate variables measured are acceptable surrogates for effects on mortality.

3.2 Feasibility

To be successful a trial must be designed to have achievable objectives. A trial which has mortality as the endpoint, but which is too large to be successfully completed, may be of less value than a well-designed smaller trial aimed at assessing impact on some intermediate endpoint. There must often be a compromise between relevance and feasibility. It is pointless to set unachievable goals, even if they look attractive in the objectives section of a proposal. Also, it may be of little value to measure the effect of an intervention on an outcome measure which is only distantly related to the measure of prime interest. The outcome measures selected will be much influenced by the resources available for the trial, the availability of skilled personnel, and necessary laboratory support to diagnose cases of disease. In many large trials every individual in the study population may have to be screened for disease or infection in a relatively short time. With such time constraints some individuals may be misdiagnosed. The consequences of reductions in diagnostic sensitivity and specificity are discussed in Section 4.2.

3.3 Acceptability

The acceptability of the measurement of an outcome variable to the study population is critical to the successful conduct of a trial. For example, the recording of birth weights may not be possible in a population that allows only close relatives access to a mother for a few weeks after the birth. The taking of venous blood samples or of repeated blood samples is unpopular in many societies. If the method for measuring the outcome involves pain or inconvenience to the participants it may be necessary to modify or abandon it. For example, an outcome whose assessment involves a long interview with participants at a time when they would otherwise be planting crops may be unacceptable and it may either have to be abbreviated or carried out at a more convenient time.

4 VARIABILITY AND QUALITY CONTROL OF OUTCOME MEASURES

4.1 Reproducibility

The extent to which different observers will make the same diagnoses or assessments on a participant, and to which observers are consistent in their classifications between participants, may have an important influence on the results of a trial. Clearly, it is desirable to choose outcome measures for which there is substantial agreement among observers with respect to the classification of participants in the trial.

For objective outcome measures, variations between observers, or by the same observer at different times, may be small and be unlikely to influence the results of a study. For outcome measures requiring some degree of subjective assessment, however, such variations may be substantial. The likely degree of such variations will influence the choice of outcome measures, as it will be preferable to select those measures that have the smallest inter- and intra-observer variations, yet still give valid measures of the impact of the intervention.

Variation among observers is often much greater than expected. If a study involves several observers, pilot studies should be conducted in order to measure the extent of such variation and, then, to seek to standardize the assessment methods to minimize the variation. With suitable training it is usually possible to reduce the variation between observers substantially.

For some outcomes independent assessment by two observers should be routine, with a third being called in to resolve disagreements. It may be costly to screen the whole trial population in this way, but a common approach is to have all suspected cases of the disease of interest examined by a second observer, mixed in with a sample of those not thought to have the disease. In this way it is possible to obtain estimates of differences of sensitivity and specificity between observers. Variable readings by the same observer may be more difficult to assess. Sometimes it is possible to have the observer examine the same individual twice, but these examinations may not be independent unless the survey is large and the observer does not remember the result of the first assessment.

It is important to make every effort to reduce variability to the greatest extent possible. Having done so, however, it is also critical to know the extent of the remaining, 'irreducible', variability for purposes of analysis. The purpose of all trials is to demonstrate differences between interventions. Knowledge of the inherent variability in diagnostic procedures is essential for this demonstration, and the best way of assessing this is through replicate measures. It is especially important to take account of between observer differences when communities are the units of randomization in a field trial. Differences between observers may produce biases if different observers are used in different villages. In such situations it is better to organize the field work so that the workload within each community is split among different observers so that differences between the observers are not confounded with the effect of the intervention.

4.2 Sensitivity and specificity

The choice of an appropriate definition of a 'case' in a field trial will be influenced by the sensitivity and specificity associated with the diagnostic criteria. *Sensitivity* is defined as the proportion of true cases who are classified as cases in the study. *Specificity* is the proportion of non-cases who are classified as non-cases in the study. A low sensitivity is associated with a reduction in the measured incidence of disease. This decreases the likelihood of observing a significant difference between two intervention groups in a study of a given size. In statistical terms, it reduces the *power* of the study (see Chapter 3, Section 2.2). If the incidence of disease in both the intervention group and the comparison group will be affected proportionately in the same way, as is usually the case, it does not bias the estimate of the relative disease incidence in the two groups, though the absolute magnitude of the difference will be less than the true difference. Thus, in the context of a vaccine trial, because protective efficacy is assessed in terms of relative differences in incidence between groups, the estimate of protective efficacy will not be biased, but the confidence limits on the estimate will be wider than they would be using a more sensitive case definition. In theory, the reduction in power associated with low sensitivity can be compensated for by increasing the trial size.

In general, a low specificity of diagnosis is a more serious problem than low sensitivity in intervention trials. A low specificity results in the disease incidence rates being estimated to be higher than they really are. Generally, the levels of inflation in the rates will be similar, in absolute terms, in the intervention and the comparison group, and thus the ratio of the measured rates in the two groups will be less than the true ratio. Thus, in vaccine trials, for example, the vaccine efficacy estimate will be biased towards zero, though the absolute difference in the rates between intervention and control groups will not be biased (unless there is also poor sensitivity). Increasing the trial size will not affect the bias in the estimate of vaccine efficacy.

In algebraic terms, suppose the true disease rates are r_1 and r_2 in the two groups under study, the true relative rate $R = r_1/r_2$ and the true difference in disease rates $D = r_1 - r_2$. If sensitivity is less than 100 per cent (but specificity is 100 per cent) and only a proportion, k, of all cases are correctly diagnosed, the measured disease rates in the two groups will be kr_1 and kr_2; the measured relative rate will be $kr_1/(kr_2) = R$; and the measured difference in disease rates will be $kr_1 - kr_2 = k(r_1 - r_2) = kD$ (which is less than D). If specificity is less than 100 per cent (but sensitivity is 100 per cent) and the rate of false diagnoses is s, the measured rates in the two groups will be $(r_1 + s)$ and $(r_2 + s)$; the measured relative rate will be $(r_1 + s)/(r_2 + s)$ (which is less than R); and the measured difference in disease rates will be $(r_1 + s) - (r_2 + s) = D$.

In the above we have assumed that it is possible to measure the sensitivity and specificity of the diagnostic procedures used in a trial. To do this it is necessary to have a 'gold standard' for diagnosis (i.e. it is necessary to know who really is a case and who is not). Sometimes this is not possible and, even if definitive diagnostic procedures exist, it may be necessary to use imperfect procedures in a field trial for reasons of cost or logistics. In this situation, if an assessment is made of sensitivity and specificity, it is possible to evaluate the consequences for the results of a field trial, and possible even to correct for biases in efficacy estimates due to the use of a non-specific diagnostic test. Unfortunately, in many situations, there is no 'gold standard' and so the sensitivity and specificity of the diagnostic methods used may be uncertain. For example, there is no universally agreed definition of a case of clinical malaria. Most would agree that the presence of parasites in the blood is necessary (unless a potential case has taken treatment before presenting) and many would agree that the presence of fever associated with parasitaemia increases the likelihood of the disease being clinical malaria, but it is also possible that the fever is due to other causes.

The bias induced by low specificity of diagnosis is most severe for diseases that have a low incidence. A good example of this is provided by leprosy, which is both difficult to diagnose (in the early stages) and also of low incidence. Consider a vaccine trial in which the true disease incidence in the unvaccinated group is 10 per thousand over the period of the trial, and the true vaccine efficacy is 50 per cent; i.e. the true disease incidence in the vaccinated is 5 per thousand over the period of the trial. If the sensitivity of the diagnostic test used for cases is 90 per cent but the specificity is 100 per cent, the observed disease incidences would be 9.0 and 4.5 per thousand, respectively. Thus, the estimate of vaccine efficacy remains correct (50 per cent). The power of the study is reduced, however. To achieve the power that would be associated with a 'perfect' test, the trial size would have to be increased by about 11 per cent. If the specificity of the diagnostic test is as high as 99 per cent and the sensitivity is 100 per cent, the observed disease incidences would be 20 per thousand in the unvaccinated group and 15 per thousand in the vaccinated group. Thus, even with a test with 99 per cent specificity, the estimate of vaccine efficacy is reduced from the true value of 50 per cent to 25 per cent. If the specificity of the test was 90 per cent the expected estimate of vaccine efficacy would be 4 per cent.

In vaccine trials the sensitivity and specificity of the diagnostic test are of consequence in different ways at different times in the trial. When individuals are screened for entry to the trial it is important that the test used should be highly sensitive, even if it is not very specific, as substantial bias may be introduced if undiagnosed 'cases' are included in the trial and included in the vaccinated or unvaccinated groups. If the vaccine has no effect on the progression of their disease and they are detected as cases later in the trial, a falsely low estimate of efficacy will result. Thus, individuals whose diagnosis is 'doubtful' at entry to the trial should be excluded from the trial. Conversely, once individuals have been screened for entry into the trial and they are being followed for the development of disease, a highly specific test is required to avoid the bias illustrated in the example above.

In situations where there may be no clear-cut definitions of a case (for example, early leprosy, childhood tuberculosis), studies of intra-observer and inter-observer variation may be undertaken using various definitions of disease. The definition that shows least disagreement between observers and gives maximum consistency within each observer may be the appropriate one to use in a trial, but the investigator should be aware of the potential for bias discussed above.

4.3 Bias

The most powerful way to minimize bias in the assessment of the impact of an intervention is through the conduct of a double-blind and randomized trial, as discussed in Chapters 2 and 7. If these two aspects are built into a trial, an effect of an intervention is not likely to be observed if there is no true effect. However, as pointed out in Section 4.2, if the specificity of the diagnosis for the outcome of interest is poor, the estimate of the efficacy of an intervention, measured in relative terms, may be biased towards zero, even in a properly randomized, double-blind investigation.

It is highly desirable that the person making diagnoses in a trial is ignorant of which intervention the suspected cases have received. If the diagnosis is based on laboratory tests or X-ray examinations, blindness should be easy to preserve. In some circumstances it may be possible to determine from the results of a laboratory test which intervention an individual has received, as the test may be measuring some intermediate effect between the intervention and the outcome of prime interest. In such cases, those making diagnoses in the field should not be given access to the laboratory results. For example, in placebo-controlled studies of praziquantel against schistosomiasis in communities where the infection was common, those who had received the active drug would be easily detected by a rapid reduction in egg counts in stool or urine samples following treatment. If the outcome of main interest was morbidity from the disease then the egg count information should be kept from those making the assessment of morbidity. It would be inappropriate to use measures of antibodies to make diagnoses of disease following vaccination, if the vaccination itself induced antibodies. Similarly, tuberculin testing should not be part of diagnostic procedures for tuberculosis in studies of the efficacy of BCG vaccination as the vaccine alters the response to the test.

If the diagnosis of disease is based on a clinical examination, it may be necessary to take special precautions to preserve blindness. An example is given in Chapter 7, Section 3 with respect to a BCG trial against leprosy. Even if the participants know which intervention they had, it is important to try to keep this knowledge from the person making any diagnoses. Thus, participants might be instructed not to discuss the intervention with the examiner and the examiner would be similarly restricted. Such a procedure is not fail-safe, of course, but great efforts should be made to preserve blindness, if at all possible, especially if the diagnosis is made on subjective criteria.

If randomization is by community, it may be especially difficult to keep examiners ignorant of the intervention an individual received. Sometimes ways can be found of doing this, for example, by conducting surveys for disease by bringing all participants to a clinic outside of the communities. If communities are randomized to receive an improved water supply or not, one outcome measure might be the incidence of scabies infection. It may be difficult to avoid the possibility of the diagnoses of scabies being influenced by the observer's knowledge of whether or not the participant was in a village with an improved water supply. In such a case it may be best to seek other measures of impact based upon objective criteria or on laboratory measures.

4.4 Quality control issues

The sensitivity and specificity of the diagnostic procedures employed in a trial should be monitored for the duration of the trial, as they may change as the study progress. Such changes may be for the worse or for the better. With experience, diagnostic skills may improve, but also as time passes the staff may become bored and take less care. It is important that the field staff are aware that their performance is being continuously monitored. If this is done then anyone who goes 'off the rails' can be steered back or removed from the study before much harm is done. Such monitoring is important for both field and laboratory staff.

The methods used to monitor the quality of diagnostic procedures may include the re-examination of a sample of cases by a supervisor or by a more highly trained investigator and, for the laboratory, may be done by sending a sample of specimens to a reference laboratory or passing some specimens through the laboratory in duplicate, in a blinded fashion, to determine if the differences between results on the same specimen are within acceptable limits. Discussion of quality control in relation to the evaluation of a schistosomiasis control programme is given in Braun-Munzinger (1989).

If the disease under study is relatively rare it may be difficult to measure sensitivity based on small samples of individuals being examined twice. While it will be possible to check if specificity is poor (a high proportion of those classified as cases are wrongly diagnosed), checks on sensitivity may involve the examination of thousands of individuals twice to determine if cases are being missed. Fortunately, in most trials, specificity is more important than sensitivity although the relative importance can change as the survey goes on, as discussed in Section 4.2.

REFERENCES

Alonso, P. L., Bowman, A., Marsh, K., and Greenwood, B. M. (1987). The accuracy of the clinical histories given by mothers of seriously ill African children. *Annals of Tropical Paediatrics*, **7**, 187–89.

Braun-Munzinger, R. A. (1989). Quality control in schistosomiasis programmes. *Tropical Medicine and Parasitology*, **40**, 214–19.

Chandrasekar, C. and Deming, W. E. (1949). On a method of estimating birth and death rates and the extent of registration. *Journal of the American Statistical Association*, **44**, 101–15.

David, P., Bisharat. L., and Hill, A. G. (1990). *Measuring childhood mortality: a guide for simple surveys*. UNICEF Middle East and North Africa Regional Office, P.O. Box 811721, Amman, Jordan.

Greenwood, B. M., Greenwood, A. M., Bradley, A. K., Tulloch, S., Hayes, R., and Oldfield, F. S. J. (1987). Deaths in infancy and early childhood in a well vaccinated, rural, West African population. *Annals of Tropical Paediatrics*, **7**, 91–9.

Hill, A. G., and David, P. H. (1988). Monitoring changes in child mortality:

new methods for use in developing countries. *Health Policy and Planning*, **3**, 214–26.

Hill, A. G., and Aguirre, A. (1990). Childhood mortality estimates using the preceding birth technique: some applications and extensions. *Population Studies*, **44**, 317–40.

Ponnighaus, J. M., Fine, P. E. M., and Bliss, L. (1987). Certainty levels in the diagnosis of leprosy. *International Journal of Leprosy*, **55**, 454–62.

United Nations (1983). *Indirect techniques for demographic estimation.* Population Studies No. 81, Manual X. New York. (ST/ESA/Series A/81).

World Health Organization (1977). *Manual of the international classification of diseases, injuries and causes of death*, (9th revision). WHO, Geneva.

World Health Organization Malaria Action Programme (1986). Severe and complicated malaria. *Transactions of the Royal Society of Tropical Medicine and Hygiene*, **80** (Suppl.), 1–50.

World Health Organization (1989). *Tropical diseases: progress in international research, 1987-88.* UNDP/World Bank/WHO Special Programme for Research and Training in Tropical Diseases. WHO, Geneva.

Appendix 8.1

POST-MORTEM QUESTIONNAIRE

Child's Name: _____

Mother's Name: _____

Father's Name: _____

Sex: _____ Ethnic Group: _____

Village: _____

Compound: _____

ID Number:

: ___ : ___ : ___ : ___ : ___ : ___ :

CHRONOLOGY

Date of Birth   : ___ : ___ / ___ : ___ / ___ : ___ :

    Record how determined _____

Date of Death   : ___ : ___ / ___ : ___ / ___ : ___ :

Date of Interview   : ___ : ___ / ___ : ___ / ___ : ___ :

CIRCUMSTANCES OF DEATH

(a) Person interviewed
    1. Mother   2. Father   3. Guardian   : ___ :
    4. Other (specify) _____
(b) Was the child seen during their last illness by
    1. Village health worker?   Y/N : ___ :
    2. Dispenser?   Y/N : ___ :
    3. Trained nurse?   Y/N : ___ :
    4. Doctor? (specify) _____   Y/N : ___ :
    5. Traditional healer?   Y/N : ___ :
    6. Other? (specify) _____   Y/N : ___ :
(c) Was the child admitted to hospital during their final illness?
                                                       Y/N : ___ :
    If YES, specify which hospital (_____)
(d) Where did death occur?
    1. Home   2. Dispensary/Health centre   3. Hospital
    4. Other (specify) _____   : ___ :

ASK QUESTIONS FROM NEONATAL DEATH QUESTIONNAIRE
(see Appendix 8.2) AT THIS POINT IF AGE AT DEATH WAS 30
DAYS OR LESS.

RESPONDENTS ACCOUNT OF FINAL ILLNESS

DIRECT QUESTIONS

Did the child have any of the following features during his/her last illness?
If YES, indicate for how many days. If NO, leave blank.

1. Fever   : ___ : ___ : ___ :
2. Diarrhoea and/or vomiting   : ___ : ___ : ___ :
3. Cough and/or rapid respiration   : ___ : ___ : ___ :
4. Stiff neck   : ___ : ___ : ___ :
5. Fits (Convulsions)   : ___ : ___ : ___ :
6. Rash   : ___ : ___ : ___ :
7. Loss of weight   : ___ : ___ : ___ :

If you obtain a positive answer to one or more of the above questions ask
the following questions (only ask about those features for which positive
answers were obtained above).

Q1: FEVER

(a) Was the fever   1. Very severe?   2. Moderate?   3. Mild?   : ___ :
(b) Was the fever   1. Present all the time?   2. Intermittent?   : ___ :
(c) Was the fever the only feature of the illness?   Y/N   : ___ :

Q2: DIARRHOEA AND/OR VOMITING

(a) Did the child have sunken eyes?   Y/N : ___ :
(b) Did the child have diarrhoea?   Y/N : ___ :
     If YES:—
     1. Was diarrhoea   1. Present throughout illness?
                        2. Intermittent?   : ___ :
     2. Was the diarrhoea   1. Very severe?
                            2. Moderate?
                            3. Intermittent?   : ___ :
     3. When the diarrhoea was worst how often did the child pass stool?
                        1. < 5 times per day
                        2. 5–9 times per day
                        3. 10 or more times per day   : ___ :

4. When the diarrhoea was worst was the stool
                    1. Watery? 2. Soft? 3. Normal Consistency?

                                                                : ___ :

5. Did the stool ever contain blood?   Y/N : ___ :
6. Did the child have abdominal pain/colics?   Y/N : ___ :
(c) Did the child have vomiting?   Y/N : ___ :
    If YES:—
    1. Was the vomiting—1. Present throughout the illness?
                        2. Intermittent?   : ___ :
    2. Was the vomiting—1. Very severe? 2. Moderate?
                        3. Mild?   : ___ :
    3. When the vomiting was worst how often did the child vomit?
        1. < 5 times per day
        2. 5–9 times per day
        3. 10 or more times per day   : ___ :

Q3: COUGH AND/OR RAPID RESPIRATION

(a) Did the child have indrawing of chest?   Y/N : ___ :
(b) Did the child have wheezing?   Y/N : ___ :
(c) Did the child have grunting respiration?   Y/N : ___ :
(d) Was the child using his/her alae nasae?   Y/N : ___ :
(e) Did the child have a cough?   Y/N : ___ :
    If YES:—
    1. Was this 1. Very severe? 2. Moderate? 3. Mild?   : ___ :
    2. Did the child cough up any sputum?   Y/N : ___ :
    3. Did the child cough up any blood?   Y/N : ___ :
(f) Did the child have rapid breathing?   Y/N : ___ :
    If YES:—Was breathing—1. Very rapid? 2. Moderately Rapid?
                                                            : ___ :

Q4: STIFF NECK

(a) Could the mother/guardian bend the neck?   Y/N : ___ :
(b) Was the child 1. Fully awake? 2. Drowsy?
                    3. Unconscious?   : ___ :
(c) Does the mother/guardian think that the child had
     meningitis?   Y/N : ___ :

Q5: FITS OR CONVULSIONS

(a) How many fits did the child have? 1. <5 2. 5–9
                                        3. 10 or more   : ___ :

(b) Were the fits   1. Small twitching?   2. Major movements?   : ____ :

(c) Did the fits involve   1. Face?   Y/N   : ____ :
                            2. Neck?   Y/N   : ____ :
                            3. Arms?   Y/N   : ____ :
                            4. Legs?   Y/N   : ____ :

(d) Between fits was the child
     1. Fully awake?   2. Drowsy?   3. Unconscious?   : ____ :

Q6: RASH

(a) Was the rash present on   1. Face?   Y/N   : ____ :
                               2. Neck?   Y/N   : ____ :
                               3. Arms?   Y/N   : ____ :
                               4. Palms?   Y/N   : ____ :
                               5. Legs?   Y/N   : ____ :

(b) What were the features of the rash?
     1. Flat patches   2. Bumps   3. Bumps with Fluid
     4. Bumps with pus   5. Other (describe) _____   : ____ :

(c) Did the child have sore, red eyes?   Y/N   : ____ :

Q7: LOSS OF WEIGHT

(a) Was the child thinner than he should have been?
                      1. Just during final illness
                      2. Before the final illness   : ____ :
     If answer to above is 2.
        Had the child been thinner than normal
        1. Since birth?   2. Since weaning?   3. Neither?   : ____ :

(b) Was the child smaller (shorter) than he/she should have
     been: Y/N   : ____ :

     If YES:—Has the child been smaller than usual since
     birth?   Y/N   : ____ :

(c) Did the child have a normal appetite?   Y/N   : ____ :

(d) Did the child have swelling of the feet?   Y/N   : ____ :

(e) Did the child have flaky skin?   Y/N   : ____ :

FAMILY HISTORY

(a) Were any other children in the compound seriously ill
     at the time that the child died?   Y/N   : ____ :

(b) If YES, describe what kind of illness they had.

(c) Had any other children in the compound recently had
     measles?   Y/N   : ____ :

NUTRITION HISTORY

(a) Had the child been weaned?   Y/N : ___ :

(b) If YES, how many months before death?   : ___ : ___ :

HEALTH CARD AND OTHER RECORDS

(a) Can the child's health card be found?   Y/N : ___ :

    If NOT, specify why not _____

(b) Health card photocopied?   Y/N : ___ :

(c) Are there any hospital records of child's illness? Y/N : ___ :

(d) Hospital records photocopied?   Y/N : ___ :

GENERAL COMMENTS

INTERVIEWER'S DIAGNOSIS

Main cause of death _____

Contributory cause of death _____

Signature: _____   : ___ : ___ :

Appendix 8.2

NEONATAL DEATH QUESTIONNAIRE

Complete the questions below when the age of the infant at death was 30 days or less.

1. Is the mother of the neonate alive?   Y/N   : ___ :
2. If no, how many days after the delivery did she die?   : ___ : ___ :
3. Age of the mother in years   : ___ : ___ :

I–PREGNANCY:

4. How many months was the mother pregnant with this
    child?   : ___ : ___ :
5. How many infants were born of this pregnancy?   : ___ : ___ :
6. How many other deliveries has she had before?   : ___ : ___ :
7. How many children to the mother are now alive?   : ___ : ___ :
8. What is the age of the last child? (in months)   : ___ : ___ :
9. Did she attend antenatal clinic when pregnant with the
    infant who died?   Y/N   : ___ :
    ASK FOR THE ANTENATAL CARD . . . .
      ANTENATAL CARD AVAILABLE?   Y/N   : ___ :
         NUMBER: : ___ : ___ : ___ : ___ : ___ : ___ :
    COPY FROM THE CARD IF AVAILABLE.
    IF NOT, ASK THE MOTHER:
10. How many tetanus toxoid (TT) did she receive in this
    pregnancy?   : ___ : ___ :
11. How many TT did she receive in other pregnancies?   : ___ : ___ :
    BORROW THE HEALTH CARD TO BE PHOTOCOPIED.

II–DELIVERY:

12. Where was the child delivered?
    1. At Home   2. TBA's Compound   : ___ :
    3. Health Centre   4. Other (specify) _____
13. Who delivered the child?
    1. Trained TBA   2. Untrained TBA   3. Midwife
    4. Doctor   5. Other (specify) _____ : ___ :
14. Did the child cry immediately when he/she was born?   Y/N   : ___ :

15. What was the cord cut with?
    1. New razor   2. Old razor   3. Knife
    4. Don't know   5. Other (specify) _____ : ___ :

16. What was applied on the cord after cutting it?
    1. Bambootulo   2. Groundnut oil 3. Palm oil
    4. Medicine   5. Nothing   6. Don't know   : ___ :
    7. Other, specify _____

17. What was applied on the cord during the first week of life?
    1. Bambootulo   2. Groundnut oil 3. Palm oil
    4. Medicine   5. Nothing   6. Don't know   : ___ :
    7. Other, specify _____

III–SYMPTOMS PRECEDING INFANT'S DEATH:

18. Was the child able to suck milk after birth?   Y/N : ___ :

19. Did the infant stop sucking milk when he/she
    became ill?   Y/N : ___ :

20. How many days passed before the infant became ill?   : ___ : ___ :

CONTINUE WITH THE POST-MORTEM QUESTIONNAIRE

9
Questionnaires

1 INTRODUCTION

The collection of information by asking a series of questions to members of the study population is likely to be a component of any intervention trial that involves contact with human subjects. Such information may be relatively simple and straightforward to collect (for example, a census of the study population in which the names, age, and sex are recorded for the members of each household in the study area) or may be very difficult to elicit reliably from respondents (for example, beliefs about the causes of illness, details of sexual behaviour). Different ways of investigating the beliefs, attitudes, and practices of members of a study population are discussed in Chapter 10. The methods range from detailed anthropological studies of a small number of subjects to questionnaire surveys of large numbers of participants. The focus of this chapter is on the latter type of survey, in which data are collected by asking the same series of questions to members of the study population. The responses are recorded on questionnaires and analysed later by manual tabulations or, more usually for large surveys, after entering the information into a computer.

In literate populations questionnaires may be 'self-administered'; i.e. a questionnaire is distributed to study subjects which they are asked to complete themselves and which is then collected for analysis. This kind of questionnaire will not be discussed in this chapter as it is of limited applicability in the areas of the world in which tropical diseases predominate, where many may be illiterate. The principles of planning and designing self-administered questionnaires are similar, however, to those for the interviewer-administered questionnaires considered in this chapter. Interviews of several respondents at the same time (group interviews) are also not considered (but are discussed in Chapter 10) and attention is confined to the interview of one respondent at a time by one interviewer, which is the type most commonly used in field studies.

In addition to asking questions, an interviewer may carry out observations. For example, questions about toilet facilities in a home can be supplemented by inspection, and observations on their geographical location and state of repair might be included as records on the questionnaire.

The methods outlined in this chapter are most appropriate when information on a relatively small number of well-defined subject areas is required, for which the responses to enquiries are either numerical (for example, number of pregnancies) or may be classified into a small number of different categories (for example, current feeding mode of an infant). Even simple items of information may be difficult to elicit accurately unless adequate research has been conducted to find out how questions should be asked and phrased in the study community. The methods described in Chapter 10 to obtain such background information are very relevant.

In a particular investigation the study subjects may be interviewed once only or several times. Simple cross-sectional surveys provide an example of the former. An example of the latter would be the collection of regular information on child morbidity from the mothers of study children through weekly or fortnightly interviews for the evaluation of the efficacy of a vaccine, say, against diarrhoeal disease. In this example, the first interview may be more extensive, with a shorter list of questions asked at each subsequent interview. Intervention trials often involve an initial cross-sectional survey, followed by periodic surveys of the same population, the frequency of which will be determined by the nature of the outcome variables under study.

In this chapter the different components of a questionnaire survey are reviewed. The formulation and validation of questions to be included is considered in Section 2. Section 3 deals with the construction of the complete questionnaire, Section 4 with the interviewers, their selection, training, and standardization, and Section 5 examines factors relating to the actual interview.

As with most aspects of field research, there is no satisfactory substitute for experience to know how to formulate and administer a questionnaire satisfactorily. Thus, the inexperienced investigator would be well-advised to seek the guidance of those who have previously conducted surveys in the study area, if possible. Those with social science, statistical, and data processing skills are also likely to make important contributions.

2 THE QUESTIONS

2.1 Relation to study objectives

The questions to be included in a questionnaire should be developed to relate directly to the objectives of the study, in so far as these objectives encompass information to be obtained by interview. Usually at least an outline questionnaire will be drawn up in parallel with the formulation of the protocol for the whole study. Most grant review committees expect to see such an outline in an application for support for the investigation, and this will certainly be so if the information obtained by interview is central to any of the main objectives.

There are constraints on the information that can be sought by interview, in respect to the sensitivity of certain subjects and to the time limits on interviews. These constraints may be such that it is not possible to realize some of the planned objectives of a study, and it may be necessary to modify some of the objectives in consequence.

When a questionnaire survey is being planned, it will often seem attractive to add questions that do not relate directly to the objectives of the study but which may be of interest for other reasons. As a general rule, this temptation should be resisted, as lengthening interview schedules is likely to lead to a higher non-participation rate, and time devoted to non-relevant questions may be at the expense of time on more important questions, with a consequent lowering of the quality of the information collected on the latter. None the less, in some circumstances it may be desirable to ask non-relevant questions, if this increases the likelihood of participation in the survey or serves to divert attention away from the main questions in order to reduce the chance of biased responses. For example, it may be more acceptable to ask a few questions about sexual behaviour in the context of a more general behavioural survey than to include only questions that concern sexual behaviour. Similarly, if particular side-effects are expected from an intervention, it may be best to include questions about effects thought to be unrelated to the intervention as this may help identify any biases in response between intervention and control groups that are not directly attributable to the intervention.

2.2 Development of questions

A likely sequence for the development of the questions to be included in a questionnaire survey is as follows:

1. Defining the information that is required from the questions. Different items of information may require a single question (for example, age and sex, though in some circumstances age determination may require multiple questions – see Chapter 6, Section 4.9) or a series of questions (for example, socio-economic status).

2. Formulating draft questions. Attention to the wording of questions is very important as slight variations may result in different responses (for example, 'where do you normally seek

help when your child has diarrhoea?' or 'where did you seek help when your child last had diarrhoea?'). Box 9.1 gives a check-list of points that should be considered in drafting questions.

3. Informal testing of the questions. This may involve trying them out on different members of the study team and discussing

---

Box 9.1 A checklist of points to consider when drafting questions.

1. Keep wording informal, conversational and simple. Avoid words longer than four syllables.

2. Avoid jargon and sophisticated language; assessing understanding at the pre-test and pilot stages is important. The wording of all questions must be appropriate to the educational, social, and cultural background of the respondents.

3. Check the cultural relevance to the respondents of concepts used. Ensure mutual understanding between the interviewers and the respondents, paying attention to cultural and educational differences.

4. Avoid long questions. But vary question length.

5. It may be necessary to define a term or a concept before asking about it. If the definition is short, it can be included in the question, but otherwise it is better given separately before the question is asked.

6. Avoid leading questions (i.e. those which lead the respondent to a particular answer; for example 'do you think the improved clinic arrangements are better?').

7. Avoid open question beginning 'Why?'

8. Avoid negative questions (for example, 'do you not think. . .')

9. Avoid hypothetical question (for example, 'if the bus fare was less would you come to the clinic more often?').

10. Keep to a single subject for each question; (for example, do not say 'do the cost and times of the clinic prevent you going?').

11. Pay attention to sensitive issues. Review the inclusion of very sensitive ones. If they are to be retained pay attention to wording, the use of indirect approaches, and position in the questionnaire (see Section 3.2).

12. Check the adequacy of the lists of responses to closed questions (for example, ensure a food list covers most things normally eaten in the community concerned). Avoid a large proportion of responses being in the 'other (specify) ____' category.

them with those knowledgeable of the study area, including residents. It may be necessary to base someone in the community under study (ideally, someone with anthropological or social science skills) to investigate how different questions will be perceived, to find out if there are taboos regarding certain topics, to find out if there are local words for some illnesses or conditions and the extent to which these correspond to the investigators definitions (for example, many communities have special words for 'measles' and for 'night blindness'). The investment that is warranted in such investigational anthropological studies will depend upon local sensitivities regarding the items on which information is required. For example, it will require less work to find out how to ask questions about breast-feeding practices than to formulate appropriate questions to elicit information on aspects of sexual behaviour. As a result of such investigations the original draft questions may have to be modified. Some may even have to be abandoned if research indicates that the information required is unlikely to be elicited through a questionnaire survey.

4. Preparation of the first draft of the questionnaire for pilot testing.

5. Pilot survey in field conditions, preferably in an area adjacent to the study area and using the interviewers who will work on the main survey.

6. Analysis of the experience in the pilot survey and of the data collected.

7. Reformulation of the questionnaire and further pilot testing.

8. Finalization of the questionnaire for the main survey, along with the instruction manual for interviewers (see Section 4.4).

2.3 Types of question

Through a questionnaire information may be sought on opinions or facts. The distinction between the two is not always clear, but, in general, the collection of data on the latter is easier to plan. Local sensitivities will influence the reliability with which either kind of information may be obtained. For example, in some cultures it is considered unlucky to count children, so asking a woman 'how many children have you had?' may be too direct an approach.

2.3.1 Historical recall

Information may be sought about the present or the past (for example, 'does your child have fever now?' or 'has your child had fever in the last month?'). The advantage of asking about the present situation is that responses are not susceptible to memory lapses and, furthermore, they may be more amenable to validation (Section 2.4). The reliability of historical information decreases the further back in time the question relates to and is influenced greatly by the importance of the event concerned. Thus, deaths will be remembered better than hospital admissions, which in turn will be remembered better than morbid episodes not requiring hospital admission. To obtain reliable information on fevers, diarrhoea, or respiratory infections a recall period of more than a week is undesirable. The implication of this for longitudinal studies, in which these outcomes are of interest, is that weekly surveys of the study group will be necessary to collect reliable information on morbidity.

2.3.2 Open and closed questions

A 'closed' question is one that allows only a defined set of answers which have been anticipated (and categorized) in advance of the interviews (for example, 'do you own a radio?'). Replies to an 'open' question can take any form and are recorded as far as possible in the respondents own words (for example, 'what were the symptoms your child had before death?'). It is possible to ask a question with a closed list of responses in an open way, with the answer being assigned to one on a previously compiled list held by the interviewer (for example, 'what did you eat yesterday?', with a list of types of food on the questionnaire for the interviewer to tick off those mentioned). This may produce a different response from asking closed questions about each of the items on the list. Reading out the list will remind the respondent of the possibilities, but may also tend to produce affirmative answers as a gesture to please the interviewer. If the information is sufficiently important, both approaches can be used, the list of (other) categories being read out after an initial response without such prompting. The two responses should be recorded separately. An analogy is medical history-taking, where questions about specific signs and symptoms might be asked after an initial neutral enquiry (for example, 'what is the problem?').

In pilot investigations in a community, of an anthropological nature, open questions are likely to be preferred to determine the full range of possible responses regarding different topics. As a general rule, however, for questions that are to be administered in a large survey, closed questions are better as they pose fewer problems for coding and analysis. It is important that they are the 'right' closed questions, of course. This requires careful research and the avoidance of the premature administration of a questionnaire that may be simple to administer, code, and analyse, but which does not provide the information required to meet the study objectives.

2.3.3 Direct or indirect questioning

'Indirect questioning' may be used to obtain information on one item by asking several questions. This can be useful for sensitive issues. In some societies, a direct question about monthly income may provide sufficient information to categorize a subject's socio-economic status, but in other societies this categorization may have to be made by asking less sensitive questions about other factors such as employment, ownership of different possessions, and nature of house structure, from which a composite classification of socio-economic status might be made which, in so far as is possible, should be planned prior to the survey. It should be stressed, however, that it is not an easy task to construct such composite classifications and to be sure they are measuring what is required.

2.4 Validation

The principles underlying the validation of a questionnaire are similar to those applicable for a diagnostic test. The objective is to determine to what extent the answers given to a question correspond to the 'true' situation. Problems arise if there is no independent way of ascertaining what is 'true'. If a mother is asked 'does your child have fever now?' the temperature of a child might be measured independently and the response to the question

validated against the direct measurement (by defining temperatures above some limit as 'fever'). It will be much more difficult to
validate the responses to a question such as 'has your child had
fever in the last week?'. If a 'gold standard' exists, i.e. a means of
obtaining an independent measure of the correct response, the
sensitivity and *specificity* of a given question can be assessed. The
sensitivity is a measure of the proportion of times the question
produces a 'positive' response when the correct response is 'positive' (for example, the proportion of all children with a current
fever who are detected by questioning the mothers). The *specificity*
is a measure of the proportion of times the question produces a
'negative' response when the correct response is 'negative' (for
example, the proportion of all children without a current fever
who are so classified by questioning the mothers). The relative
importance of sensitivity and specificity in intervention trials is
discussed in Chapter 8, Section 4.2.

If there is no 'gold standard', other characteristics of the responses to questions must be evaluated to assess their usefulness in
a particular survey. A minimal requirement for a question should
be that the respondent gives the same answer to the same question
at different times if the circumstances have not changed. Also, if
different interviewers administer the same question to the same
person, the same answer should be obtained (i.e. responses should
be 'reproducible'). Reproducibility is not a guarantee of reliability,
of course. The question 'did you murder your spouse?' might be
answered consistently over time to the same interviewer and repro-
ducibly to different interviewers, but it may still be a very poor
way of detecting spouse-murderers! A man might consistently
report that his wife is his only sexual partner, even if this is not the
case. In the end, the degree to which a question is soliciting correct
responses may be a matter of judgement, bearing in mind the
consistency of the response with those to other questions included
in the questionnaire. If a question fails to induce consistent
answers either within or between interviewers, it may be because
of a fault in the question or in the interviewers. By definition, it is
not due to a fault in the respondent (unless they are being deliber-
ately unhelpful and vary their responses to compensate for being
asked the same question repeatedly by different interviewers as
part of the testing of validity!)

2.5 Translation

If the investigators speak a different language or dialect from that of the study subjects, it will be necessary to translate a questionnaire into whatever local languages are used. Any such translation should always be undertaken with great care and attention to detail, as it is very easy for the sense of a question to be changed greatly by subtle nuances in the translation process. For example, apparent differences in responses to a question asked to those in different language groups may be due entirely to variations in the translation processes. Words for some illnesses or concepts may not exist in a language, and this may necessitate major changes in the wording of questions. An 'equivalent' word may exist, but it may be used in a different way and cover a smaller or wider range of conditions than the original word. For example, there may be a variety of local words used to describe acute respiratory infections, one of which corresponds closely to what we mean by pneumonia. It is worth spending a lot of time delving into this issue before starting a survey. Conversely, difficulties may be encountered when one local word is used to describe what are, to us, very different conditions. Workers in The Gambia had difficulty in this respect in separating a 'floppy' from a 'stiff' neck (B. Greenwood, personal communication).

Once a questionnaire has been translated into a local language it should be back-translated into the original language by an independent person. Comparing the original text with the back-translated text may be very illuminating with respect to possible areas of confusion.

3 THE QUESTIONNAIRE

3.1 Length

Adequate time must be allowed for the interviewer to solicit the correct responses to all of the questions included in a questionnaire. The length of time that an interview will take may not be easy to estimate and may depend on the inherent interest of the subject matter to respondents as well as the amount of time they can spare. It can be evaluated during testing of the questionnaire. Neither the interviewer nor the respondent should feel under time-pressure to complete the interview. The questionnaire should be long enough to allow the required information to be collected but without unduly inconveniencing the respondent. The work schedule of interviewers should be planned such that they are not tempted to hurry through interviews. In general, it is an unsound policy to pay interviewers according to the number of interviews completed, unless it is certain that this does not compromise quality. Sufficient time must be allocated for each interview to allow the interviewer to explain why the survey is being conducted, to emphasize the importance of correct responses and to reassure the respondent regarding the procedures undertaken to ensure the confidentiality of any information divulged in the interview.

The choice of the time of day, month or year to conduct interviews is discussed in Section 5.1. It is desirable to avoid times when respondents have important competing demands on their time (for example, market days, the planting season).

Interviews lasting an hour or more are rarely feasible in the context of a large-scale survey and usually it is more realistic to aim for an upper maximum of around 30 minutes per interview. This may mean shortening the questionnaire by asking some questions to only a sample of respondents. For all questions in a survey, the need to put them to all respondents should be assessed and, where possible, questioning reduced to a representative sample only. Respondents may not complete an interview that is too long, and problems of compliance could grow as the interviewers' reputations go before them. Brevity may be relatively more important if repeated contact with respondents is planned.

It is a good strategy to have the interviewers record the time that each interview starts and finishes. This is one way of checking how interviewers spend their days (though it is obviously susceptible to manipulation) and, more importantly, it provides a measure of whether different degrees of attention are being given to those in the intervention or control groups with a consequent possibility of bias.

3.2 Order of questions

The initial questions in an interview will seek to verify the identity of the respondent (to ensure the correct person is being questioned) and to collect basic demographic information (for example, age, sex, marital status). The most sensitive questions should usually be asked near the end of the questionnaire. This is done to give the interviewer time to establish a rapport with the respondent and also so that if the respondent should be upset by the questions and withdraws from the interview, at least this happens after most other information has been collected (though questions that result in this action should have been weeded out during pilot testing). Questions which are not judged to be sensitive should tend to be asked in their order of importance (to the study objectives), the most important ones being asked first, to minimize the losses due to the premature cessation of an interview.

Responses to some questions may condition the responses to other questions and this should be taken into account in their ordering. For example, a question asking if the respondent is generally 'well' which produces a 'yes' response may bias questions about specific illnesses if the respondent feels obliged to justify their overall 'wellness'. If the interest of the study is in specific diseases it might be better to focus on these first, before questions about general health.

Some questions may seek to obtain the same information in different ways as a validation procedure. If this is done the questions should be separated in the questionnaire so they are not asked too close together.

3.3 Layout

A questionnaire should be able to be used in the field without other than infrequent reference to other manuals or instructions. Thus, it should provide the interviewer with sufficient information to conduct the interview smoothly and without difficulty, after suitable training (Section 4.2). At the same time, it should not be too bulky a document as this may alarm the respondent (in terms of the time they think it will take to complete) and it will also add to the problem of storage if the survey is large. Instructions to interviewers may be distinguished from questions to respondents by printing them in a different typeface. Each interviewer should be issued with an interviewers manual (Section 4.4) which contains information to supplement any instructions to interviewers given on the questionnaire.

It is especially important that the initial introduction that the interviewer gives a respondent is clear and consistent from interview to interview. It is common for the text of this introduction to be printed on the top of the questionnaire. Usually interviewers will be instructed to ask questions exactly as they are written, using the text that it printed for each question. This is an important way to achieve greater reproducibility and standardization between interviewers.

The questionnaire should be designed so that it is pleasing to look at. The paper size and quality should be chosen to suit field conditions. Cards are often easier to work with in the field than paper sheets, but are unsuitable if more than one is required for an interview and they are also bulky to carry about. The layout of the questionnaire should be sufficiently spaced to allow those with large handwriting to record all the required information. If some questions are optional this should be indicated on the questionnaire with clear instructions and appropriate branch and jump explanations. All questions should be assigned a number. For questions that are repeated several times such as questions about each of a mother's children, a tabular layout can be used, but this should be designed with care as such a layout puts more demands on the interviewer.

To facilitate later checking and coding it may be useful to include on the questionnaire the names that variables are going to be assigned for computer processing (see Chapter 13, Section 3.4). These might be in capital letters, placed adjacent to the coding boxes on the questionnaire.

3.4 Coding

Coding is discussed in Chapter 13 (Sections 4.2 and 5.1), and only a few points pertinent to questionnaire design are covered here. Coding is the process of converting the recorded answers to questions to a numerical or alphabetical code. The answers may be numeric (for example, age or date), or be the replies to closed questions. For closed questions there are two possible ways of coding, depending upon whether only one answer out of the list of possible responses can be given, or whether several are possible. Examples of the former are any 'yes/no/don't know' answers or answers to questions such as relationship to head of household (for example, may be one of wife, child, brother, sister, and so on, but cannot be more than one). An example of the latter is food consumed on the previous day, when several kinds of food could have been consumed. In the first case, the possible responses are each given a code, usually a letter or a digit, and a respondent's answer is coded accordingly. In the second, each possible response must be coded for the answer 'yes' or 'no' (often coded as '1' or '2', respectively, or as 'Y' or 'N') or 'don't know' (if applicable) (often coded as '9'), and the codes for each of them will make up the respondent's reply.

It is important to allow codes for 'don't know'. Answers to questions that are skipped (i.e. which are not relevant) are normally left blank during the interview. It may be convenient to leave the codes blank as well, or a specific code for 'not applicable' (for example, '8') can be used. The choice depends on data processing requirements (see Chapter 13). With lists of possible responses, a category 'other' is often included, and needs to have its own code. There should be space on the questionnaire to write in the actual reply, but the pre-testing and pilot work should ensure that the 'other' category is seldom used for a reply.

The codes are commonly written into 'boxes' in the questionnaire. Boxes are usually put in a column down the right hand side of the form (for languages written left to right). Though this is not essential, it simplifies the data entry process. These conventions were more important before recent developments in data-entry computer software. Such software permits a mimic of the entire questionnaire to be displayed on the screen for the data-entry clerk, so that picking out where information is to be entered is easy, without having to copy it beforehand to one side of the document.

Important in questionnaire design is the decision as to when coding is to be done, and by whom. With a simple coding scheme, the data can be recorded during the interview. This has the advantage of involving less transcription, reducing the possibility of transcription errors, but has the disadvantage that the interviewer's attention may be focused on the coding process rather than on the respondent.

Alternatively, the interviewer may record answers (apart from numeric ones) by ticks against, or circles around, the relevant response. If ticks are used the questionnaire must be so designed and completed such that there is little chance of ambiguity as to which response has been ticked. The ticks or circles are converted to codes later, though as soon as possible after the interview. An advantage of this procedure is that the questionnaire is inspected soon after the interview for discrepancies. This should be done anyway, but the need to code forces attention on the replies more than does a simple inspection.

Interviewers might be instructed to write notes or make comments next to any questions that cannot be answered according to the instructions. This will assist the supervisor in the detection and checking of apparent errors and may highlight deficiencies in the questionnaire.

Appendices 9.1 to 9.6 give some examples of different ways of designing a questionnaire and examples of different types of questions.

Advice on the design of forms to facilitate entry of data into a microcomputer, with special references to studies in the tropics, is given in Byass (1986).

4 THE INTERVIEWERS

4.1 Selection

Interviewers should be selected with careful attention to the tasks they will be expected to perform. It is important that they are accorded an appropriate level of respect by the study subjects. They must be seen as individuals who can be trusted to hold possibly sensitive and confidential information. They must be of pleasant disposition, be well-mannered, well-dressed, reliable, and punctual. They must not make promises to respondents that they do not honour (for example, if they say they will return on a given day they must do so, or at least send a message in advance to explain and apologize if they cannot). The study investigator must attempt to assess whether potential interviewers have these characteristics during selection interviews and pilot-testing exercises. Only in exceptional circumstances should an interviewer be offered a contract of employment for the duration of the study in advance of a probationary period during which their suitability is assessed.

Even after this there must be provision for removing an interviewer from field work if their performance is unsatisfactory.

If possible, interviewers should speak the same language as the respondents, otherwise interviews will have to be conducted through interpreters, which is usually an unsatisfactory procedure (for the reasons outlined in Section 2), although it is sometimes unavoidable.

The sex, age, and normal place of residence of an interviewer may be important. In some societies male interviewers are less likely to get reliable information from mothers and may even be unable to interview them at all. If interviewers clearly belong to the health services, replies may be biased towards support for those services. Extensively educated interviewers may not be best for interviews with less-educated respondents. Differences of social class, and often of sex, between interviewer and respondent may be best avoided. Young interviewers may not be regarded as reliable or trustworthy recipients of sensitive information. Also, sometimes sensitive information may be more readily given to a stranger than to a member of the same community, provided the respondents are assured of confidentiality, or the reverse may be the case.

The most skilled and reliable interviewers are not always the most intelligent or highly educated. Indeed, highly educated interviewers may be more likely to become bored with repeated administration of the same interview schedule.

4.2 Training

The training of interviewers might initially be done as a group exercise, with classroom-type teaching. This must be supplemented with practical exercises. These might consist of one interviewer administering the survey questionnaire to another interviewer while others look on, followed by a critical evaluation and discussion of the interview with the group.

The interviewers manual (Section 4.4) should be used extensively in the training process, so that by the end of training the interviewer should be familiar with all aspects of the manual and know which parts to consult for advice on queries about particular questions or aspects of field procedures.

Only after interviewers have been through a preliminary training should they be allowed to try out interviews in the community. Initially such interviews might be done by pairs of interviewers in the presence of a trainer, with detailed 'post-mortems' being conducted after each interview or series of interviews. The training process will merge with the processes of standardization (Section 4.3) and validation (Section 2.4).

Throughout a survey it is important to monitor the performance of each interviewer and to institute corrective training if required. One means of quality control is to organize for a proportion of respondents (selected at random) to be re-interviewed by another interviewer. Discrepancies in the two interviews may identify deficiencies in the interview methods of one or other interviewer. (It is not an uncommon experience in large surveys that some interviewers complete some questionnaires without ever having seen the 'respondents'. A good system of checking, supervision, and quality control is necessary to prevent this, or at least to detect it soon after it occurs so that remedial action can be taken.)

4.3 Standardization

As discussed in Section 2.4, an interview must be reproducible. That is, interviewing the same person again, or interviewing another respondent whose answers should be the same, should produce answers that are the same. Standardization of interview technique within and between interviewers is necessary for reproducibility. Interviewers must be instructed and trained to follow instructions on the questionnaire, as well as all other instructions, exactly. This extends to asking all questions exactly as written, if this is appropriate. As well as questions, the introduction to the interview, explanations and definitions made to the respondent, and transition statements that explain a change of subject of the questions, should be said as written. The points in the interview to use probes and prompts to get the respondent to reply more fully should also be clearly specified.

Standardization may also apply to the place and time of interviews. For example, to mix interviews in homes and in a health centre will, in some circumstances, produce different responses between the two.

It is not realistic, however, to insist on interviewers being merely 'transcription machines'. They must have some leeway to add extra explanations and guidance when it is clear that a respondent does not understand a question and its definition. Interviewer training should cover this and detail the extent to which this is permissible. There must remain a definite stress on following the written wording throughout.

Standardization needs a certain degree of regimentation and this can act against rapport and personal contact. Since the wording of questions is laid down in advance, it is important to ensure that it is friendly and does not alienate the respondent. If different interviewers are getting different responses to the same questions, it is important to investigate why. For example, one of the interviewers may be deviating from the interview schedule and giving undue emphasis to part of a question. Different interviewers attempting to collect the same information from one respondent at different times will normally be a part of the validation of standardization procedures (see Section 2.4).

No matter how well interviewers are trained and standardized against each other, it is as well to assume in the design of a survey that some differences will exist in the responses obtained by different interviewers. This will influence the way different interviewers are deployed for field work. Not only is it important to record on the interview schedule who conducts each interview, so that analyses can be conducted to look at differences between interviewers, but also interviewers should be deployed in a 'balanced' way so that interviewer differences are not confounded with other differences of potential interest. For example, in an intervention trial, each interviewer should question similar numbers of subjects from the intervention and control groups. The worst situation would be for one interviewer to question those in the intervention group and another interviewer to question those in the control group.

4.4 Interviewer manuals

During the development of a questionnaire, and in the course of the training programme for interviewers, a manual should be developed for use during the field survey. The manual will give detailed instructions regarding how individuals are selected and approached for inclusion in the study and will detail any special instruction regarding each question in the questionnaire and the responses that may be given. It will include guidance on how to deal with unusual situations and how to code unusual responses. It will also outline what checks are to be conducted on completed questionnaires and how and when completed questionnaires should be submitted for data processing or analysis. The first response to any question from the interviewer to the study organizer should be 'is this covered in the manual?'. If it is not, the manual may need updating.

During the conduct of field work regular meetings should be held of interviewers to discuss progress and queries. When new problems arise the solutions should be incorporated into the field manual so that there is consistency in dealing with the problem in the future and so that a permanent record is kept of the solution adopted. The manuals held by each interviewer should be updated regularly and, if possible, the text should be kept on a word processor to facilitate this.

5 THE INTERVIEW

An interview should be a conversation between interviewer and respondent and must not be an interrogation. Good rapport between the two is vital and the onus is entirely on the project team to assure this.

5.1 Who, where, and when

In studies of children, the best informant regarding their health or behaviour is likely to be their mother. Thus, only as a last resort should someone other than the mother be interviewed for this purpose. This may necessitate repeated visits to a household until the mother is at home. Other than for children, proxy informants should be avoided if possible.

The choice of the place of interview will be influenced by logistic considerations and the nature of the information to be collected. Usually the place will have to be chosen for the convenience of the respondent rather than for that of the interviewer. Privacy will be easier to ensure in a hospital or a clinic than in a village setting, but special arrangements may be made to ensure greater privacy in a village. If interviews are to be conducted in subjects' homes, the time must be chosen to fit the convenience of the residents. If possible, they should be consulted, or at the very least informed, in advance regarding when an interview will take place. Preliminary investigations, before the main survey, should be made to ascertain when the most generally convenient time will be for interviews. During planting or harvesting seasons evening interviews may be preferred. But if interviews take place after dark, poor lighting may be a problem and attention to clear printing and a well-spaced layout for the questionnaire becomes more important (as well as the provision of torches and batteries to interviewers). In some areas security after dark may also be a significant problem, and interviewing at that time may be inadvisable.

5.2 Non-response

Non-respondents in a study are rarely representative of the total study population. They are a biased group and thus their exclusion introduces bias into the results of a survey to a degree that is usually not directly measurable. Thus if a high proportion of the target population for interviews are not interviewed, the valid interpretation of the results on those who are interviewed, and in particular the generalization of these results to the whole community, may be open to serious question. Therefore, great care must be taken to ensure that the response rate is high. This may be achieved in several ways. First, the questions included in the questionnaire should be thoroughly tested in a pilot study so that those which a significant proportion of respondents cannot answer adequately are weeded out. Second, the appropriate explanation of the survey to study participants should be given in advance of the main survey, and any false suspicions they have about the motives or intentions of the investigators must be dispelled. Third, interviewers must be selected who are persistent yet polite and who will probe for a correct response to a question and not accept a 'don't know' response too readily. The interviewer training should emphasize this also. Fourth, interviewers must be instructed to call back repeatedly if a house is empty or a respondent is away before abandoning an interview. Their work schedule should take into account the necessity for such return visits.

Even in the most well-conducted surveys a 100 per cent response rate is rare. As much information as possible should be obtained about non-respondents, possibly from proxy informants, so that in the analysis of a study characteristics on which information is available (for example, age and sex) may be compared with that available on responders. This may give clues to the extent of possible biases resulting from their exclusion.

REFERENCES

Byass, P. (1986). The design of computer forms for tropical medical research. *Methods of Information in Medicine*, **25,** 229–32.

Appendix 9.1

RECORDING THE RESPONSE TO A SINGLE QUESTION

			CODE FOR COMPUTER
(1) Q27.	Do you usually listen to the radio every day? (CIRCLE RESPONSE)	Yes.......1 No........2	☐
(2) Q27.	Do you usually listen to the radio every day? (TICK RESPONSE)	Yes (1) ___ No (2) ___	☐
(3) Q27.	Do you usually listen to the radio every day? (YES=1; NO=2)		☐
(4) Q27.	Do you usually listen to the radio every day? (YES=Y; NO=N)		☐

Note: Using (1) or (2) the response might be entered into the computer directly, by the data-entry clerk, entering whichever response was circled or ticked. More usually, the response is coded into the box on the right-hand side, possibly at the end of the day or at the end of the interview (so that the interviewer can check that the question was not missed) and the data-entry clerk only looks at the boxes when entering data into the computer. Using (3) or (4), the interviewer codes straight into the boxes with no intermediate step. Ticking responses, as in (2), may cause problems if the questionnaire is closely spaced, when it may be unclear exactly which response is ticked. If there is a danger of this happening it is better to adopt the system whereby the number or letter corresponding to the response is circled, as in (1), or that in which the response is directly coded, as in (3) and (4). Whichever system is adopted it is advisable to use the same system throughout the questionnaire to avoid any possibility of confusion of the interviewers.

Appendix 9.2

PRE-CODED RESPONSES WHICH ARE MUTUALLY EXCLUSIVE

Q49. What is the major source of drinking water for members of your household? (CIRCLE ONE RESPONSE)	CODE FOR COMPUTER
	⊔⊔
Piped into residence 01	
Piped into yard or plot 02	
Public tap 03	
Well with hand-pump 04	
Well without hand-pump 05	
River, spring, surface water 06	
Tanker truck, other vendor............................. 07	
Rain-water 08	
Other _____ .... 09 (specify)	

Note that 2 boxes are allocated for the computer code, but only 9 choices are given. This is done in case it is decided to subdivide any of the responses in the 'other' category in the analysis. This would necessitate that all the questionnaires coded '09' were re-examined and the responses given new codes (for example, 10, 11, 12, and so on).

Appendix 9.3

PRE-CODED RESPONSES WHICH ARE NOT MUTUALLY EXCLUSIVE

Q33. Which of the following items does your household own? (TICK RESPONSES)	CODE FOR COMPUTER (YES=1; NO=2)
Radio _____	☐
Television _____	☐
Bicycle _____	☐
Car _____	☐
Tractor _____	☐

Appendix 9.4

QUESTIONS ILLUSTRATING A 'SKIP' INSTRUCTION

	CODE FOR COMPUTER
Q39. Have you ever had any live-born children? (TICK RESPONSE) Yes (1) ___ No (2) ___ →GO TO Q41.	☐
Q40. How many of these are: still alive? _____	☐☐
dead? _____	☐☐
Q41. Is your mother still alive? (TICK RESPONSE) Yes (1) _____ No (2) _____	☐

Appendix 9.5

RECORDING OF MULTIPLE ITEMS OF INFORMATION FOR DIRECT COMPUTER ENTRY

Q93. For all your children who were born alive, give the following details: (starting with the first born).

No.	Name	Alive(A) or Dead(D)?	Sex (M or F)	Age* Years	Months
⊟	_____	☐	☐	⊟	⊟
⊟	_____	☐	☐	⊟	⊟
⊟	_____	☐	☐	⊟	⊟
⊟	_____	☐	☐	⊟	⊟
⊟	_____	☐	☐	⊟	⊟
⊟	_____	☐	☐	⊟	⊟
⊟	_____	☐	☐	⊟	⊟
⊟	_____	☐	☐	⊟	⊟
⊟	_____	☐	☐	⊟	⊟
⊟	_____	☐	☐	⊟	⊟
⊟	_____	☐	☐	⊟	⊟
⊟	_____	☐	☐	⊟	⊟
⊟	_____	☐	☐	⊟	⊟
⊟	_____	☐	☐	⊟	⊟
⊟	_____	☐	☐	⊟	⊟

IF NO. OF CHILDREN IS DIFFERENT FROM NO. RECORDED IN Q40, PROBE AND RECONCILE.

* IF DEAD, GIVE AGE AT DEATH.
  RECORD AGE IN <u>COMPLETED</u> MONTHS YEARS.
  IF AGE LESS THAN ONE MONTH (OR DIED BEFORE ONE MONTH) RECORD AS '00' MONTHS.

Note: In this example the letters of each name have not been allocated separate boxes (as is sometimes done), but the data entry clerk will be instructed to type into the computer the first, say 14 characters, of each name. Earlier on in the questionnaire the woman was asked to give the number of liveborn children who had died and the number who were still alive. The interviewer is instructed to cross-check that the responses to the two questions are consistent and, if not, to make the appropriate correction.

Appendix 9.6

AN 'OPEN' QUESTION

Q3. What do you do when your child has diarrhoea?
(RECORD MOTHER'S RESPONSE)

(PROMPT: DOES SHE INCREASE OR DECREASE FLUID INTAKE?)

(PROMPT: IF SHE SEEKS OTHER HELP, WHO DOES SHE GO TO FIRST?)

Note: The prompts are included so that the interviewer is asked to enquire about these aspects if the mother does not volunteer the information spontaneously. The coding of the information for analysis on the computer (if this is to be done) might be worked out when the questionnaires have all been completed and the range of different responses can be assessed. This may be a lot of work if the survey is large and it is usually better to have worked out this in pilot studies and to have asked as much as possible in the form of closed questions.

10
Qualitative research in field trials

1 INTRODUCTION

This chapter describes how qualitative research methods may be used in the development and conduct of field trials and in the interpretation of the results. The basic assumptions underlying qualitative research approaches are reviewed, the principal methods are presented and the strengths and weaknesses of each method are summarized. Methods of managing and analysing the kinds of data collected in such investigations are also outlined. It should be emphasized that the proper application of the methods described requires substantial training and experience, such as that of a skilled anthropologist or sociologist. In unwary or unskilled hands, the approaches may produce misleading information. The material in this chapter does no more than provide a brief guide to the methods used in qualitative research and more details are given in some of the references cited. A useful annotated bibliography on qualitative research methods has recently been published (Jefremovas 1995).

Qualitative research is intended to produce information on the language and belief systems of the study population, including their methods of categorizing events, illnesses, etc. It also provides information on behaviour through the observation of events and activities. The emphasis is on gathering open-ended textual data, in the words and phrases of the local people, particularly to gain information on the context of behaviour and the belief systems that influence behaviour. Such data can provide much more information about how and why people behave as they do than can simple quantitative surveys, and may be used to devise strategies to modify behaviour.

The research techniques employed may provide rich contextual information relevant for the successful completion of intervention trials. They may suggest explanations for findings which are unexpected, provoke new hypotheses and provide a basis for bridging conceptual and attitudinal differences between the community and the research team.

Qualitative research should be an integral part of intervention trials. Such studies may be useful before, during and after an intervention study. The contribution is likely to be greatest if qualitative information gathering forms an integral part of the design of the intervention study, and social scientists are members of the research team. They are thus well placed to identify the need for qualitative research during the course of the study.

Intervention trials must be both culturally appropriate and acceptable to the community in which the trial is to be conducted. The community should be involved in such a way that the commitment of community members to the project is obtained. These issues are discussed in more depth in Chapter 5.

2 QUALITATIVE RESEARCH APPROACHES

Qualitative research methods involve a set of *techniques* and an *approach* for their use in conducting research. The techniques of qualitative research have been described in a number of books and articles

(Pelto and Pelto 1978; Spradley 1979; Bernard 1986; Bernard 1994) and include interviewing key informants, focus group discussions (and other types of group techniques), different forms of systematic data collection and analysis (for example, pile or triad sorts and ranking—see Section 3.4) and the direct observation of behaviours. The relatively open-ended nature of these techniques make them ideal for exploring beliefs and behaviours from the insider's ('emic') point of view. They provide information relevant to devising alternative communication strategies, on obstacles to co-operation, and on ways to increase acceptance of new interventions. The techniques can be used to explore new or sensitive topics, such as reproductive health and sexual behaviour, and may suggest new research questions, as well as assisting in the design of effective data collection instruments.

Qualitative research approaches embody four key concepts: *explorative flexibility*, *iteration*, *triangulation* and *contextualization*. The researcher has specific topics to be explored, but it is assumed that new questions will emerge frequently as the research progresses. Specific techniques and associated data collection methods are refined and modified throughout the research process. A *flexible* approach is adopted, whereby unproductive forms of data collection are dropped and new methods developed, without losing sight of the original research objectives. There is an emphasis on in-depth investigation. Key informants and other respondents are interviewed repeatedly, each new interview building upon the previous one with increasing refinement and focus. This *iterative* process applies not only to specific methods, but to the qualitative research process as a whole.

Quantitative studies of behaviour commonly utilize a single form of data collection (that is, the survey), whereas qualitative research may employ multiple data collection strategies, including one-to-one conversation (for example, key informant interviewing), group discussion (for example, focus groups) and observations of actual behaviour (for example, structured direct observations). This *triangulation* approach, seeking information through different routes, has many advantages, particularly in the enhancement of data validity (Jick 1979).

Attempts are made to describe the *context* of the topic under consideration by using in-depth and open-ended data-gathering techniques. For example, in the planning of a specific intervention trial, issues relating to the trial need to be put into the general context of the behaviour and belief systems operating in the community.

3 MAIN QUALITATIVE METHODS

In this section, summaries are given of the nature and uses of the most common qualitative data collection methods and their strengths and weaknesses. The descriptions are necessarily brief and references are given which provide more details of the various methods.

3.1 Unstructured observations

Unstructured observations include both traditional ethnographic participant observation, as well as more structured focused observations (Bernard 1994). *Participant observation* is the classical method of social anthropology. The investigator endeavours to become a functioning member of a community and engages in activities or ceremonies of interest, watches carefully what others do and how they react to the investigator's own behaviour. The purpose is to view the community from the perspective of a participating member rather than as an outsider. Observations are recorded in detailed notes taken down following the activity. Participant observation is appropriate in the initial stages of research, when a context or problem is not well understood, or when the research subject is complex, such as exploring patterns of health-seeking behaviour.

Focused observations are a more systematic description of activities in which the observer is not directly part of the activity under study (Bentley *et al.* 1994). Focused observations may concentrate on an individual (for example, a pregnant woman), location (for example, the kitchen), or event (for example, a wedding party). The observer attempts to record as much behaviour as possible, including actions, conversations, description of the physical locale, and other features of interest. Focused observations often require some preliminary examination of the activity or location to prepare the observer. For example, the investigator may have a general impression of the interior of a rural house, but may not know the kind and quantity of cooking utensils, nor how they are washed or stored. Some research questions require detailed observations on how a procedure is actually carried out. For example, how a mother mixes water with rehydration salts at home for the treatment of diarrhoea. Such observations may be used in the design of questionnaires and to confirm or refine data collected through interviews.

The strengths and weaknesses of these techniques, together with those of other methods discussed below, are summarized in Table 10.1.

Table 10.1.   Strengths and weaknesses of different qualitative research methods.

Study method	Strengths	Weaknesses
Unstructured observations	Gives a record of actual, as opposed to reported or recalled, behaviour Participant observation can be less reactive and can help build rapport with local people Permits recording of the temporal sequence of behaviours, so causal linkages may be examined	Potential reactivity on the part of persons being observed for focused observations (less of a problem for children) Less useful for exploring people's beliefs and perceptions Requires much time to conduct and write up Difficult and time-consuming to train data collectors
Structured observations	Gives a record of actual, as opposed to reported or recalled, behaviour Easier to administer and to train data collectors than less structured observational methods As results are collected using standardized methods and are amenable to quantification, results easier to compare over time or between communities	Considerably more time-consuming than surveys Some behaviours difficult or sensitive to observe (for example, sexual behaviour, defecation) Focusing on a specific subset of behaviours may miss new or infrequent behaviours of importance

Table 10.1.   Continued

Study method	Strengths	Weaknesses
Unstructured and semi-structured interviewing	Iterative, in-depth interviewing can cover a large number of topics in great depth Issues can be explored within a socio-cultural context Especially useful for determining the language of discourse (terminology, concerns and perceptions) surrounding a particular topic area, including those culturally-defined categories (domains) of key importance from the local perspective	Number of informants (sample size) generally small due to the costliness and time-consuming nature of this type of interviewing Requires highly skilled interviewers
Systematic interviewing	Data are collected in a systematic way and may be easily compared in different sites Standard data collection instruments are used, which may be administered by lay interviewers Can be analysed using statistical analysis software, such as ANTHROPAC (Borgatti 1992)	If cultural domains have been improperly determined during preliminary interviews with informants, respondents may not understand the exercise Some respondents may feel they are being 'tested'

Table 10.1.   Continued

Study method	Strengths	Weaknesses
Focus groups	Provides data on consensus, mainstream opinions	Does not pick up the full range of beliefs and behaviours surrounding a particular topic, especially if the topic is deemed sensitive according to local standards
	Encourages debate and discussion by local people around a key topic	
	Can be used to assess feasibility of intervention	Logistic problems in getting groups of people together at specific times are common
Participatory rural appraisal	Local people create and own the data. The data are not extracted from the community, but subsist and are used within the community	Often difficult to include all members of the community, and therefore may be unrepresentative
	A high level of rapport is built between outsiders (the investigators) and local people	An emphasis is placed on public, less sensitive knowledge, and so the methods may be less likely to obtain information on highly sensitive topics, such as sexual behaviour and fertility history, particularly if used in groups

3.2 Structured observations

Structured observations involve the recording of behaviours, or the outcomes of behaviours, by trained observers, through the use of a pre-coded or partly coded data collection instrument (Bentley *et al.* 1994). Structured observation methods include continuous monitoring and spot checks. Structured observational approaches are used when the behaviours that are to be studied in detail have been identified (possibly through participant observation) and it is clear what information is needed (for example, time of day, frequency and types of behaviour).

The researcher observes, as unobtrusively as possible, occurrences of events or behaviours. A dilemma faced by every observer is where to focus attention and what details to record. The data collection instruments are designed to help concentrate the researcher's attention on matters of greatest relevance to the research problem. Predetermined structure limits discovery but assures relevance and consistency. The complexity of structured observation instruments vary. Some studies focus on detailed description of one or two events of interest, breaking them into fine units of activities, noting who performs them, where, with what tools and for how long. For example, Stanton and Clemens (1987a) studied hand washing and use of the sari for cleansing in Bangladesh. Observations of food preparation might be done in this way. Unlike most methods described in this chapter, structured observation may yield data amenable to statistical analysis and which can be repeated to monitor behavioural change over time.

3.3 Unstructured and semi-structured interviewing

Both unstructured and semi-structured interviewing techniques emphasize an open-ended approach, where uncovering the informant's terminology and understanding about how and why things work are the focus of the interaction. Emphasis is placed initially on building rapport between interviewer and respondent. One of the characteristics of both of these methods is that they seize on new pieces of information and dart off in unplanned directions. Informants are encouraged to give detailed responses through the use of probing. Unstructured interviewing can resemble an informal conversation, as the investigator usually does not take notes during the interview process, and both asks questions and responds to questions from the informant.

The semi-structured interview is a more systematic type of in-depth interviewing, in which the interviewer uses a list of guiding questions (or topics) to orient the interview, and takes notes or tapes the interview for later transcription. Unlike a structured survey, the interview guide serves only as an *aide-memoire* (Caldwell 1988). The discussions are guided by the particular interests of the researcher and by what the informant desires to communicate.

In-depth interviews are time-consuming and can be conducted with only a few individuals in a community. Depending on the objectives of the study, respondents for unstructured or semi-structured interviews may be 'key informants' or more objectively selected individuals representing particular characteristics of interest (for example, mothers who have lost a child, migrants). Key informants tend to be of three different types: administrators/community leaders or other persons in positions of power, community health workers, and individuals in the community with specialized areas of expertise or experience (for example, traditional birth attendants, traditional healers). Key informants are identified through casual inquiry of formal and informal leaders and other pivotal community members, or through more systematic methods, such as consensus analysis or social network analysis (Johnson 1990). Informants become 'key' because they are more co-operative and accessible than other respondents and often are interviewed on multiple occasions. They serve to inform the investigator about selected aspects of their culture and may be used to provide information throughout the course of the study.

In-depth interviews frequently make use of specialized techniques to focus discussions. Life history or case study approaches may be especially useful in providing the context for interpreting intervention studies. A 'case' may consist of a single individual, groups of individuals or even institutions, on which information is compiled on the basis of one or more interviews. These typically take a historical perspective on the development of an event (for example, an illness episode) or characteristic central to the research, and usually include a number of related issues which may have important explanatory value.

3.4 Systematic interviewing

Systematic interviewing techniques include a variety of methods derived from the field of cognitive anthropology used for identifying and exploring the underlying beliefs and assumptions (also termed 'grammars' or 'rules') that organize people's thinking and guide their behaviour (Weller and Romney 1988). These methods were developed largely for exploring 'cultural domains of knowledge' (Spradley 1979) through the elicitation of items and terms in domains (for example, through free lists), understanding how these items are categorized (for example, through pile sorts), and how they are ordered (for example, through ranking). Most of the data can be collected using semi-structured data collection forms. Data are gathered from a large number of respondents who may be randomly selected.

Free listing is a structured data collection technique in which an informant is asked to list all the different items in a particular cultural domain (for example, all the different illnesses of children). The results from a sample of informants are tabulated to obtain a list of 'cognizant' items. This constitutes the preliminary exploration of a cultural or cognitive 'domain'.

Pile sorting is a structured data collection technique that elicits indigenous categories and groupings of domain items by asking informants to group a set of domain items either 'freely' (according to what they think is important) or according to predetermined criteria. Respondents are usually asked to sort cards on which the items have been drawn or the names written. *Triad sorting* is often used as an alternative to pile sorting, which can prove difficult for illiterate informants. Informants are presented with groups of three domain items at a time and are asked to identify the item that does not belong, or is the most different, from the others.

Ranking is a method used to order items within a domain along a dimension either determined by the investigator or by respondents. For example, the respondent may be asked to order items according to relative 'tastiness' or 'healthiness'. Paired comparisons are used as an alternative to ranking, which can prove difficult for illiterate informants or a large number of items.

3.5 Multiple informant interviewing

3.5.1 Focus groups

In a focus group discussion, a small group of participants (usually six to twelve), under the guidance of a moderator, talk about topics which are thought to be of special importance to the respondents and to the investigation (Morgan 1988). Topic guides are utilized by the moderator to stimulate discussions around areas of interest. Participants are selected from specific target groups, whose ideas and experiences are germane to the study. Participants in a focus group are chosen to be relatively 'homogenous', to avoid conflict and power differentials that could disrupt the discussion. Generally, participants are of the same sex and age group, but similarity in other characteristics may be important in different settings, such as ethnicity, socio-economic status and marital status. It is important, but difficult, to ensure that participants are comfortable with one another and that there are no 'experts', whose opinions would be held in higher regard than others, and who might dominate the discussion.

The focus group method assumes that informants will be more forthcoming in discussing local beliefs and practices if they can discuss the information together rather than in a one-to-one interview. A group discussion helps the investigator to determine what is truly common knowledge or practice and what is idiosyncratic. For discussions to be productive, the facilitator must have skill in group dynamics and motivation and must steer the discussion to reduce the amount of time spent on irrelevant matters. It is useful to have an observer who makes notes and is alert for non-verbal cues.

Subjects for discussion can be introduced through direct questions, general statements or by techniques such as 'dilemma tales' in which a social problem related to a topic of relevance to the intervention is posed and the participants asked what advice they would give. Highly sensitive and difficult subjects should usually be avoided in group discussions. If possible, a focus group discussion should be tape-recorded but if this inhibits open discussion, detailed notes should be taken by an observer. The number of focus groups held will depend on the number of different relevant groups in the community. Focus group sessions usually last for at least an hour and continue until the facilitator considers that all the participants have expressed their opinions adequately on the topics under investigation.

A useful guide to the use of focus groups in health research is that by Dawson *et al.* (1993), which is available in both English and French from the WHO Tropical Diseases Research Programme.

3.5.2 *Participatory rural appraisal*

Participatory rural appraisal is 'a semi-structured process of learning from, with and by rural people about rural conditions' (Chambers 1992; Mascarenhas 1992), though it can be used in non-rural settings involving groups which perceive themselves as different or disadvantaged. The core philosophy entails a genuine respect for those living in a rural setting and methods are used that rely on participation of the people themselves to describe and communicate their behaviour and belief systems. Appropriate local materials and data collection methods are used, which permit the people to express and share their knowledge. Methods tend to be visual, and conducted in groups. There is an emphasis on relative ranking according to local standards (for example, more or less time spent breast feeding than on doing laundry during the day), rather than on measurement according to an external set of standards (for example, number of minutes spent breast feeding in a day).

One of the main methods involves asking the participants to create a map of their community, using locally available materials, termed 'participatory mapping'. They are encouraged to include any elements in the map they consider relevant and important. In rural villages, community maps commonly include the locations of all the households (and sometimes their relative sizes). Villagers in India will commonly indicate the castes of households by using different coloured powders. Community members may be asked to indicate specific kinds of households (for example, those with diarrhoea cases, malnourished children, pregnant women). Other types of products created by community members using this approach include seasonal work diagrams, rankings of wealth, well-being and control of local resources.

4 REPRESENTATIVENESS, RELIABILITY AND VALIDITY

Representativeness, reliability (or repeatability) and validity of findings from small-scale qualitative studies are generally of greater concern than those from large-scale structured surveys. It has been argued that since qualitative studies tend to be small-scale, their conclusions are not easily applied to other groups. Borman *et al.* (1986) argue that findings from qualitative studies can be generalized to other settings if investigators adhere closely to standards of translatability (where 'methods, categories and characteristics of phenomena and groups be identified so explicitly that comparisons can be made across groups and disciplines with confidence') and comparability (which requires the use of standard and non-idiosyncratic terminology).

In qualitative research, the distinction is made between researcher-imposed (etic) and subject-generated (emic) meanings. By considering the perspective of both kinds of constructs, investigators can reduce the tendency to impose their own constructs upon the field (Borman *et al.* 1986). While proof of validity of qualitative conclusions can be difficult, the depth and intensity of the qualitative approach gives a degree of reassurance about findings, provided they are appropriately documented by the recording instruments.

Measures are listed in Box 10.1 that can be taken to increase the representativeness of individuals or groups selected and to enhance the validity of the information obtained.

Box 10.1.   Measures which may be taken to increase representativeness in qualitative research studies

1. Randomly select participants from a larger survey or from a census-type enumeration.
2. Ensure that all major sectors of the study population are represented, for example, by holding separate group discussions for each sector.
3. Compare the results of several different approaches to check on their mutual consistency (triangulation).
4. Independently interpret tape-recorded interviews or discussions, including interpretation by local community members.
5. Make special efforts not to confine data collection to the more accessible and co-operative members of the study population.

---

5   MANAGEMENT AND ANALYSIS OF QUALITATIVE DATA

Data recording is a critical component of any kind of research. For qualitative research, the methods used for recording data play an important role in analysis and validation. Recording can take many forms: notes in a book, tape recordings, photographs, videotape recordings, and maps. It is essential that qualitative data be managed properly so they can be easily and efficiently searched during analysis. Hundreds of pages of written (or 'expanded') field notes may be generated, based on interviews with key informants, transcripts of focus group sessions, observations of behaviours and events, secondary data (such as clinic records and genealogy charts), and the researcher's comments and thoughts about what the data mean.

If the textual data collected exceed about 200 pages, it is recommended that a microcomputer-based system of textual data management be used because of its greatly enhanced speed and efficiency (Fielding and Lee 1991; Tesch 1993). A variety of text retrieval and management software programs are available, such as ZyINDEX, dtSearch, GOFER, NOTEBOOK PLUS, TEXTBASE ALPHA and ETHNOGRAPH. The relative merits of many of these programs have been reviewed elsewhere (Weitzman and Miles 1995). A guide for managing, coding and retrieving qualitative data is outlined in Table 10.2, which has been adapted from Gittelsohn (1992).

Brief field notes should be expanded using a word processor. Alternatively, expanded field notes can be written up for typing into a word processor. Each data file should have a unique, meaningful filename and each file should represent a discrete data collection unit: for example, one interview, one observation of a key event, one focus group session.

Expanded notes should be reviewed, and a preliminary coding list derived. The notes should be coded within the word processing program. Once the preliminary coding process is complete, the notes can

Table 10.2. Managing qualitative data using a microcomputer

Process	Method used
Raw field notes	Hand-written and/or tape recorded
Expanded field notes	Expanded in long-hand to be typed into word processor or expanded as typed into word processor
Spell-checking	Word processor
Review of expanded field notes and derivation of preliminary codes	Word processor and word processor macros, TEXTBASE ALPHA
Coding of expanded field notes	Word processor and word processor macros, TEXTBASE ALPHA
Indexing expanded field notes and codes	Analysis program (for example ZyINDEX, dtSearch, TEXTBASE ALPHA)
Searching through expanded field notes and codes	Analysis program (for example ZyINDEX, dtSearch, TEXTBASE ALPHA)

be indexed. Preliminary searches of the data should be conducted at this stage. If the investigator is still in the field, these preliminary searches assist in identifying gaps in the data (that is, areas for continued research). The coding list should be refined and expanded at this point as well.

A code is an 'abbreviation or symbol applied to a segment of words... in order to *classify* the words... they usually derive from research questions, hypotheses, key concepts or important themes' (Miles and Huberman 1994). Codes have a number of different functions relating to textual data, including organization, retrieval of information, assembly and reduction of data into analysable units. They can be applied to data at several *levels of abstraction*. Miles and Huberman (1994) describe three coding levels, descriptive, interpretive, and explanatory. At the lowest level are codes that describe things as they are found in the data set (descriptive), at a higher level codes represent judgements by the coder about what is happening in the data (interpretive), and at the highest level they relate important concepts according to emergent themes, patterns, or explanations (explanatory).

All textual data should be entered into a word-processing program. Codes should be clearly marked as separate from the textual data (for example, capitals, in bold face, in brackets and with symbols at each end—for example, **[#STATUS OF WOMEN#]**), which allows search exclusive or inclusive of the code. To save time, it is possible to use macros, whereby codes are inserted into the text in response to one or two keystrokes. It is generally best to place the codes immediately following the text they relate to. Locating appropriate places to insert codes can be a lengthy process involving reading and rereading field notes. Text management programs can be used to hasten this process, by permitting rapid searching for potential 'coding points'.

Once a computerized textual database has been created and coded, the user can access the data to address specific research questions. The procedures for searching the indexed database differ depending on the type of research question asked. As a general rule of thumb, it makes sense to start with the simple questions. If these basic questions cannot be answered by the material in the database, it makes no sense to move onto more complex questions. Systematic searches may be conducted in a qualitative database, which can lead to an analytic assessment of key patterns in the data (for further discussion and examples, see Miles and Huberman, 1994). Products of qualitative data analysis include quotes, tables, matrices, taxonomies, maps, multidimensional scales and complex models (Miles and Huberman 1994).

6 QUALITATIVE RESEARCH AND FIELD TRIALS

6.1 Designing the study

From the earliest stages in the planning of a trial, qualitative information can be used to design more appropriate and effective field trials. Investigators should seek out existing qualitative data sets on the community/region/ethnic group of interest. In-depth ethnographic studies have been conducted in thousands of cultures and subcultures around the world. A good place to start is the *Atlas of World Cultures* (Price 1990). More intensive searching by subject area can be conducted in the *Human Relations Area Files* (Murdock 1971), a set of ethnographic materials which have been extensively coded by topic area. These files are available in some libraries in microfiche or disk form.

Information from previously existing qualitative data sets should be complemented with preliminary qualitative data-gathering in the communities of interest. This data-gathering can contribute to the initial stages in the design of a field trial in several ways, including assisting with the definition of variables, instrument design and sampling.

Qualitative data can provide information crucial for the definition of key variables. Variables defined using qualitative information have high internal validity, because they represent or are constructed from categories which the study population consider important. For example, many field trials attempt to initiate behavioural change at the household level. But what is a household? From work in a variety of cultural settings, it appears that while households share one or more features (for example, co-residence, joint production, shared consumption and kinship links), no particular feature or combination of features can be used for a universal definition of a 'household'. The concept of the household will vary from culture to culture and may vary within cultures as well. Preliminary qualitative research can help identify local concepts of the household that are useful for defining this unit. Another example lies in defining 'economic status'. In most rural settings, simple measures such as income and land-holdings are insufficient means by which to differentiate households by economic status. Taking a qualitative approach would involve asking local people how they differentiate richer from poorer people, and/or by conducting direct observations in the local communities. For example, in rural Nepal, patterns of wealth differ by caste level, with higher castes tending to have greater wealth in terms of land and material possessions, while lower castes have relatively greater wealth in animals (Gittelsohn 1989).

Preliminary qualitative research can assist in instrument design in several ways. First and foremost, qualitative methods emphasize learning terminology and categories in the local language (Coreil *et al.* 1989). How do local people express and organize their own knowledge about the world around them? By learning these basics, we can learn what questions should or should not be asked, how to ask a question politely, how to ask a question to obtain a valid response and how to position questions in a survey. The classic study by Stone and Campbell (1986) in Nepal illustrates how a survey developed without this kind of input yielded grossly erroneous results. The relationship between local terminology and survey instrument terminology can be clarified. For example, linkages can be made between local illness terms and biomedical disease terms, permitting more accurate reporting of morbidity histories.

Finally, preliminary qualitative data can help investigators develop their sampling strategy by identifying locally defined significant subgroups in the population. This is particularly important when attempting to develop a stratified sampling scheme. While the researcher may divide subgroups ethnically, geographically and economically, community members may divide their population by clan, lineage, occupation and caste. The local system of categorization may be more meaningful for the intervention's success. Qualitative information can assist in appropriate sampling when multiple communities are being studied, to determine the extent of their similarities or differences in social, economic or demographic terms. If the community is the unit of application for the intervention, more detailed qualitative studies of the distribution of the key variables may be necessary for stratifying prior to randomization.

6.2 Developing the intervention

The use of qualitative research to develop interventions is most commonly termed *formative research*, and has a large literature (Atkin and

Freimuth 1991; Helitzer-Allen *et al.* 1993; Lloyd *et al.* 1994). Formative research is most successfully used in developing interventions which have a large behavioural component. Qualitative methods are appropriate for identifying both positive and negative health behaviours, and in describing the context of these behaviours. It is not always apparent which particular behaviours place a population at increased risk for a health problem. Qualitative research can help the investigator identify target behaviours to modify. For example, iodine deficiency is a public health problem in many regions of Nepal, even in those regions that receive an ample supply of iodized salt. After a small study, a few unstructured observations were sufficient to reveal the cause of this problem. Food preparers commonly wash the salt (in rock crystal form) before adding it to food, removing the iodine, which had been sprayed on. Qualitative data collection can even give a rough sense of the prevalence of a particular behaviour across sites. Discussions with local people and additional observations revealed that this practice is performed by most households in the area (B.K. Dahal, personal communication).

As well as assisting the investigator to identify key behaviours, qualitative information can help in the formulation of intervention strategies. Qualitative interviewing techniques allow discovery of appropriate terminology and modes for communication. Some of the main uses of qualitative information for this purpose are summarized in Table 10.3, which includes specific examples. Also indicated are the qualitative methods discussed which would provide the most relevant information for the purpose.

Finally, qualitative information can also contribute to process evaluation in which the proper deployment of interventions is assessed while they are being implemented.

6.3 Studies initiated during a field trial

Qualitative research should be considered from the earliest stages of conducting a field trial. The methods continue to be of value throughout a trial and may be deployed in several ways during the intervention delivery: (i) to investigate a set of variables which have already been found to be important and which require in-depth investigation. For example, assessment of water contact in schistosomiasis control programmes often involves observing when and how rivers and streams are used, and by whom; (ii) to study in-depth one or several

Table 10.3.   Uses of qualitative research methods to develop intervention strategies

Objective	Examples (references)	Qualitative research approach
Conduct a 'needs assessment' in the community	To build rapport and community support for the research-intervention process [community health needs assessment in Tanzania (Rifkin *et al.* 1992)]	Focus groups, individual interviews
Identify key behaviours which place populations at risk	Describing preferential allocation of foods that favours males over females and adults over children [to improve nutritional status within the household: Nepal intra-household food allocation (Gittelsohn 1991); Nepal vitamin A deficiency (Shankar 1995)]	Direct observation of behaviour, reports of behaviour
	Recording how and when people wash their hands, clean and bathe their children, prepare infant foods, etc. [Bangladesh sanitation (Stanton and Clemens 1987b)]	
Ascertain feasibility of modifying risk behaviours	Determining which behaviours are modifiable. Assessing how modifying a particular behaviour will effect other factors	In-depth interviews, focus group discussions
	Determining what are the culturally and financially acceptable alternatives to the behaviours	
Select appropriate language and terminology for health communications	Determining what are the appropriate (recognizable, consistently applied) illness or symptom terms to communicate to mothers [Gambia acute respiratory infection study (Gittelsohn *et al.* 1991)]	In-depth interviews, free lists

Table 10.3.   Continued

Objective	Examples (references)	Qualitative research approach
	Selecting the appropriate systems of food classification that will encourage child care-givers to prepare a beneficial food	
Determine culturally appropriate metaphors to communicate key concepts	Determining which concepts local people are familiar with and knowledgeable about. For example, in many rural communities, agriculture and farming provide understandable analogies/ metaphors for communication [South India nutrition education (Nichter 1989a, 1989b)]	In-depth interviews, focus groups
Develop a set of guiding principles for health messages	Determining which beneficial beliefs or behaviours currently practised should be reinforced [Ojibwa-Cree diabetes prevention (Gittelsohn 1995)]	In-depth interviews, focus groups
	Using existing beliefs in ways that will help people identify healthy alternatives for risk behaviours [promotion of oral rehydration therapy in Pakistan (Herman *et al.* 1992)]	
Organize health education in ways that are meaningful to community	Utilize the local system for categorizing insects, to design intervention against vector borne disease	Pile sorts, other grouping techniques, in-depth interviews
	Promote increased consumption of healthful foods, acknowledging and using local patterns of food classification	

Table 10.3. Continued

Objective	Examples (references)	Qualitative research approach
Define the message for health communications	Identifying phrases/expressions in local terminology which are most meaningful to community members [water boiling in Sri Lanka (Nichter 1985); prevention of vitamin A deficiency in Thailand (Smitasiri *et al.* 1993)]	In-depth interviews, focus groups
Decide target groups for health communications	Determining whether interventions should be community-wide, neighbourhood-based, school-based, and/or targeted to high risk individuals [diabetes prevention among the Oji-Cree (B. Zinman, personal communication)]	Direct observation of behaviour, in-depth interviews, focus groups
Select the most appropriate media for health communications	Determining whether mass media or one-on-one (role model) approaches are likely to be more effective	Direct observation, focus groups
	Determining which form of mass media is likely to be most effective [prevention of vitamin A deficiency in Thailand (Smitasiri 1993)]	
	Deciding the appropriate target group for messages [weaning project in Manoff (Griffiths 1992)]	
Identify constraints to appropriate health-seeking behaviour	Determining why some health messages/projects have not worked [hygiene/nutrition intervention in Sri Lanka (Nichter 1985)]	In-depth interviewing, focus groups
Ascertain local perceptions and classifications of disease	Determining the local beliefs and perceptions of disease aetiology [South India folk dietetics (Nichter 1987)]	Pile sorting, key informant interviews

Table 10.3.   Continued

Objective	Examples (references)	Qualitative research approach
	Determining the differences and similarities between the perceptions of community members and those of health providers	
	Determining how community members describe health problems, to assist with appropriate diagnosis and treatment [female reproductive tract infections in India (Kanani 1992)]	
Get community feedback on proposed interventions	Determining if health messages are likely to be understood by local community	Focus groups, participatory rural appraisal
	Learning how best to modify interventions to make them acceptable and timed to take account of local constraints and schedules	

variables or relationships discovered to be important during the course of the study. Often such investigations are related to understanding behaviour such as personal hygiene practices which would be difficult to study using other research methods; (iii) to investigate new areas which emerge in response to the changing needs of the study. For example, a study may be necessary to suggest reasons for, and possible solutions to, a problem such as a community's change of attitude towards participating in a trial.

6.4 Use in analysis and interpretation of trial results

Qualitative research may be used at the end of an intervention trial as an aid in the interpretation of findings (Miles and Huberman 1994). Such information may be used: to provide guidance in proper analytic procedures; to provide explanations for unexpected findings; and to confirm the results of the quantitative analysis. Qualitative information can assist in the process of conducting quantitative analysis in several ways, including the selection of items appropriate to include in a scale (for example, socio-economic status). Qualitative data may be used to help interpret quantitative findings that are contrary to expectation or appear to lack internal consistency and also provide a contextual base on which to judge the soundness of findings obtained from quantitative methods.

REFERENCES

Atkin, C.K. and Freimuth, V. (1991). Formative evaluation research in campaign design. Chapter 6 in: *Public Communication Campaigns*. (2nd ed), (ed. Rice, R.E. and Atkin, C.K.). Sage Publications, Newbury Park.

Bentley, M.E., Boot, M.T., Gittelsohn, J. and Stallings, R.Y. (1994). *The use of structured observations in the study of health behaviour*. Occasional Paper No. 27, IRC International Water and Sanitation Centre, The Hague, The Netherlands.

Bernard, H.R. (1986). The construction of primary data in cultural anthropology. *Current Anthropology*, **27**, 382–96.

Bernard, H.R. (1994). *Research methods in anthropology: qualitative and quantitative approaches*. (2nd ed), Sage Publications, Thousand Oaks.

Borgatti, S. (1992). *ANTHROPAC 4.0*. Analytic Technologies, Columbia, South Carolina.

Borman, K.M., LeCompte, M.D. and Goetz, J.P. (1986). Ethnographic and qualitative research design and why it doesn't work. *American Behavioral Scientist*, **30**, 42–57.

Caldwell, J.C. (1988). Micro-approaches: similarities and differences, strengths and weaknesses. In *Micro-approaches to demographic research*. (ed. Caldwell, J.C., Hill, A.G. and Hull, V.S.). pp. 458–70. Kegan Paul International, London.

Chambers, R. (1992). *Rural appraisal: rapid, relaxed and participatory*. Discussion Paper 311, Institute of Development Studies, University of Sussex.

Coreil, J., Augustin, A., Holt, E. and Halsey, N.A. (1989). Use of ethnographic research for instrument development in a case–control study of immunization use in Haiti. *International Journal of Epidemiology*, **18** (Suppl 2), S33–7.

Dawson, S., Manderson, L. and Tallo,V.L. (1993). *A manual for the use of focus groups*. International Nutrition Foundation for Developing Countries, Boston.

Fielding, N.G. and Lee, R.M. (1991). *Using computers in qualitative research*. Sage Publications, Newbury Park.

Gittelsohn, J. (1989). *Intrahousehold food distribution in rural Nepal*. Doctoral Dissertation, University of Connecticut. University Microfilms, Ann Arbor.

Gittelsohn, J. (1991). Opening the box: intrahousehold food distribution in rural Nepal. *Social Science and Medicine*, **33**, 1141–54.

Gittelsohn, J., Sillah, B. and Sanneh, K. (1991). *An ethnographic study of acute respiratory infections in The Gambia. Vol 2: Data analyses of the core and confirmatory studies*. Report prepared for UNICEF/Banjul, August.

Gittelsohn, J. (1992). An approach to the management and coding of qualitative data using microcomputers. *The Indian Journal of Social Work*, **53**, 611–20.

Gittelsohn, J., Harris, S., Burris, K., Kakegamic, L., Landman, L.T., Sharma, A., Wolever, T., Logan, A., Barnie, A. and Zinman, B. (1995). Use of ethnographic methods for applied research on diabetes among Ojibway-Cree Indians in Northern Ontario. *Health Education Quarterly* (in press).

Griffiths, M. (1992). Understanding infant feeding practices: qualitative research methodologies used in the weaning project. In *Rapid assessment procedures: qualitative methodologies for planning and evaluation of health-related programmes*. (ed. Scrimshaw, N.S. and Gleason, G.R.). International Nutrition Foundation for Developing Countries, Boston.

Helitzer-Allen, D., Kendall, C. and Wirima, J. (1993). The role of ethnographic research in malaria control: an example from Malawi. *Research in the Sociology of Health Care*, **10**, 269–86.

Herman, E., Bentley, M., Sultana, F., Hamzah, M., Huzaifah, S., Masreah, S., Pelto, G. and Pelto, P. (1992). Beyond data collection: facilitating the application and use of ethnographic information to guide health programmes and further research. In *Rapid assessment procedures: qualitative methodologies for planning and evaluation of health-related programmes*. (ed. Scrimshaw, N.S. and Gleason, G.R.). International Nutrition Foundation for Developing Countries, Boston.

Jefremovas,V. (1995). *Qualitative research methods: an annotated bibliography*. International Development Research Centre, Canada.

Jick, T.D. (1979). Mixing qualitative and quantitative methods: triangulation in action. *Administrative Science Quarterly*, **24**, 602–11.

Johnson, J.C. (1990). *Selecting ethnographic informants*. Qualitative Research Methods Series 22. Sage Publications, Newbury Park.

Kanani, S. (1992). Application of rapid assessment procedures in the context of women's morbidity: experiences of a non-governmental organization in India. In *Rapid assessment procedures: qualitative methodologies for planning and evaluation of health-related programmes.* (ed. Scrimshaw, N.S. and Gleason, G.R.). International Nutrition Foundation for Developing Countries, Boston.

Lloyd, L.S., Winch, P., Ortega-Canto, J. and Kendall, C. (1994). The design of a community-based health education intervention for the control of *Aedes Aegypti. American Journal of Tropical Medicine and Hygiene*, **50**, 401–11.

Mascarenhas, J. (1992). Participatory rural appraisal and participatory learning methods: recent experiences from Myrada and South India. In *Rapid assessment procedures: qualitative methodologies for planning and evaluation of health-related programmes.* (ed. Scrimshaw, N.S. and Gleason, G.R.). International Nutrition Foundation for Developing Countries, Boston.

Miles, M.B. and Huberman, A.M. (1994). *Qualitative data analysis: an expanded sourcebook.* (2nd ed.). Sage Publications, Newbury Park.

Murdock, G.P. (1971). *Outline of cultural materials.* (4th edition), Human Relation Area Files. New Haven, Connecticut.

Nichter, M. (1985). Drink boiled water: a cultural analysis of a health education message. *Social Science and Medicine*, **21**, 667–9.

Nichter, M. (1987). The ethnophysiology and folk dietetics of pregnancy: a case study from South India. *Human Organization*, **42**, 235–46.

Nichter, M. (1989a). Cultural interpretations of states of malnutrition among children: A South Indian case study. In *Anthropology and International Health: South Asian Case Studies.* Kluwer Academic Publishers, Boston.

Nichter, M. and Nichter, M. (1989b). Education by appropriate analogy. In *Anthropology and International Health: South Asian Case Studies.* Kluwer Academic Publishers, Boston.

Pelto, P.J. and Pelto, G.M. (1978). *Anthropological research: the structure of inquiry.* Cambridge University Press.

Price, D.H. (1990). *Atlas of world cultures.* Sage Publications, Newbury Park.

Rifkin, S., Annett, H. and Tabibzadeh, I. (1992). Rapid appraisal to assess community health needs: a focus on the urban poor. In *Rapid assessment procedures: qualitative methodologies for planning and evaluation of health-related programmes.* (ed. Scrimshaw, N.S. and Gleason, G.R.). International Nutrition Foundation for Developing Countries, Boston.

Scrimshaw, S.C.M. and Hurtado, E. (1987). *Rapid assessment procedures for nutrition and primary health care.* The United Nations University, Tokyo. UNICEF and UCLA Latin American Center Publications, University of California, Los Angeles.

Shankar, A.V. (1995). *In search of the light of your eyes: anthropological and epidemiological perspectives of vitamin A deficiency in Nepali children.* PhD dissertation, Case Western Reserve University. University Microfilms, Ann Arbor.

Smitasiri, S., Attig, G.A., Valyasevi, A., Dhanamitta, S. and Tontisirin, K. (1993). *Social marketing vitamin A rich foods in Thailand: a model nutrition communication for behaviour change process.* UNICEF, Bangkok.

Spradley, J.P. (1979). *The Ethnographic Interview.* Holt, Rinehart and Winston Inc., Chicago.

Stanton, B. and Clemens, J. (1987a). Twenty-four hour recall, knowledge–attitude practices questionnaires, and direct observation of sanitary practices: a comparative study. *Bulletin of the World Health Organization,* **2**, 217–22.

Stanton, B. and Clemens, J. (1987b). An educational intervention for altering water-sanitation behaviors to reduce childhood diarrhoea in urban Bangladesh: formulation, preparation and delivery of the educational intervention. *Social Science and Medicine,* **24**, 275–83.

Stone, L. and Campbell, J.G. (1984). The use and misuse of surveys in international development: an experiment from Nepal. *Human Organization,* **43**, 27–37.

Tesch, R. (1993). Personal computers in qualitative research. In *Ethnography and qualitative design in educational research.* (2nd ed), (ed. LeCompte, M.D. and Preissle, J.). pp. 279–314. Academic Press, San Diego, California.

Weitzman, E.A. and Miles, M.B. (1995). *Computer programs for qualitative data analysis.* Sage Publications, Thousand Oaks.

Weller, S.C. and Romney, A.K. (1988). *Systematic data collection.* Qualitative Research Methods Series No. 10, Sage Publications, Newbury Park.

11
Field organization

1 INTRODUCTION

The complexity of the organization of a field trial will depend largely on the size of the study population, the frequency of follow-up, its expected duration, and its location. For example, a trial of a leprosy vaccine may involve a population of tens or even hundreds of thousands of participants, living in a relatively remote rural area, in which repeat follow-up examinations are required every two to three years for over a decade. Such a trial will be a much more complex undertaking than, say, a trial of a new measles vaccine, involving only a few hundred subjects, conducted in or near a major population centre, and completed within a year or two.

Whether a trial is small or large, however, it is important to plan the organizational aspects of the investigation in great detail before starting any substantial field activities. The design of the trial must be reviewed to identify all the procedures and tasks that must be undertaken to meet the study objectives, and the logistics developed to carry out these procedures and tasks in a timely fashion. During this planning it may become clear that compromises have to be made between what is theoretically desirable and what is logistically possible. For example, in a vaccine trial, it may be of great interest to relate the immune response to vaccination to subsequent protection against disease on an individual-by-individual basis. This would involve collecting a blood sample from all participants before, and shortly after, vaccination, and possibly at repeated intervals thereafter. In practice, it may be feasible to do this only for a sample of participants (for reasons of cost, or because the study population would not accept repeated blood samples being taken) and thus relating protection to individual responses to vaccination would have to be excluded from the trial objectives.

A check-list of some of the items that it may be necessary to consider when planning a field trial is given in Appendix 11.1 at the end of this chapter. It is included to give guidance as to what such a list should contain, but it will generally be necessary to draw up a more detailed list tailored to the requirements for a particular trial.

The field team must understand, and be sensitive to, local customs and cultures. This will be facilitated if many of the field team members are from the same locality. The planning for the trial must take into account cultural practices that may affect both the acceptability of the trial and the organizational arrangements for conducting it.

The requirements for field organization in an intervention trial have much in common with the need for field organization in a military campaign. In each case, it is most important to keep in mind the overall objectives of the activities, as specified for the field trial in the study protocol. Detailed planning should start at an early stage in the trial as once activities get under way it is easy to 'lose sight of the wood for trees' unless there is a clear plan of activities made beforehand. A check-list which covers some of the organization aspects of field trials is given in Appendix 11.2.

2 MANUAL OF FIELD OPERATIONS AND STUDY DIARY

The tasks and procedures necessary to achieve each objective of a trial should be listed. A manual of field operations should be prepared in which each procedure to be carried out is fully detailed and each task fully described (for example, step by step instructions for the administration and completion of questionnaires, the method to be used for weighing infants, including maintenance procedures for the weighing scales, check-lists for equipment and materials required for each procedure). Each fieldworker should be given a copy of the manual, or of the relevant parts of the manual, and care should be taken to make sure these are updated if changes are made to procedures as the trial progresses. Not only should such a manual provide a clear set of rules for actions under different circumstances, but it can also serve as a long-term record of the detailed design aspects of the trial. This latter feature may be of special value in trials of long duration, where there is the possibility of changes in the investigators or failures in memory.

In addition to the field manual it is very valuable to maintain a trial diary in which the progress of the trial is recorded, problems which are encountered are noted, and the solutions adopted recorded. This will be useful in maintaining consistency of decisions throughout the trial. Some of the notes may be of value when final reports on the trial are being written, in which it may be necessary to document some of the unpredicted events during the course of the trial (for example, recording exactly when a particular disease epidemic took place or when fieldwork had to stop because of adverse weather conditions).

To guard against loss it may be worth maintaining the diary on a computer file rather than just in a notebook, but this will be largely a matter of personal preference. The latest version of the field manual is best stored on a computer file so that it can be updated and modified easily.

3 PERSONNEL ISSUES

Field trials may involve a large number of personnel, often for considerable periods of time, working under difficult conditions, and the staffing arrangements must be well organized. Each person should know what they have to do and when they have to do it, to whom they should report, and when, where and how they should report.

A job description should be prepared for each position, incorporating the set of tasks as specified in the field manual. Preparing such descriptions forces the investigator to work out in advance what each individual will do, and the descriptions inform each worker what is expected of him or her. The job description should specify not only the tasks to be undertaken, but also the workload (for example, the approximate number of the thick and thin blood films to be collecᴛᵉd per day) and the quality of work expected. An estimate should be made of the minimum educational levels and training required for each position. On the basis of the job descriptions, personnel for the posts must be recruited and trained for the specific tasks. Managerial and supervisory activities, with appropriate hierarchical relationships and lines of authority, need to be established. An organizational chart illustrating the lines of authority may be useful. Each staff member should be familiar with the responsibilities of other staff.

For some kinds of study a field team might include, typically, a driver, a census registration clerk, an interviewer, an assistant to take temperatures and to measure height and weight, or to test eyes, a nurse or medical assistant, a physician for physical examinations and the application of the intervention procedures, a laboratory technician to collect blood, urine, or stool specimens for laboratory tests, and a medical assistant or nurse for dispensing medications. A constraint on the size of a field team may be the number of persons who can be accommodated in a vehicle with the equipment they must use in the field. It will be useful to draw up an organizational plan outlining the activities and functions of the members of such a team with a diagram showing how the team will operate in the field. A section from the manual of procedure used in field surveys conducted by the Onchocerciasis Control Programme is given in Appendix 11.3, which also shows the physical set-up, and the planned flow of people, and forms during the examinations. Detailed descriptions of the procedures to be followed for each of the activities should be included in the field manual (for example, how the census form should be completed, how the items on the form should be checked, what should be done with the form at the end of the day).

Good financial management is essential for staff morale. Salaries and allowances should be paid on time, and petty cash should be available when required. A detailed record of expenditures should be kept together with receipts, as a senior staff member will have to account for all funds issued and spent. For large studies it will be essential to employ an administrator to take care of these aspects as they may be very time-consuming.

4   PHYSICAL LOCATION AND FACILITIES

An issue to be resolved early in the planning of a field trial is whether the study participants should be examined at a central location, at a series of local collecting points, or be visited for examination on a house-to-house basis. The decision will depend upon the procedures to be carried out, the nature of equipment required, the time the examination procedure takes, the population size, density and distribution, and the environmental and physical conditions.

A central collecting point may be most efficient for the study team, since more people can be seen in a day than in a house-to-house survey. If heavy or delicate non-portable equipment must be used, then a central gathering point for examinations cannot be avoided. Even if some of the examinations have to be done at a central location, however, it may be advisable to conduct the census and perhaps the questionnaire interviews at participants' houses.

The advantage of a house-to-house survey is that it is possible to be reasonably sure of having listed most of those who are eligible for entry into a trial. Any persons who do not report to a central testing point can then be identified and, if necessary, attempts made to find them. Chasing up the missing can be costly and time-consuming, however, and decisions about the benefits of doing this, as compared to the time and effort required, need to be considered in the planning phase. Also, the likely magnitude of 'non-response' may need to be estimated during the pilot phase.

Careful planning of the physical layout for the flow of people from one station to the next is important. Special attention may have to be given for carrying out the physical examination in order to ensure both privacy and adequate light. Usually there is little difficulty about making such arrangements when the examinations are conducted at a central collecting point, but for more mobile surveys special arrangements may be necessary, ranging from simple screening under a shady tree to the use of a chief's lodge with special lighting.

In addition to whatever arrangements are made for the interviewing, examinations, and specimen collection from study subjects, there are supporting functions that will require physical facilities. These include a headquarters for administration, a room for team meetings, briefings, and review of activities and problems on a daily basis, space for computer processing of data, file storage space, laboratory accommodation, stores for equipment and supplies, and transport garaging. The various components may be needed at one place, or at several places, or may need to be mobile.

If the field team must live away from home for long periods they may be able to obtain local accommodation, but other accommodation might have to be provided (for example, tents). Accommodation and cooking facilities should be arranged in advance and employment of a cook will save on staff time. Food may need careful storage and cooking in order to avoid food poisoning. Water for drinking may need to be purified, filtered, or boiled. Refuse disposal and toilets may also be needed if survey staff stay in rural areas.

5 EQUIPMENT AND SUPPLIES

The major items of equipment and reagents required must be specified in the study protocol. The choice of what equipment to buy should be influenced by what others in the area have used and whether they have found it satisfactory (and this will include servicing arrangements). It may be important to order a basic supply of spare parts at the same time as ordering equipment, if local availability is in doubt.

The field manual should include lists of all the equipment required for each of the trial procedures (for example, record cards, questionnaires, needles and syringes, laboratory supplies) and for the support of those procedures (for example, vehicles, files, benches, tents). Maintenance and quality control must be carried out (see Chapter 12).

Provision for transport is essential in most developing countries. Transporting people and equipment will require careful planning. Extra time should be allowed for possible mishaps. If possible, back-up transport should be available in case of emergencies. Maintenance of vehicles and close supervision of their use is vital. Control and discipline of vehicle use are key factors in the conduct of almost all field trials. Particular problems may arise if field staff are issued with vehicles (for example, motor cycles) that they keep at home rather than return to a central park on a daily basis. Maintenance, fuel supply, and the use of vehicles for purposes other than those for which they were intended can pose substantial problems.

Loss of stores and supplies can be a major problem, particularly due to theft. It is best to appoint one staff member as storekeeper to be solely in charge of stores, maintaining inventories, and issuing items.

6 TIMETABLE FOR FIELD ACTIVITIES

An organizational timetable should be constructed which shows all of the field activities and indicates when each will be under-

TIMETABLE OF ACTIVITIES

Activity	J('89)	A	S	O	N	D	J('90)	F	M	A	M	J	J	A	S	O	N	D	J('91)	F	M	A	M	J	J	A	S	O	N	D	J('92)	F	M
Design of survey instruments	●	●	●																														
Pilot study			●																														
Building works			●	●	●																												
Delivery/installation of equipment				●	●	●																											
Finalizing methods and data-processing systems				●	●	●																											
Recruitment of field staff						●																											
Mapping and enumeration							●																										
Zone A Baseline							●	●																									
Dosing cycles									●			●			●		●																
Follow-up											●	●	●	●	●	●	●	●	●	●	●												
Zone B Baseline							●	●																									
Dosing cycles									●			●							●			●											
Follow-up												●	●	●	●	●	●	●	●	●	●	●											
Data entry							●	●	●	●	●	●	●	●	●	●	●	●	●	●	●	●	●	●									
Preliminary analysis																									●	●	●	●					
Detailed analysis																													●	●	●	●	●
Reports to sponsors and Ministry of Health													●													●							●

Fig. 11.1 Example of an organizational timetable for a field trial.

taken. An example of such a timetable, for a trial of the effect of regular vitamin A supplementation on episodes of diarrhoea and respiratory infections, is shown in Fig. 11.1 (B. Kirkwood, personal communication). The dates for fieldwork may have to be fixed some time in advance. The time required for preparations and pilot testing may overlap with training, but all three must be completed before the start of the main fieldwork. Similarly, analysis and consultations should be completed before the final report is produced.

The planning of trial activities must take account of climatic and seasonal factors. These may affect access to the trial area (for example, flooding) and the activities of those in the area such as to make them difficult to survey (for example, seasonal migrations for work, working on farms during the planting or harvesting seasons). It may be important to plan activities to take into account market days, local holidays and festivals, and activities of the local medical services (for example, antenatal clinics). Also, adequate plans must be made to allow for staff leave and sickness absences. The former should fit into local practices if possible (for example, if most people do not work at weekends it may be best to plan the study to fit in with this practice).

Appendix 11.1

A CHECK-LIST FOR PLANNING A FIELD TRIAL

1. Proposed trial

Title
Purpose
Type
Population included: location and numbers involved
Expected duration of trial
Persons in charge: both central and field
Address and phone/fax numbers of trial headquarters

2. Clearances: legal and ethical

Local authority – District health officers
                     – Local government
Police
Government – Ministry of Health
                   – others as appropriate
Local population – informed consent procedures

3. Location

Climate
Geographical features
Maps
Road conditions
River conditions
Airstrips

4. Data collection and storage

Type
Regularity
Timing
Logistics

5. Staff requirements

Functional categories
Number

Existing/new staff
Training

6. Accommodation

Location
Survey team
Support group
Females/males
Tents/housing arrangements
Electricity
Water

7. Supplies

Immediate
Replenishments
Stockpile
Order/indents – logistics
Food/cooking
Water/purification
Petrol
Refrigeration

8. Transportation

Vehicles, bicycles
Boats
Aircraft
Maintenance
Tools
Spares

9. Equipment

Field
Laboratory
Survey equipment
Record forms
Questionnaires
Computer hardware
Computer software
Stationery
Chemicals
Generator

Water-proofing
Other equipment

10. Specimens

Reception
Pick-up schedules
Refrigeration
Containers
Instruction slips
Labelling procedures

11. Special points

Emergencies
Data entry
Back-ups
Communications
Medical care for staff
Medicines and drugs
Records
Photographic equipment
Tape recorders

Appendix 11.2

A CHECK-LIST OF ORGANIZATIONAL ACTIVITIES FOR A
FIELD TRIAL

The activities are listed in the order in which they might be done:

Planning

Develop preliminary study design that includes purpose and estimates of
population size and duration of trial.
Consult with Ministry of Health officials at headquarters and district
levels.
Consult people with the relevant experience in local district government,
community leaders and health workers.
Visit local communities to discuss the trial and learn about the local
situation, their needs and perceptions and how the proposed trial would fit
into their priorities.
Choose an appropriate population sample.
Decide which observations and measurements are needed and standardize
the techniques.
Design and pilot-test record forms and questionnaires.
Make arrangements for staff, training, equipment, transport, finance,
accommodation.

Organization

Obtain co-operation from local leaders.
Develop manual of field operations.
Train survey staff.
Arrange for laboratory procedures.
Draw up a daily work plan for all staff.
Pilot-test all organizational details.

During the fieldwork

Supervise and provide feedback to all staff to ensure a high standard.
Monitor participant compliance and follow-up with local leaders.

Make random checks on staff at the survey centre and interviewers during household visits.

Conduct regular staff seminars for reporting progress, discussion of problems, maintaining morale.

Analysis and communications

Analyse the data as soon as possible, preferably daily, for ongoing operational analysis.

Discuss results and their meaning with health workers and community leaders to obtain their comments.

Write report, incorporating comments, and make recommendations for new or improved health programmes.

Distribute report, discuss recommendations with relevant local committees and organizations and with local media, as appropriate.

Take steps to ensure that appropriate action based on trial outcome, at central and local levels.

Plan to evaluate any changes introduced as a result of the trial and to estimate their effectiveness.

Appendix 11.3

EXTRACT FROM THE MANUAL OF PROCEDURES FOR THE 'SIMPLE EPIDEMIOLOGICAL EVALUATION' FOR ONCHOCERCIASIS SURVEYS CONDUCTED BY THE ONCHOCERCIASIS CONTROL PROGRAMME

(Reproduced with the permission of the Director of the Onchocerciasis Control Programme.)

1 PREPARATION OF THE TRIP

In preparing the plan for a simple evaluation round the team leader should bear the following points in mind:

1.1. Evaluation must be conducted during the dry season. In the rainy season farmers are busy in the fields and only a few people would be available for examination. Moreover, some villages are inaccessible at that time of year.

1.2. To ensure maximum collaboration by the population, village authorities should be apprised of the impending evaluation and if possible of the precise date of the team's arrival.

1.3. The team should arrive in each village during the afternoon of the day preceding the evaluation in order to mobilize the population.

1.4. Even an experienced team cannot examine more than 300 people in a day.

1.5. A pattern of one day's travel alternating with one day of evaluation is ideal unless the evaluation of one or more villages with populations of over 300 is planned.

1.6. Information should be collected on the negotiability of roads and tracks so that travel times can be calculated realistically.

1.7. In case of a follow-up evaluation obtain from the statistical unit the list of all people examined during the baseline survey of all villages included in the travel plan and carry those lists in the field.

2 APPROACH TO THE VILLAGE

2.1. As soon as the team arrives in a village, the Chief and the Secretary of the village should be contacted, together with any other persons of note (for example, teacher or health assistant) who are present. Explain to them the purpose of the evaluation and mention that treatment of all sick people will be given free of charge at the end of each day's work.

2.2. In most villages the key person will be the Secretary, whose responsibility it will be to inform heads of families of the impending examination and arrange for them to be present the following morning with all the members of their families.

2.3. If the village is being evaluated for the first time, collect information on the number of families, their size and duration of their residence in the village from the Secretary, and compile a list of families selected for the examination following the criteria expressed elsewhere. In the case of a follow-up evaluation this information and the list will be available from the previous survey forms.

2.4. Give the list of families to be examined to the Secretary and ask him to contact the head of families included in the list and arrange for them to be present the following day early in the morning (at least by 8.00 a.m.) at the survey site (for the choice of the survey site see paragraph 3.1) with all members of their family.

2.5. If the village is too large for the survey to be completed in one day, make sure that the families convened for the next morning do not total more than 300 individuals, leaving the rest to be examined the day after.

Note: Because of the longitudinal nature of the study (villages are followed for 15 years), it is essential to impress upon the team's census officers, upon the village Chief and Secretary, and upon heads of families the need to examine the entirety of the population selected in each village. If the percentage of non-attendance is too high, the data collected will be meaningless. An additional extra effort should be made to examine all individuals in each village that are included in the list of all people examined during the baseline survey.

3 SET-UP OF THE TEAM FOR AN EVALUATION

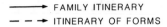

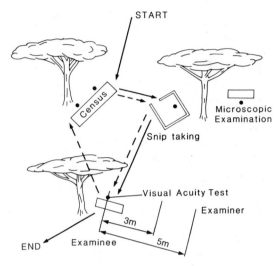

3.1. Use a shady outdoor area or the school building or a combination of both.

3.2. Families will be called one at a time, but some may contain over 100 people so leave sufficient space between the different examination posts.

12
Field laboratory methods

1 INTRODUCTION

Laboratory tests may provide the definitive basis for the measurement of outcome variables in field trials, either directly by demonstration of the presence of the pathogenic agent, or indirectly by demonstration of a host reaction to the pathogen or of biochemical changes due to the pathogen. They may also provide evidence of the action of the intervention, either directly by measuring the drug or metabolic by-products, or indirectly by measuring an immune response to a vaccine. In addition, they may be used to detect, or confirm the presence of adverse reactions.

The organization and operation of a field laboratory for the support of a field trial are different from those of a routine medical laboratory. In field trials the emphasis is often on the collection and processing of large numbers of samples on which only a few specific tests will be performed. Because of the repetitive nature of the collection and processing of the samples, it is essential to include appropriate quality control procedures at all stages.

General aspects of the setting up and running of a field laboratory are discussed in this chapter. For information on specific laboratory tests and specific laboratory methods other literature should be consulted. Useful general texts containing relevant information for the operation of a field laboratory and for collecting specimens include WHO (1980), Cheesbrough (1981) and Brouard *et al.* (1989).

2 SAMPLE COLLECTION

2.1 Types of specimen

The kinds of specimen which are commonly collected in field trials on which laboratory tests may be performed include:

1. Human specimens, including blood, stool, urine, sputum, skin snips and other tissue biopsies, and swabs or smears collected from skin or mucosal surfaces.
2. Entomological specimens for studies of vectors, and animal or malacological specimens for studies of intermediate hosts, related to effects on transmission.

3. Food, water and environmental samples.

This chapter will discuss specimens collected from humans.

2.2 Handling specimens

The collection of samples for laboratory studies will usually involve the following steps:

(1) collection of specimens from the study participants;
(2) placement in a suitable container;
(3) labelling of the container;
(4) temporary store at appropriate temperature;
(5) initial processing (for example, serum separation from whole blood), with appropriate relabelling;
(6) transport to intermediate or final destination for further processing, testing, and storage.

The procedures for collecting and processing samples must be unambiguously specified, including to where they are to be transported and how they will be labelled. All aspects of the collection, transport, and processing of samples must be piloted. Often much attention is paid to the proper design and testing of questionnaires, but much less care is taken to find the most appropriate and culturally acceptable methods for the collection of blood, stool, urine, or tissue samples. This may be crucial to ensure sustained community involvement and participation.

2.3 Blood collection

The usual methods by which blood is collected in field surveys are by venepuncture or by finger or heel pricks. In most, but not all, communities it is easier to persuade individuals to donate a finger-prick sample, and this will be the principal means of blood collection in many trials. This method of collection provides an adequate volume of blood for many laboratory tests. 'Micro-techniques' have been, or are being, developed for many assays, and investigations should be conducted before a study starts to find out the latest availability of such techniques (for example, by contact or correspondence with those in a central or reference laboratory). It is important to verify that the methods have been adequately validated. Some tests require larger quantities of blood, however, and it will often be desirable to collect blood by venepuncture from at least a sample of the population.

After collection, blood can be separated into several components including serum, plasma, red cells, and white cells. The separation must be done shortly after the blood has been collected and it is common for this procedure to be carried out close to where the samples have been collected or in a nearby field laboratory.

A sample of blood taken from a finger-prick may be collected in one of several ways, including:

(1) collection into narrow glass tubes, by capillary action;

(2) dropping onto a glass slide for direct examination of the blood smear; or

(3) dropping onto strips or disks of absorbent paper (filter paper).

A detailed discussion is given in Brouard *et al.* (1989) of the method to use for puncturing the skin and of the relative advantages and disadvantages of collection by capillary tube as compared to absorbent paper.

A specimen of blood obtained from a finger-prick may be sufficient in volume to use for several purposes. For example, when a very small amount of Hemolube® (silicon grease) is applied to the finger tip before pricking, sufficient blood can be obtained to allow the first drop to be wiped off, to obtain drops for 2 thick and 2 thin malaria smears, to do one or two haematocrits ($50\,\mu l$), and to collect $50–100\,\mu l$ blood in a microtube or Microtainer® for serum and to place a drop on filter paper (WHO 1980). After the haematocrits have been read, the tubes can be broken at the interface to the packed cells and both ends sealed with plasticine (plastic modelling clay). (It should be noted, however, that there are safety concerns regarding such procedures – see Section 8.) The tube with the plasma can be stored in a freezer or in liquid nitrogen. The amounts of plasma and serum recovered from finger-prick samples will be sufficient to perform various ELISA-based serological tests and is sufficient for the determination of some micronutrients such as vitamin A or zinc (minimum serum requirements $25–40\,\mu l$).

If repeated blood sampling is to be undertaken during the course of a study it is likely to be easier to maintain the co-operation of most study populations if finger-prick, rather than venous blood, sampling is used. For many purposes, filter paper samples are just as satisfactory as blood samples collected in capillary tubes, and the former are easier to handle, label, and store (Brouard *et al.* 1989). For some assays, however, larger samples are currently needed (for example, tests for cell-mediated immunity or HLA typing) and venous blood sampling will be required.

All blood samples should be considered to be potentially infectious and appropriate handling procedures must be employed to safeguard all those who will come into contact with the specimens during their collection, processing, analysis, or storage (Brouard *et al.* 1989). Special precautions should be taken when collecting blood by finger-prick. If possible disposable gloves should be worn and other safety measures should be employed. At the very least, a bucket containing water and detergent should be available for use by those taking blood.

2.4 Stool and urine collection

A summary of different methods that may be used for collecting urine and stool samples, with details of different container types, is given in WHO (1980). The methods considered for use in a particular survey should be discussed with those knowledgeable of local customs and taboos. In some cultures sensitivity regarding the collection, or public display, of stool specimens may be greater than that for blood. A container which is technically appropriate may not be acceptable in a particular study community (for example, due to colour, transparency, resemblance to cultural motif). In advance of a survey the proposed stool and urine containers should be shown to the village leaders and the proposed methods of sample collection discussed. As with all field procedures, it is important to undertake pilot testing to ensure that the procedures planned will be acceptable (both to the investigator and to the study population).

As stool samples can rarely be collected 'on the spot' it is usually necessary to leave the container with an individual overnight and to arrange to pick up the specimen on the following day. A potential hazard in doing this is that containers may be exchanged between individuals or, for example, one person may provide a sample for the whole family. It is difficult to rule out this possibility completely, but it is important for fieldworkers to stress the importance of participants adhering to the correct procedures and to be on the look out for possible cheating.

2.5 Sputum collection

The WHO (1980) manual gives a concise description of recommended methods of collecting sputum samples using different kinds of jars, boxes, and containers including transport media. Two points merit special attention:

(1) all sputum samples should be considered potentially infectious;
(2) careful attention should be given to the cold-chain requirements if sputum samples have to be sent for culture to another laboratory.

3 LABELLING AND STORAGE

3.1 Labelling

Proper labelling of samples is essential. The labelling scheme should be made as simple as possible, consistent with the study objectives, and must take due account of the size of containers and how the specimens will be handled, transferred, and stored. Self-adhesive, preprinted labels (possibly prepared using a microcomputer), with the individual identification numbers duplicated on data sheets, can speed processing. Also, labels in a variety of materials suitable for differing storage conditions, and with each number duplicated several times, are available commercially (for example, from W. H. Brady & Co Ltd., Daventry Road Industrial Estate, Banbury, Oxfordshire OX16 7JU, UK, or Shamrock Scientific, 34 Davis Drive, Bellwood, Illinois 60104, USA, or Thomas Scientific, 99 High Hill Road, Swedesboro, New Jersey 08085, USA).

The information recorded on a label will vary according to particular requirements. It may include just a single number or code which is utilized during laboratory processing and which may be linked back to an individual by reference to records kept at the time the sample was taken. In some circumstances it will be appropriate to include on the label a record of the date of collection, the type of specimen, if not evident, and possibly the name of the village. Individual names may also be recorded but this can create problems with blinding and confidentiality, and often names are not a unique identifier as several individuals may have the same name.

Containers should usually be labelled using water-proof marker pens (but see note 1, below), writing directly onto the container labelling area or onto adhesive labels attached to the container. If the container has a cap, the marking should be on the body of the container (and possibly on the cap as well, but never on the cap only).

A 'flag' can be attached to *capillary tubes*, made from an adhesive strip, for the identification information, written with a waterproof marker pen, or tubes may be stored in labelled envelopes as they are collected in the field. Alternatively, capillary tubes which are 75 mm long will fit into an ordinary microscope slide box. The tubes can be put into a numbered sequence according to subject, and multiple tubes may be taken from a subject and stored together. The box facilitates transport and obviates the need for flags, which are awkward and may have to be removed before spinning. Staff need to be careful, however, to record and maintain the correct numbering and not invert or tip the box. Packing with cotton wool will keep the tubes in place.

Filter paper can be written on directly.

It is not possible to recommend a single standardized form of labelling for different sample containers that will be appropriate in all circumstances. It will be necessary in a particular study to establish a method that guarantees the reliability of the labelling from the time the sample is first collected, through transportation, processing, analysis, and storage. Useful advice on these aspects is given in Brouard *et al.* (1989). Using sets of labels with series of identical numbers on them, for coding samples and associated record forms, reduces the chances of labelling errors.

A few warnings are appropriate.

1. If the transport cold chain includes a stage where samples are frozen in salt-alcohol mixtures, *never* use felt pens (even water-proof ones). Always use plain pencils.

2. Numbers and letters must be written in a clear and standard-ized form (for example, 191 looks the same as 161 upside-down!). Advice on some of these aspects is given in Chapter 13, Section 4.2.

3. The methods to be used for collection, storage, and transport of specimens should be pilot tested. This testing should include evaluation of how labels stick under the varying conditions (for example, freezing), how pen and pencil writing is conserved from the field collection to the final place of analysis and storage, and where there is the possibility of transcription errors. Labelling of specimens with commercially available self-adhesive labels should be undertaken with care. They often curl off plastic tubes and sometimes inscriptions on them rub off with frequent handling or wetness, even if waterproof markers have been used. Some workers have found that fixing transparent adhesive tape around the labels helps to overcome these problems, in the absence of better labels. Special containers and labels are required if samples are to be stored in liquid nitrogen.

Quality control procedures in the laboratory are likely to require that some samples are stored and coded in replicate, both for checking analysis and handling procedures and for establishing the variability of tests (see Section 6). Procedures for dividing and labelling such samples should be devised and laid down in the field procedures.

3.2 Storage

The storage area of a field laboratory should be designed to be adequate for a particular study (or studies). This will require estimation of the rate at which samples will be collected and processed and for how long they must be stored before being transported on to another location (for example, for processing or storage in the base laboratory). Serum and plasma samples should be frozen as soon as possible after separation, and storage in a field laboratory at $-20°C$ is adequate for most purposes, at least for several weeks. For only a few tests is immediate storage at less than $-70°C$ required.

Stool, urine, and tissue samples may be stored under various conditions using appropriate fixatives and stabilizers; different possibilities are summarized in WHO (1980).

3.3 Aliquoting

Biological samples are easily damaged by repeated freezing and thawing. This can be avoided if samples are divided into small portions before freezing. Ideally, the size of aliquots should be chosen so that there is just sufficient material in each aliquot to perform the tests required at a particular time. This is not always possible and, in practice, compromise procedures may have to be adopted (for example, on grounds of cost). It is important that the laboratory recording procedures are such that the histories of each aliquot are adequately documented (especially recording how many times each one has been thawed and re-frozen) so that any recipient of the samples can be given detailed information about their preparation (for example, whether volumes are precisely measured or are approximate).

3.4 Storage system

When large numbers of samples are collected and stored, a storage and record system must be devised that allows the rapid retrieval of particular samples. If this is not done, sorting through large numbers of samples can be a very time-consuming activity. The particular storage system used should be tailored to the design of the specific study. In general, it is appropriate to store samples in batches according to the date they were collected or frozen, with a careful record being kept of the contents of each batch. This information can be recorded on a microcomputer so that, if necessary, a computer search can be made to find the location (batch) of a particular specimen.

4 DOCUMENTATION OF LABORATORY PROCEDURES

There should be clear and explicit documentation of all laboratory procedures to ensure reproducibility and to enable appropriate comparisons to be made with results from other laboratories. Records should be made of equipment maintenance, the batches of supplies and reagents used at different times, the detailed test procedures and the duties and responsibilities of staff members. Records should also be made of unusual events that may affect the results of a test (for example, power failures—though in some circumstances these may not be 'unusual').

Depending on the size of the laboratory and the variety of tests and procedures undertaken, the documentation should be arranged in a single, or several, log-books that are arranged chronologically.

4.1 Supplies

The laboratory log-book should provide information on: the reagents, test kits, laboratory equipment (including brand names), the shelf-life of reagents, storage conditions, batch or lot numbers, and the relevant re-ordering arrangements (for example, when, how much, by and through whom).

4.2 Equipment maintenance

Regular checks should be made on each piece of equipment to ensure that it is in good working order. Such checks should be recorded and, for some items, publicly displayed. Among items that should be checked regularly are:

(1) daily (morning and evening) recording of temperatures of refrigerators, freezers, and cool-rooms, using maxima and minima thermometers;

(2) checking on the position of the cap and the level of nitrogen in liquid nitrogen containers;

(3) regular and systematic inspection of all items of equipment which require clean lenses (for example, microscopes) and checks on focus and adjustment of light sources;

(4) periodic checks on the position of centrifuge rotors (tight centre bolts) and regular cleaning;

(5) regular zero-line/level calibration of balances and cleaning of balance pans;

(6) checking the filters and calibration of spectrometers and varipipettes.

In moist areas of the tropics fungus may grow on glass lenses and damage microscopes and similar equipment. In these circumstances it may be worth storing microscopes, cameras, and similar equipment in a 'light-box' (a box containing, and heated by, a low-wattage electric light bulb) to prevent condensation, or with silica-gel (as a dessicant) in air-tight boxes for lenses.

Maintenance procedures are usually described in the instruction booklets for the relevant equipment, but these are often inadequate. Complete maintenance instructions for each piece of equipment should be incorporated into a manual and a log-book with check-lists kept for each piece of equipment. The supervisor should review these log-books regularly with the appropriate members of the laboratory team.

4.3 Procedures and staff duties

Every laboratory procedure should have detailed, step-by-step, instructions described in a manual (i.e. what to do with specimens from their receipt in the laboratory to the storage of specimens and the communication of the results). Each step should be clearly detailed and the responsibility of each staff member indicated. In addition, staff members need to know to whom they should report and how they should record results, additional observations, mistakes, and other unusual events. These include any change of: kit or batch number of sera, media, preservatives, and so on; working arrangements, such as a new brand of glassware, changes in incubation time or temperature; and coding procedures for samples and results. Staff members involved in distinct sequences of the procedures should be indicated on relevant flow charts and these should be written into the log-book(s).

4.4 Unusual events

The log-book(s) should be used to keep a record of errors in test procedures, and in the preparation of reagents, power failures, temperature and humidity changes that might influence the results of the tests or the quality of stored samples.

5 QUALITY CONTROL

Quality control is an inherent component of a good study. A comprehensive work plan will facilitate the systematic implementation of quality control mechanisms. Appropriate references on quality control include Braun-Munzinger (1989), Goddard (1980), Russell (1974), and Tonks (1972).

5.1 Reproducibility of test results

The reliability of data should be tested by regular checks on its reproducibility. There is no general rule for an acceptable level. This will depend on the test involved and on the test conditions, and information on these aspects should be sought in manuals or papers in which test procedures are described.

In addition to ensuring that all procedures are carried out in accordance with the instructions as detailed in the manuals, that all equipment is in good working order, and that materials are properly stored and kept up-to-date, the basis of the approach to internal quality control is through checking on the reproducibility of test results. Many test systems have inbuilt controls using standardized reagents for this purpose of known concentration or quantity. The use of such standard controls is necessary but not sufficient to monitor the quality of test procedures. Whenever possible, coded duplicate samples should be tested. The frequency with which such duplicates are included depends upon how smoothly the laboratory is running and how long it has been doing the test. Typically, when a test is first introduced, a high frequency of such checking may be appropriate, with a decreased frequency as the procedures become more familiar. In many circumstances it will be appropriate to ensure that duplicate analyses are done on between 5 and 10 per cent of samples on a routine basis.

Reproducibility should be checked within batches, between batches and from day-to-day or week-to-week by the use of appropriate controls. Intra-observer variation can be determined by having duplicate samples processed by the same observer at different times, and inter-observer variations measured by having the same samples processed independently by two different staff members. Inter-product variation is tested by comparing new batches of staining solutions, media, reagents, and so on with the old on a group of the same samples.

5.2 Internal quality control

Two types of quality control can be distinguished, 'internal' and 'external'. Internal quality control comprises procedures that are introduced within the field laboratory. External quality control involves external monitoring, such as the duplicate testing of samples in another laboratory to serve as a 'gold standard'.

The essence of internal quality lies in a tight circle of checks, reporting, evaluation, and action. It is essential to have detailed manuals of every procedure, with a check-list to be consulted each time the procedure is run. Well-kept records with regular review by the supervisors are key elements in quality control. Quality control procedures must be an integral part of the work-plan for the study.

5.3 External quality control

A major reason for having specimens sent to external laboratories is to check the accuracy of test results. Reproducibility can be assessed adequately by internal quality control procedures, but checks on accuracy are best done, for many tests, in collaboration with other laboratories. The results from a laboratory may be highly reproducible within that laboratory, but might be consistently incorrect. Arrangements with other laboratories should be organized well in advance and should be included in the work plan. The actual checking procedures involved are similar to those for internal reproducibility checks as outlined above.

Samples that are sent should be accompanied by an investigation request form and every effort should be made to ensure that transport conditions are appropriate and the same for all samples (for example, route, packing conditions, type of container). The field laboratory may make arrangements with the main laboratory to have samples sent to an external laboratory, rather than sending them direct, but these samples should have been tested by the field laboratory within its routine programme. At the beginning of a field study and during training phases this part of quality control activities should be strengthened.

6 LINKS WITH OTHER LABORATORIES

A field laboratory may be set up specifically for the conduct of a particular study and may have no regular links with other laboratories. Often, however, there will be a link to another laboratory in the home-based institution at which some of the laboratory tests may be checked or performed. There should be a clear specification in the study protocol of which procedures and checks will be performed at which laboratory, of how arrangements will be made for transport of specimens and supplies between them, and how and which records will be interchanged. Links with an external reference laboratory may be desirable for independent checks and quality control procedures or for the conduct of new or specialized tests.

If samples are to be sent to other laboratories for further storage, processing, or analysis (for example, blood, sera, slides), it may be important to give attention to the suggestions listed below:

1. It is unwise to send all samples to another laboratory at the same time. Duplicates should be kept, even when storage facilities are limited, to guard against loss during shipment.

2. Samples should not be sent to another laboratory without a clear agreement as to what analyses will be done and how these will be reported back. It is essential to know *who does what, with what, and when* ('the rule of the 5W's'). This point is very important. A laboratory may be tempted to do more tests on samples than are requested (for example, to try out a new test on a variety of samples), but it must be made clear that this should only be done if there is prior agreement for this. No tests should be performed other than those previously agreed. It is always a very sound policy to send samples to another laboratory in such a way that they are analysed 'blind' (for example, no details are sent of which intervention group the samples are from or of the age and sex of the individual subjects). Agreement with respect to publication procedures should also be made before specimens are sent.

The arrangements agreed between the field and other laboratories should be part of the study protocol, in which the division of responsibilities should be specified. All parties must also adhere to the provisions of the agreement to undertake the study (for example, local research clearance, ethical clearance).

7 CODING AND LINKAGE OF RESULTS

The coding of specimens is discussed in Chapter 7. In order to remove the possibility of bias, those in the laboratory should not know which intervention group any sample is from, and it should not be possible for this to be deduced from the labelling system employed. Specimens must be labelled in such a way, however, that each is identified uniquely and any test results can be linked back later to records of the individual from whom the specimen was taken. While this seems to be stating the obvious, the problems that arise with these aspects in large studies are often substantial. Special care is necessary in longitudinal studies where individuals may be followed for many years, in studies involving many different research groups or laboratories, and in studies where results need to be linked with census information that may be updated over time (for example, individuals may move house and this may cause problems if the coding system for individuals is too closely linked to a house code).

Laboratory results will usually be recorded in laboratory books or on specially prepared forms to facilitate computer entry. For such recording it will be important to develop result codes that identify particular problems or features. For example, codes might be developed to indicate lost and broken samples, technical problems with batches of samples (for example, staining, storage, transport), and the identification of the technicians involved with each test (to check variations between observers).

If the study uses laboratory numbers in addition to individual identification numbers (as is often the case), both numbers should be entered on a computer form for data entry so that cross-checks can be made in the computer.

If multiple laboratory tests are being performed on samples from the trial population, it may be best to wait until all the results have been assembled and collated before entering them into the computer so that the checking and linkage back to other data on each individual can be done in relatively few steps. This will depend on how the computing system is organized, but repeated processing of many small sets of data is liable to lead to confusion and may be unnecessarily time-consuming.

8 LABORATORY SAFETY

Detailed attention to safety aspects is as important in a field laboratory as in any kind of laboratory. Indeed, this is of special importance in field laboratories as there may be much greater accessibility by the public than is usual in a laboratory. It is important to ensure that proper procedures are documented and implemented for activities such as the disposal of needles, blood, stool, urine, and sputum samples, and of used reagents, chemicals, and detergents. Special attention should be paid to precautions concerning the transmission of blood-borne infections such as hepatitis B and HIV (WHO 1988).

Shattering of packed cell volume (PCV) tubes in a microhaematocrit centrifuge is likely to carry special hazards and, if possible, the centrifuge should be put in a hood. Also, cutting PCV tubes with a diamond to obtain serum is very hazardous and should be discouraged.

Laboratory safety guidelines are given in WHO (1980). Safety procedures should be reviewed regularly by laboratory supervisors and all staff concerned.

REFERENCES

Braun-Munzinger, R. A. (1989). Quality control in schistosomiasis programmes. *Tropical Medicine and Parasitology*, **40**, 214–9.

Brouard, Y. J., Blackwell, J. M., and Fine, P. E. M. (1989). *Blood collection, fractionation and storage methods: a practical manual for immuno-epidemiological studies with emphasis on work in developing countries*. Ross Institute Bulletin No. 15, London School of Hygiene and Tropical Medicine, London.

Cheesbrough, M. (1981). *Medical laboratory manual for tropical countries*. Austin & Sons Ltd, Hertford, England.

Goddard, M. J. (1980). A statistical procedure for quality control in diagnostic laboratories. *Bulletin of the World Health Organization*, **58**, 313–20.

Russell, R. L. (1974). Quality control in the microbiological laboratory. In *Manual of clinical microbiology* (2nd ed), (ed. Lenette, E. H., Spauling, E. H., and Truant, J. P.) pp. 862–70. American Society for Microbiology, Washington.

Tonks, D. B. (1972). *Quality control in clinical laboratories*. Warner-Chilcott, Scarborough, Ontario.

World Health Organization (1980). *Manual of basic techniques for a health laboratory*. WHO, Geneva.

World Health Organization (1988). *Guidelines on sterilization and high-level disinfection methods effective against human immunodeficiency virus* (HIV). WHO AIDS Series 2, Geneva.

13
Data processing

1 Introduction

2 Computing requirements
   2.1 Software
   2.2 Computers
   2.3 Printers and storage devices
   2.4 Uninterruptible power supply
   2.5 Air conditioners
   2.6 Staff

3 Planning the data-processing system
   3.1 List of data sources
   3.2 Data flow
   3.3 Form preparation
   3.4 Computer files

4 Data recording in the field
   4.1 Quality control
   4.2 Practical aspects of recording
   4.3 Computer recording devices

5 Coding
   5.1 During and after data collection
   5.2 Grouping of responses
   5.3 Common errors

6. Data entry
   6.1 When and where to do
   6.2 Entry and verification
   6.3 Data cleaning
   6.4 Updating and storage

7 Preparing data for analysis
   7.1 Recoding variables
   7.2 Computing new variables
   7.3 Combining data from several files

1 INTRODUCTION

All field trials involve the collection of data on the study population, on the effects of the interventions and on factors that may affect the impact of the interventions. For small trials it may be sufficient to record these data in a notebook or on cards and analysis may consist of a simple hand-tabulation of the recorded information. For most field trials, however, more information is likely to be collected than can be processed easily in this way. Although it is advisable to undertake 'hand' analyses while a trial is in progress to monitor that it is being conducted satisfactorily, the main analyses for the trial will involve summarizing large quantities of data using a computer.

Data processing is the conversion of field notes, questionnaires and laboratory forms into data in computer files which are ready for statistical analysis. It involves setting up appropriate data collection systems as well as coding, entering, cleaning and editing the data.

Over the last two decades tremendous advances have taken place in computer technology. In the late 1970s and early 1980s most computing was done on 'main-frame' computers. These were large and expensive machines, located in universities or research centres, that required considerable maintenance and expertise to use. The development of microcomputers has revolutionized this situation, and now powerful and small machines can be purchased from about a thousand dollars that have the data processing capacity to meet the requirements of virtually all field trials. Machines that run off the normal electricity supply (mains-powered) can be installed wherever there is a source of such power in a relatively cool and dust-free environment (for example, an air-conditioned room). Alternatively, battery-powered portable computers (lap-top computers) will work for several hours before recharging from a mains source is necessary (and some will work off car batteries). Furthermore, computer programs (software) have been developed that are simple to use so that only minimal training is required before a research worker can begin to process and analyse data.

In the computer processing of data it is important to remember the 'GIGO' principle, that is 'garbage in, garbage out'! The information that comes out of a computer is only as good as the information that goes in. Thus, while computer developments have made the processing and analysis of data much easier, it is still necessary to pay careful attention to the way in which the original data are collected and recorded in the field and transferred to the computer. Not only must the survey instruments (questionnaires, laboratory methods, and so on) be properly validated and quality control procedures maintained throughout a trial, but care must also be taken in the design of data forms, with the recording of the data and with its transfer into a computer. These data processing aspects are the focus of this chapter.

The choice of hardware and software for use in a trial, and staffing requirements, are discussed in Section 2. The planning of the data processing, from the field collection of data to computer entry, is covered in Section 3. Methods of recording data in the field and of coding are considered in Sections 4 and 5, respectively, and in Section 6 the entry of data from field forms into a computer and the checking and correcting ('cleaning') of these data are examined. Finally, in Section 8, advice is given on how data should be prepared for analysis.

2 COMPUTING REQUIREMENTS

Microcomputers are now relatively inexpensive and will be used for data handling in most field trials, whether these involve a few hundred subjects or tens of thousands. The range of machines and software available changes so rapidly that recommendations on which to choose are soon outdated. Some general principles that should govern choice will be outlined, however, and more specific recommendations made which, though relevant in 1996, may be outdated in a few years. The choice will be much influenced by the skills available to the project for data processing and statistical data analysis. Particularly for field trials in developing countries, it is safer to be 'conservative' and to go for 'tried and tested' products, especially in situations where technical back-up may not be readily available.

2.1 Software

For most field studies, word-processing software (such as Word Perfect or Word), a good database package, a spread-sheet and a statistical package are the minimum requirements. FoxPro, dBase or Access are good choices for the database. SPSS/PC+, SAS/PC or BMDP-PC are suitable for most statistical work; the first is more widely used and has advantages for this reason. For fitting statistical models and for statistical inference, a user-friendly package is EGRET. If the project team includes a statistician, STATA, S+ or GLIM are likely to be useful. Sometimes it may be necessary to transfer data between one software package and another. If there is not a facility within the packages to import data from other programs, a file translation program, such as BMS Copy, may be required.

A useful general purpose package (called Epi Info – Version 6) for word processing, questionnaire design, data entry and validation, and simple tabulations and statistical analysis has been developed by workers at the Centers for Disease Control and Prevention in the United States in collaboration with the Global Programme on AIDS at the World Health Organization in Geneva. Attractive features of this package are that it is designed specifically for epidemiological studies, its comprehensive facilities enable problems of transferring between different software packages to be avoided and it is distributed free of charge (apart from a small charge for postage and materials). Details can be obtained from USD Incorporated (2075A West Park Place, Stone Mountain, GA 30087, USA, telephone +1 404 469 4098). The software may also be freely copied to or from others. Epi Info is particularly useful for small and medium-sized studies. For those involving many thousands of individuals or complex data structures, a package with more sophisticated data management capabilities, such as FoxPro, may be required. Further software may be chosen on the basis of what members of the project team are familiar with using, and after receiving specialist advice with respect to particular applications.

Until recently, most IBM-type microcomputers used the 'DOS' operating system, which allows one program to be run at a time. With the advent of more powerful machines, the 'Windows' operating system has become much more commonly used. This has several significant advantages. Several programs may be kept active at the same time and it is much easier to move data, text and figures between one program and another. Also, the mouse-based system is easier to use and does not require command instructions to be remembered. As Windows becomes more widely available, updated and improved versions of software are being developed for use with the Windows system only and, thus, DOS-based software is likely to become increasingly outdated.

There is frequently a need to transfer data between computers and an efficient way of doing this is via a cable link, which goes between the serial or parallel ports of the two machines (note that transfer between parallel ports is significantly faster, but requires a special cable). Software will be needed to drive the transfer of data, such as LapLink. Data can be transferred more quickly this way than via a floppy disk. Also, floppy disk drives sometimes fail (especially in dusty environments) and in such circumstances, a cable link may be the only way of getting data out of the damaged machine, short of replacing the defective drive.

Computer viruses can cause havoc once they get into a data processing facility. Stringent precautions should be taken to prevent machines becoming contaminated by such viruses and to detect such contamination if a virus slips through. A virus checking software package, resident in the memory of each computer, facilitates routine checking for the introduction of viruses. Any floppy disks that are brought by visitors, or which are brought in from outside the project, should be scanned for viruses before being read into the computer. New viruses continue to be developed and the software package purchased should be one for which the user is automatically provided with periodic updates, so that the virus software on each machine can be kept up-to-date. The package should also be one that enables viruses to be 'cleaned' from the computer once they have been detected.

2.2 Computers

At the present time (1996) the machines in most common use are those based on the 486 and Pentium microprocessors ('chips'), using the MS DOS or Windows operating systems. Such machines are produced by many different manufacturers and the price ranges, for computers with the same basic specifications, are considerable. It is important that computers are completely IBM-compatible, so that it will be straightforward to use software that has been developed for the IBM specification. Microcomputers come in a range of capacities as regards processing speed and data storage, and it is advisable to purchase machines which are larger than initially thought necessary to allow for errors in the estimate of the capacity required (which occurs commonly!). The marginal increase in cost for such increases in capacity is relatively small. In general, the 'hard disk' (or 'hard drive') capacity should be at least 500 megabytes (Mb), especially if Windows-based software is to be used, as these programs tend to be large (for example, SAS/Windows requires 50Mb). Hard disks speed up the processing of data in the computer and, in addition, are better sealed against dust than are floppy disks. At least 4Mb of random access memory (RAM) is standard on most new machines, but if Windows is to be used, at least 8Mb is desirable.

If possible, professional advice, from a statistician or a systems analyst, should be sought regarding the computing capacity required (for example, the number and type of computers, printers, data storage back-up devices, the size of hard disks). An important determinant of the make of computer bought should be the availability of good local servicing and repair facilities (or good access to remote servicing facilities). It is worth making enquiries in the locality where the machines will be based regarding other groups using microcomputers. Such groups may have expertise that can be called upon if there are computing problems during the course of the project. They can also advise on the experience they have had with reliability and servicing of their machines. It is always better to base the choice of machines on the performance and servicing as experienced by local users, than on that promised by a computer salesperson! The cheapest machines may not be the best choice.

Although the reliability of microcomputers has increased greatly since their first introduction, they are still far from being totally dependable and it must be anticipated that they will sometimes break down. In such circumstances, it may take days, weeks or months to have them repaired, depending on the availability of spare parts and of appropriate technical help. It may be catastrophic for the processing of data from a field study to be delayed for this long, and it is important, therefore, that such events are anticipated in the study plan. Some duplication of equipment is essential. It is dangerous to rely on one computer and a strong case can be made for having at least two identical machines capable of all the data-processing tasks. Similar considerations apply to other essential computing equipment (for example, uninterruptible power supplies, printers, air-conditioners).

A common cause of hardware problems in tropical environments is dust. Regular cleaning of disk drives, using kits that can be bought specifically for this purpose, and regular internal cleaning of computers, can reduce the risk of such damage. If a hardware problem does arise, it is worth removing the back of the computer and cleaning the machine before assuming the problem is more serious and sending it away for repair.

Linking computers together in 'networks' is becoming increasingly common. It enables several machines to share the same software and printers, and different users can have simultaneous access to the same data set. A disadvantage is that if the network 'goes down', all those connected to it may be prevented from working until the fault is repaired. This problem is avoided if each user has a 'stand-alone' machine or has the facility to use their machine as a stand-alone machine in the event of network failure. Whether or not networking will make a significant difference to data processing will depend on the nature of the research project. It is likely to be most useful when several users require access to the same large data set at the same time—such as might be required when several data entry clerks are trying to update data on individuals in a trial, as a result of the follow-up of a trial population.

2.3 Printers and storage devices

Printers are subject to heavy mechanical wear and are thus subject to breakdown. For most purposes, dot-matrix printers are sufficient and the 24-pin printers give high quality output. Ink-jet printers generally give good quality output, but tend to be slower. The highest quality of output is obtained from laser printers, which are more costly than other printers and have relatively high running costs. Dot-matrix printers tend to be the most robust and are probably most appropriate in remote situations, far from servicing facilities, but laser and ink-jet printers now have good reliability and may be preferred because of the better output they give.

Similar considerations apply to the choice of printers as for computers regarding choosing 'tried and tested' models for which local servicing facilities are available. An important consideration is also the local availability of replacement ribbons, ink and paper. More printers than are immediately needed should be purchased to provide back-up for equipment failure. This may be crucial if the printers are required to print survey forms for the conduct of a study. It is generally advisable to purchase printers that have both 'sheet-feed' and 'tractor-feed' facilities and at least one (and preferably two) printers with a wide carriage should be purchased if forms for a study are to be printed in landscape rather than portrait mode. Printer switch boxes are relatively cheap and allow several users to share the same printer.

Professional advice should be sought on what kinds of data storage devices are required, as rapid advances are taking place in this area. Floppy disks may be sufficient for the storage of data from small studies, but hard drives are now the norm. A hard-disk will hold hundreds of millions of items of information in the computer for quick access. Interchangeable hard-disk units (such as 'Bernoulli-boxes') may be needed for very large data sets.

Data stored on hard disks may be 'lost' and regular back-up of the information on the disk is essential, on a daily or weekly basis. All the information in the computer should be copied onto some other storage device to guard against losing information in the event of hard disk or computer failure. This may be done using floppy disks, but for large amounts of data, this method of back-up will be slow and it is better to use a 'tape-streamer', which enables the data in the computer to be copied rapidly onto a small magnetic tape. Floppy disks are also more prone to damage from dust or heat. These aspects are discussed further in Section 6.4.

Some equipment may be difficult to service in developing countries (for example, Bernoulli-boxes and tape-streamers) and this should be taken into account in designing the computer system for a trial.

2.4 Uninterruptible power supply

In many developing countries the power supply is subject to considerable voltage fluctuation and interruption. The former may cause extensive damage to computing equipment and the latter may result in the loss of information that has been entered into the computer. It is vital, therefore, to take adequate precautions against an unreliable power supply. Generally, voltage stabilizers, surge protectors, line filters and similar devices offer little protection against the poor quality of power found in some developing countries, and no protection against loss of data in the event of power failure. Uninterruptible power supplies (UPS) are designed to connect between the power supply and the computing equipment and to isolate hardware from irregularities in the mains supply. They consist of a three-function unit: a mains-powered battery charger, a battery and a battery-powered inverter that generates power at mains voltage and frequency. Thus, the computer runs off the inverter output, which will be stable. Also, if the incoming mains supply fails, the inverter will continue to supply power until the battery discharges, say for 30 minutes or more depending on load and specification. This should be sufficient time to finish ongoing tasks and to shut down the computer in an orderly fashion with no loss of information. If there are concerns about possible failures of the power supply, a UPS is essential (and, for the reasons, outlined above, at least two are desirable as they are also not failure-free). Their cost is comparable with that of a simple micro-computer. It is important to use a UPS that has sufficient power output (expressed in volt-amps or watts) for its intended load of computers, monitors and printers. Several computers may be run off a single UPS if it is sufficiently powerful. If the power supply is reliable (for example, from a small generator whose fuel supply is maintained), but the voltage fluctuates, a voltage stabilizer may offer sufficient protection.

Some UPS devices are designed to cope with voltage surges which are smaller than those commonly experienced in some developing countries. It is worthwhile to enquire whether there is a locally manu-factured UPS available, which will have been designed to deal with the local power supply and will also be easier to have repaired in the event of failure or damage. A 'belt and braces' approach, which has been found necessary in some situations, is to have a voltage stabilizer in the power supply to the UPS, but there is, of course, a correspond-ing increase in the cost for such precautions.

Portable microcomputers operate off rechargeable batteries and are thus relatively protected from power fluctuations and failures. However, power surges can damage the adapter that charges the com-puter battery from the mains power supply. It is safest to charge up the computer battery and to run the computer disconnected from the mains power supply until it becomes necessary to recharge the battery again. This also prolongs the useful life of the battery as rechargeable batteries last longer if they are fully discharged before being recharged. The cost of portable computers is slightly greater than that of desk-top machines but some of them have equivalent computing capacity (for example, 200 Mb hard-disk built in) and they avoid the need for a UPS, which may cost as much as an extra portable machine. Their portability does make them more susceptible to theft, however, and the screens on some of them are more tiring to look at for long periods than those on desk-top machines, though most port-ables can be connected to full-screen monitors.

Unless suitable protection has been installed, such as lightning-strike interrupters, it is advisable to disconnect computers and similar equipment from the power supply during storms and, for similar reasons, to disconnect the machines when they are not in use.

2.5 Air conditioners

It is advisable to set up desk-top microcomputers in an air-conditioned room to ensure that they do not overheat (which they may do if the day-time temperature exceeds 25°C), that they are in a relatively dust-free environment and that the humidity is controlled (less than 80 per cent humidity is desirable). Modern computers can be used in normal ambient conditions, at least for short periods, but they should be well protected from moisture and dust. Portable computers are fairly robust and, in general, do not need an air-conditioned environment.

2.6 Staff

Staff must be recruited and trained to enter data into the computers and to manipulate the data in the computers using software packages. The most important attributes are conscientiousness, reliability and attention to detail. It may be necessary to train data entry clerks who have had no previous experience of such work. Sometimes, field workers can be trained to be good data entry clerks. This has the advantage that they will be familiar with the kind of data being collected and the forms that are being used. They will also be aware of the problems that may arise in the collection of data in the field. The intellectual demands of the job are not great. Simple typing skills must be acquired, or recruitment might be targeted at those with such skills. Careful supervision will be necessary, especially during the initial work period.

If large quantities of data are to be handled, a data processing manager should be recruited, with previous experience of the kind of work to be undertaken. He or she must work in close co-operation with the project statistician or statistical advisor in the design of the data processing system, and must also liaise closely with field supervisors regarding the way in which data and queries will be transmitted to and from the computing facilities. It is an added advantage if the data processing manager can also undertake some computer fault-finding and is able to identify and replace faulty components. In case the data manager is sick, or moves away for any reason, a deputy should be trained to be familiar with the data management system and to be able to take over in an emergency, at least for short periods.

A supervisor may be required for every four to six data entry clerks, to control the quality of their work, to ensure a proper and equitable distribution and flow of work and to ensure that all data and forms are correctly processed and stored. A good way to identify persons who might be trained as supervisors may be to select them from among the data entry clerks, based on their performance and aptitude for this work, although the ability to type data quickly and reliably does not necessarily provide a good indication that an individual will make a good supervisor. This will depend to some extent on the level of education of those performing these tasks.

Pilot studies may be necessary to determine how much data can be processed by a clerk in a day, to know how many such individuals to budget for in the study plan. As the work is repetitive, not intellectually demanding but requiring considerable care, it is advisable to plan that any clerk should not be entering data for more than five or six hours a day. Data entry may be interspersed with filing tasks to maintain variety in the work.

If a project is large, substantial numbers of forms may accumulate quickly and the design of an appropriate filing system (such that individual forms can be retrieved if needed) is important. The employment of filing clerks will also be necessary.

Data entry and filing are inherently boring tasks and it is important to devise ways of maintaining staff morale so as to ensure high quality work. Working out career development structures within the project may be important (for example, the progression from filing clerk or field worker to data entry clerk to supervisor). Also training in new techniques and the use of computer packages may be appropriate. Individuals must be aware that their work is considered important, that its quality is monitored and that bad work is detected and that good work is noticed and rewarded (see also Section 4.1).

The data processing staff must be made to feel that they are an integral part of the project. Appropriate measures should be installed to allow field and data processing staff to liaise with each other so that they consider themselves part of the same team. Field staff must understand the problems that errors in data collection cause in the processing and analysis of data, and data processing staff must appreciate the obstacles to high quality data collection in the field. Visits by computing staff to the field can do much to aid such mutual understanding, as can field staff spending periods working in the data processing office.

3 PLANNING THE DATA PROCESSING SYSTEM

The data processing system for a field study must be planned, in detail, at the study design stage, well *before* the data collection process starts, so that the budget for the study makes adequate provision for the required hardware and software. Deficiencies found in the middle of a study may have serious consequences for the conduct or analysis of the study. It is not an uncommon experience for a data processing facility to become swamped by record forms from the field because inadequate consideration was given to the quantities of data accumulating and to the speed with which they must be entered into the computer. In surveys which involve multiple visits to the same subjects, an effective use of computers is to prepare the field forms for the next survey round or to produce labels that may be affixed to survey forms giving identification information on the person to be examined. The build-up of a back-log of survey forms for data processing in these circumstances could have serious repercussions on field-work activities. Examples of the use of a microcomputer to manage the follow-up and related activities in a field trial are given in Byass *et al.* (1988), Rowan *et al.* (1987) and Stephens *et al.* (1989).

3.1 List of data sources

A list should be made of all the data sources that will require processing, such as questionnaires, laboratory forms and field observation records. For each, the size of the data record, the number of persons, specimens or other units of observation and the frequency of application (for example, once, weekly, yearly) must be determined. Many kinds of data forms may be generated in a large study. For example, initially a census may be conducted, collecting information on the names, ages and sexes of the members of each household. A household survey form may record items about each household (for example, water and sanitation facilities, house construction methods, cash crops grown). Baseline data may be collected on children who are to be the focus of an intervention. Assessment may include the recording weekly of information on weight and diarrhoea incidence, whereas length and feeding practices may be assessed monthly. Some members of the population may be specially monitored and information on behaviour recorded. A detailed evaluation of all subjects in the study may be conducted at the end. Thus, many different data collection forms will have been generated, and unless these are carefully designed, and appropriate numbering and computer filing systems are set up at the start of the study, subsequent data processing may be, at best, inefficient and, at worst, chaotic.

In many studies, information is collected relating to different hierarchical levels. Information may be collected on whole villages (for example, population, distance to hospital), on houses (type of building, water supply), on families (type of family, occupation of the head), on individuals (age, sex, schooling) and on disease episodes (duration, signs, management). Adequate systems of numbering and recording of the units at each level must be devised and systems to link the information in appropriate ways must be designed (for example, houses within villages, families within houses, individuals within houses, episodes of sickness within individuals).

3.2 Data flow

Plans should be drawn up for the flow of data from the time they are collected to when they are entered into computer files. The plans should include provision for supervision, coding, transport of completed forms, error checking, recording of throughput, and routine tallying and tabulation. Each separate data recording form should be described in the plan.

Data should be entered into a computer as soon as possible after they have been collected and the number of times information is copied manually from one form to another should be minimal (preferably never!). As far as possible, interviewers should write answers and code them on the questionnaire used in the field and further copying should be avoided. The questionnaire should be the document from which data are entered into the computer. Hand-copying is error-prone, however carefully done. The data entered into the computer provide duplicate records in the event of forms being lost.

The organization of data processing will depend on circumstances, such as the nature (length and number) of the forms, number and remoteness of the data collection places, distance from the computers used for data entry, how often the data-gatherers send forms to the computer centre, and whether facilities to set up (temporary) offices at remote locations exist. An example of the organization of data flow, from interviews carried out by a team of interviewers remote from the computer, is given in Box 13.1.

Box 13.1.   Example of the organization of data flow from field to computer centre in a field trial

(1) interviews;
(2) daily checking and coding of interview schedules by each interviewer;
(3) day's work of whole team tallied to summary tables;
(4) recording of numbers of forms completed and the identification numbers of respondents;
(5) collection and checking of forms by supervisors, weekly;
(6) dispatch of forms to computer site, weekly;
(7) numbers of forms and identification numbers checked on arrival;
(8) double-entry of data into computer;
(9) validation and any necessary correction of double-entered data;
(10) range and consistency checks on computer;
(11) lists of errors and inconsistencies returned to field supervisors for checking and correction;
(12) storage of forms and back-up copies of computer files;
(13) editing of computer data files when corrections notified by supervisor.

Data managers should establish regular procedures to return queries to the field staff and to discuss problems with them. Close links and interaction between those collecting the data and those processing and analysing them are essential for ongoing quality control.

If large numbers of forms have to be processed, a suitable storage system must be devised that will enable a particular form to be located quickly, should it be necessary to examine it later, for example to check on an apparent recording error. The storage system used will be much influenced by the way in which forms are accumulated. It may be appropriate to file them according to the identification numbers or codes associated with the study subjects to which each form refers. This may involve extensive sorting of forms if they do not come into the data centre in this order. An alternative system is to assemble a set of forms (say, those completed by a field-worker in a day) into a 'batch' and to allocate all the forms in the batch the same 'batch number', stamping this number on each form. The batch number is also entered into the computer record with each form. Thus, if the forms are stored by batch, no additional sorting is necessary and reference to the computer record will enable the location of a particular form to be narrowed down to a batch quickly. If more than one kind of form is being processed at the same time, it will usually be advisable to sort them by form type before making up batches, keeping forms of the same type in the same batch. Such sorting will also be necessary for data entry into the computers.

3.3 Form preparation

All forms to be used for recording data collected in a trial should be carefully designed to ensure that the relevant data are collected and that they may be easily extracted for data processing. This is described for interview questionnaires in Chapter 9. Such design can be a lengthy process that should start early in the planning of the trial. Design of the other forms, for field observation and laboratory results, should follow the same principles regarding adequate definition of each item of data to be entered and coded (see Section 6).

As well as the data to be recorded, each form should include the following items:

(1) form number (indicating which type of form);
(2) identification number of respondent or unit of observation;
(3) form serial number, or laboratory number (for specimens);
(4) date;
(5) interviewer's/observer's code number;
(6) interviewer's signature.

(1) to (4) are required to link the data in the computer with other information on the same individual and (5) and (6) are required for checking and quality control purposes.

For hierarchical data, it may be necessary to record more than one identification number (for example, of house, family and person). If

possible, all identification numbers should incorporate a check digit
(see Chapter 6, Section 4.5). This is usually the last digit, and takes a
value dependent on the other digits following a defined rule.

The forms may be printed on cards or paper. Cards may be preferred
when repeated visits are planned and new information is to be added to
an existing record. However, they are heavier and therefore harder to
carry than paper sheets, especially if several thousands must be carried.

In general, it is better to have separate forms for each individual
rather than to use one form for several subjects (such as those in the
same household). For example, if one subject is present and another is
absent, the form for the first subject can be completed and sent for
processing and the form for the second subject kept for a later visit,
rather than holding a household form in the field until everyone in the
household has been seen. A household census form may be an excep-
tion to this rule. One form for each household is generally preferable
for an initial census, which might be updated to record changes of
household composition in later censuses.

3.4 Computer files

For each type of data collection form, a computer file will be created
to contain the data. Entry of data into a file is usually done through a
database package. Database packages allow a representation of the
form or questionnaire to be presented to the operator on the computer
screen to facilitate data entry. Consistency and range checks can be
designed into these 'data entry screens' so that the data entry clerk is
alerted immediately to likely errors in what is being entered. The clerk
should be instructed how to respond to different kinds of error, as
some may be due to simple mistyping in the data entry process, but
others may be due to data recording errors in the field.

Names for the variables for which data are recorded must be chosen
for use in computer processing. Variables may be identified by numbers (such as VAR001 or VAR147, for variables 1 or 147, respectively), but this makes later analysis of the data cumbersome. It is better
to use abbreviated names that describe the variables, such as AGE,
BIRTHWT, MATEDUC (for maternal education). The software packages used will constrain the number of characters allowed in a name,
but most allow at least 8 characters. A good general rule is to use no
more characters than are allowed by the most restrictive (in terms of
number of characters) computer package that is likely to be used.

If data are required from two or more different files for a particular analysis or report, it is much better to make a temporary link between the files within the data base package than to copy data from one file to another (to avoid having to change multiple files when information on a variable is updated). Database packages allow files to be 'related' using a unique identity number for each individual which appears in each file.

In follow-up studies, in which different data may be collected for each individual in different survey rounds, or in a survey in which data relating to the same individual may be collected via different routes (for example, some data may be collected in the field and some may come from the laboratory analysis of a blood sample taken from that individual), it is better to store the information from each source or round in a separate file, rather than trying to edit the data from one source into the file created for the data from the other source. Data base packages make it straightforward to link data from different files using a common person identifying code.

If some information collected in a study is common to several individuals, whereas other information is specific to the individual, these two kinds of data should be kept in separate computer files. For example, a 'household' file may contain data about the size of the compound and materials used for construction. This information could be linked to that for each individual in the household by recording the household number in the computer file containing the information on each individual in the study. The manipulation of hierarchical data of this kind is now straightforward in most data base packages, using the 'standard query language' (SQL).

A manual with the names and details of all the variables (what the variable is, meaning of codes, allowed values, etc.) and primary computer files (files in which data collected in the field are entered and stored) should be maintained and given to all data processing and data collection personnel. It should be updated on a regular basis, as necessary.

4 DATA RECORDING IN THE FIELD

4.1 Quality control

The importance of quality control for data collection and recording activities cannot be over-emphasized. The components to effective quality control include system design, form design, training, team-work and supportive supervision. All components must work together to provide timely feedback and reinforcement for high quality performance. System design should include built-in checks, random replicate measures by the interviewer, co-worker and/or supervisor, and routine review measures by the work team to provide regular and rapid feedback. Form design should include fail-safe procedures in recording and coding as described below. Training must focus on accuracy and completeness with an emphasis on how and why the work of the entire project is dependent upon the quality of the data recorded. Each member of the team should understand what all others are doing, the problems they face and why and in what ways each is dependent upon the others. Supervision should be of a supportive, non-threatening nature to be most effective and generally should be directly linked with continuing education and training. Successful work must be seen as a team effort. Quantitative and objective quality scores (for example, number of records completed without errors per day) and performance ratings for the work completed by the team should be kept and reviewed regularly (for example, weekly). Rewards and reprimands likewise should be on a team basis. When things go wrong, the fault is often with the system design and not due to an individual worker. The ideas of continuous quality improvement with their focus on process (doing the right things in the right way at the right time) and through team work with clearly defined quantita-tive performance indicators and rapid feedback have proven effective in manufacturing industries, and increasingly in service industries, and are appropriate for the work of field research teams. Members of the team must know their responsibilities and participate regularly in the planning and review of their activities as part of the team. They must know that their work, as well as that of their colleagues, will be monitored through the use of quantitative indicators by the team on a regular and continuing basis. Thus, they should know, for example, that their task is to ensure that forms are being correctly completed, that the information is recorded legibly and that the weighing scales are being calibrated daily. The team must be enabled to carry out these tasks.

A hand-tally of important variables into tables on a regular basis (for example, age by disease status, absences of family members dur-ing follow-up) assists in the detection of problems. A shift in the pat-tern of data will signal the need to check on particular aspects (for example, one interviewer whose refusal rate is much higher than others). All, or at least a sample of, field forms should be checked daily so that errors are detected early, the reasons for the errors identified and a solution to the problem worked out. Regular team meetings, probably weekly in the early months of a project, must be held to monitor progress and work towards reducing or eliminating any problems identified.

4.2 Practical aspects of recording

When different forms are required for different individuals (for example, special forms for pregnant women or for persons with a recent disease episode), it is essential to ensure that all field workers know which forms to complete for each person. Using different coloured paper for different forms may be helpful.

Procedures for minimizing recording errors should be devised and tested. For example, measurements, such as weight, might be read aloud and written down by a different field worker immediately after they are taken. It is easy to forget a child's weight, for example, if it is not recorded until the end of an interview.

Special attention should be given to coding or recording responses in questionnaires to distinguish 'not known' from 'not recorded' from 'not relevant'. Wherever possible, the leaving of 'blanks' should be avoided (for example, record 'not appropriate' rather than leave blank). Different interviewers might interpret a blank in any of the three ways noted above. It is also advisable to avoid using a dash '–' as a code for a response and better to allocate a specific alphabetical or numerical code for each possible response (for example, 1 = yes; 2 = no; 3 = not known; 8 = not relevant; 9 = not recorded). A common error is for interviewers to supply the current year when filling in information on dates (such as when recording the date of birth). Attention to such errors should be given in pilot surveys and training sessions and throughout the main survey.

Field workers should be trained to record data in the right place on the form and to use legible writing (a test for the legibility of their writing should be one of the selection criteria used for employing field workers). Some investigators prefer field workers to record information in pencil, using pencils with built in erasers for correcting any mistakes. Others insist that ball point pens are used (say, blue for field workers and red for supervisors, so that supervisor corrections can be distinguished) and that errors are corrected by deletion and writing the correct response above or below the original response but *never* writing over the incorrect response to make it correct. The use of correcting fluid ('liquid paper') to obliterate incorrect responses should be discouraged in most circumstances, probably to the extent of banning its use in the field. Supervisors should ensure that field workers always have an adequate supply of writing implements (and a pencil-sharpener, if necessary).

Field workers should be instructed how to write numbers and letters so that the coding and data entry clerks have no difficulty in reading the forms. Some letters and numbers are frequently confused and special instructions should be given regarding these. Examples are given in Table 13.1. Data entry clerks should be warned, however, that although recording clerks have been instructed to write numbers and letters in a certain way they may lapse into their old habits!

Instructions relevant to the field workers (such as those in Table 13.1) should be included in their field instruction manual.

4.3 Computer recording devices

A recent innovation in the recording of field data has been the use of small portable computers, not much larger than a calculator, to record information directly in the field. A questionnaire can be programmed into the machine so that the interviewer is prompted to ask each question. Data are entered into the machine throughout the day, for example during house-to-house surveys, and each evening the recorded information is transferred, using a cable link, directly into a micro-computer. Thus there is never any written record and the step of transferring data from forms into a computer by data entry clerks is avoided completely. These portable computers can be programmed to check for range and consistency errors. Therefore if a date is entered as 27/32/88 it will not be accepted and the interviewer is instructed to re-enter correct information. Of course, not all data entry errors can be detected by such checks, and checking and correcting recorded data is not as straightforward as for a written document.

This technology holds great promise for the future but it has not been fully 'tried and tested'. Thus it cannot be recommended for general use, but early experience with its use in Africa is encouraging, where it was found to result in significantly fewer errors in recording

Table 13.1. Characters commonly confused in handwritten forms
and some suggested solutions to avoid confusion

Characters confused	Solution
1 and 7	This confusion arises if ones are written with an initial upward stroke (for example 1). If this is the situation, then always write sevens with a horizontal line through them (as do the French), that is 7. A simpler solution may be to insist that ones are written with a single stroke (for example I)
O (oh) and 0 (zero)	Note (1). Write 0 (zeros) with a line through them, that is θ
4 and 9	Write 4 as 4
4 and 7	These digits may be confused if sevens are written with a horizontal line through them! Instruct field-workers to make sure that the top of the seven is written horizontally
6 and 9 (upside-down)	Relevant when coding laboratory specimens (for example, is it 61 or 19?). Draw a horizontal line under all numbers, for example <u>19</u>
2 and Z	Note (1). Always write Z with a horizontal line through it, that is $\mathbb{Z}$
5 and S	Note (1). Always write 5 using 2 pen strokes
O (oh) and Q	Note (1)
I and 1	Note (1). Always write I with 'hat and shoes', not as a single stroke, that is I not I
U and V	Avoid both letters as codes as far as possible (will be needed for names)

Note (1).   Avoid using the alphabetical character in data fields that may
contain alphabetical or numerical information.

than conventional paper and pencil methods (Forster *et al.* 1991,
1995). It is likely, for the next several years at least, that pen and
paper recording will continue to be the method of choice, offering the
most reliable recording system for most field data.

5 CODING

'Coding' is the name given to the procedure used to convert data from a questionnaire or record into a form that is ready for entry into a computer. Instructions on coding are given on most questionnaires and other data recording forms (for example, record exact number of children, if not known code as '99'). Data on many variables collected in field studies need no further coding beyond that done by the field worker who collected the data, as the information recorded is either numerical (for example, number of siblings) or, in the case of categorical variables, the possible answers have been assigned codes at the time of collection. Problems arise when an answer does not fit into the pre-coded options and the field worker writes out the response, in full, on the questionnaire. Such answers should not occur frequently (except in qualitative research investigations, see Chapter 10) if the questionnaire has been adequately tested (see Chapter 9), but those that do occur more than a few times can be given additional codes, and the remaining grouped together in the 'other' category. It is useful to survey a sizeable batch of questionnaires before deciding how to make up additional codes. Separate notes should be kept of answers coded as 'other', with the questionnaire numbers and dates, to review them at the time of analysis. Changes in coding should be noted in the instruction manual.

5.1 During and after data collection

The questionnaires or forms may be designed so that the field worker writes out the 'pre-coded' answers in a space ready for reading and computer entry by the data entry clerk. This approach has the advantage of minimizing transcription errors, but later coding is still required for 'open' questions or for answers which do not fit in the pre-coded categories.

An alternative approach is for the interviewer, or supervisor, to code the information after the questionnaire has been completed. The questionnaires are divided by a vertical line; the questions and space for the recorded responses occupy the larger section on the left-hand side and the coding form occupies the vertical column on the right. The latter is drawn so as to resemble the screen on a data entry program (for example, Epi Info or FoxPro). During the interview, the field workers ignore the right-hand side of the form and fill in the answers in the spaces provided on the left-hand side. At the end of a working day, information is transferred from the left-hand side to the right. This allows a check that all questions have been answered. In the case of blank answers, the field worker may still remember what the answer was, or may have to return the next day to collect more information. Open questions (if any) are coded according to the instructions, or left blank for later coding in the study headquarters. The field worker may also realize that there are inconsistencies in the data which should be corrected. In addition, readability of the letters and numbers is generally improved when transferring the field-collected data to the right-hand side of the form in the quieter surroundings of the study base. Coding on the same day as the interview has been shown to be a useful tool for quality control. Similar considerations apply to forms for field observations and laboratory data. Examples of the design of questionnaires for computer processing are given in Chapter 9.

5.2 Grouping of responses

A left-over from the time when punched cards and counter-sorter machines were the main computing tools to analyse survey data is the tendency to record information in groups. For example, the number of pregnancies a woman has had might be recorded as in one of the groups 0, 1–2, 3–6, 7+ as this is the way it was anticipated the data would be analysed. If it is decided later that it would be of interest to look at women with only one pregnancy as a special group, it is impossible because of the way the information was recorded.

With modern computing capabilities there is no reason to group data in this way prior to putting it into the computer. Information should be recorded in full detail rather than in pre-determined groups. This preserves the possibility of using various groupings in analyses should this be appropriate.

5.3 Common errors

A common practice when devising coding instructions is to require that a specific code be recorded if a particular question is not applicable to a respondent (for example, number of pregnancies for a man) for which the responses are left blank during the interview (for example, the instruction might be to fill the data field with eights). A common error is for the coding clerk to use 0 or blanks where the instructions call for eights or another specific code.

This error may be so common and difficult to correct that the most rational solution may be to assume that it will happen some of the time and to program the analyses such that the data field is ignored if it is not applicable (using another data field, for example, that for sex, to identify such subjects). This strategy may not be possible for all variables, and for those for which it is not, special checking of suspicious codes (for example, all blanks and zeros) may be necessary.

Another common error is to use more digits than are allowed in a numeric field where the value exceeds the number of digits allocated, for example when a respondent's age is 100 years or more and the data form allows for only two digits, as persons of this age were not anticipated. This may cause the data entry clerk to insert an extra number and to displace all following digits. The appropriate action would be to assign the code 98 to signify '98 or over' (reserving '99' for 'not known'). (Note: the use of this device to reduce the digits (that is, grouping at the end) should be confined to unusual events, as in this example).

6 DATA ENTRY

6.1 When and where to do

After coding, the information on the forms is ready to be entered into a computer. Unlike coding, which should generally be carried out in the field, entry of data into a computer may be carried out at a later stage. Special care should be taken to ensure that the delay in processing the information does not result in questionnaires being lost or damaged in transit or storage. The time between data collection and computer entry should be kept as short as possible. This is partly to reduce the chance of data being lost, but also so that range and consistency checking programs can be run on the data as soon as possible. Errors revealed can be rapidly referred back to field workers for correction, and simple tabulations of important variables may be made to facilitate monitoring the progress of the study.

In a trial that covers a large geographical area, there are potential advantages if the data entry computers are close to the field work to permit more rapid transfer of field data into the computers and consequent rapid feedback to field workers of queries and errors found through consistency and other checks. Problems of a suitable environment and power supply may preclude this, but portable machines may be suitable for this purpose.

6.2 Entry and verification

Each data set collected in a study should be entered into the computer *twice*. The second entry should be independent of the first and should preferably be done by a different data entry clerk. After this, the two files of data in the computer are compared, using a computer program (for example Epi Info has this facility), and any differences indicated, so that the original records can be checked to determine which file, if either, is correct. The incorrect file(s) should be altered (edited) appropriately. The program to compare the files is then run again and the editing process repeated until no differences between the files are found. There should then be reasonable assurance that the data recorded in the computer correspond to those on the original forms.

Some data entry software allows for data to be entered a second time by the same clerk immediately following the first entry as a method of checking data entry. The danger with the use of such a system is that a careless or tired data entry clerk may be inclined to ignore discrepancies that are thrown up on the screen or may repeat the same mistake. For this reason, it is recommended that the first system described be used.

The importance of double entry of data must be stressed. It is tempting, especially when large amounts of data have been collected or there is a back log of data to be entered into the computer, to enter data only once. Even the best data entry clerks cannot avoid making errors (a low error rate would be 1 per 1000 characters) and if these errors are not detected until the data are analysed, great inconvenience is likely to be caused (as finding and correcting such errors during an analysis is time-consuming). Some errors can be detected through consistency and range checking (described in Section 6.4) but some cannot.

A common error in data entry is to skip a field, so that all following figures are displaced to the left (the reverse, that is inserting an extra field, may also occur). When using 'data field-based' packages for data entry, these errors are likely to be found when the end of the form is reached and the record is either over-full or incomplete. They will also be detected by range or consistency checks when these are applied at the time of entry, or when the same data are entered a second time and the files are compared.

6.3 Data cleaning

A powerful way to detect errors in data entry, or in the recording on the original field record, is to run programs that conduct range and consistency checks on data files, either as they are entered into the computer or once they have been entered and verified. Range checks, applied to each data item, verify that the entered values are in an allowed range. For example, codes for sex other than 'M' or 'F', and heights above 2.5 m would be flagged as errors. Identification numbers might also be checked to verify that any check digit or character was correct. Consistency checks seek contradictory values for different variables, such as persons entered as males breast feeding, adults having a morbidity record applicable only to children, a child aged 6 years having a weight of 75 kg. They can be applied to data in the same file only, or to data from several files for mutual consistency, particularly with hierarchical data. If data are entered by experienced, rapid typists, it will be better to carry out range and consistency checks by running programs at a later stage ('in batch'), as checks carried out at the time of entry ('interactive') will cause delays if a supervisor has to be consulted to sort out errors. A situation in which interactive checking may be preferable, however, is when data are entered at the end of the day by the field staff who collected them. They are likely to be slow typists and, having the interviews fresh in their minds, are likely to be able to correct errors at the time.

Interim tabulations of data are also recommended as a way of detecting data errors. Scatter plots of quantitative variables, such as height against weight, are effective in revealing unlikely outlying observations. Special checks might be made on observations that are more than two or three standard deviations from the mean. Such observations should be checked individually as they are not impossible, merely unlikely.

Some data base packages do not allow two individuals to be entered with the same identification number. Others permit such erroneous recording (which may be due to a mistake in the field or during data entry) and this can lead to problems when linking different sets of data on the same individual. It is worthwhile to develop programs to check for such erroneous duplication of identification numbers.

Correcting errors is often straightforward. Inspection of the data recording form may show poorly written codes, or it may be clear from the context (based on data elsewhere in the same form or from other forms) what the correct value is, or it may be possible to return the record to the field for correction. Sometimes, however, particularly if it is some time since the data were collected, discovering the correct values may be impossible. In these cases, missing value codes must be used. The number of times this is done should be kept as small as possible.

Errors in the data are likely to be found after the fieldwork is complete and when the main data analysis is under way. It is useful, at some stage, to make the formal decision that the data are now 'closed' for more corrections, or a stable set of analyses will be impossible to achieve. This should not be done before finding errors has become uncommon.

6.4 Updating and storage

Back-up copies of data should be made regularly (at least weekly and possibly daily) on floppy disks or other storage devices as soon as data entry starts. At least two back-up copies of data that are in the computer should always exist. The copies should be updated regularly and frequently, although it is a good idea to keep some old versions as well, as errors are sometimes found in the more recent ones that make it necessary to restart data entry from a previous copy. Some of the copies should be stored in a geographically separate location in a dry and relatively dust-free environment (such as in a sealed plastic bag). Complete records should be kept of what data are in all files on all stored disks and tapes, and should also be recorded in duplicate or triplicate at more than one location.

The questionnaires and other data forms should also be stored, at least until the project is finished and preferably well beyond. Due attention must be paid to security against hazards such as rot, insects and theft (all of which may be non-trivial risks in some tropical environments). Questionnaires and forms should be stored in batches or in serial order (either by date of collection or by identification number) so as to facilitate their retrieval for checking apparent errors detected in records on computer (see Section 3.2). They should be kept tidy in folders or file boxes which are properly labelled.

7 PREPARING DATA FOR ANALYSIS

The 'raw materials' for data analysis are the data files used for the production of cross-tabulations of frequencies and of averages and standard deviations. The variables as measured and entered as raw data are not always the ones directly suitable for data analysis. Recoding and computing of new variables is likely to be necessary. It is useful to give different names to consecutive versions of the same file (for example, FOLLUP1, FOLLUP2, FOLLUP3, etc.). It is advisable to keep copies of earlier versions of the files and of the commands used to update them (the 'log' files) as it may be necessary to rebuild files from the earlier files in order to make corrections or additions to the basic data.

7.1 Recoding variables

Quantitative variables may be treated as such in the analysis, or may be recoded into categories. This latter approach often makes it easier to understand the data and, in particular, to look for non-linear associations. There are some rules of thumb that are useful to guide decisions on recoding quantitative variables. The number of categories should usually be between 3 and 6, depending partly on the total number of observations. In a large study, more categories might be used. Each category should include a reasonable number of observations (say, not less than 10 per cent of the total), unless there is a clear reason for keeping a small group separate (for example, mothers with no schooling should probably not be grouped with those with 1 year of education). It will usually be best to examine the distribution of the raw data (or in many 'fine' groups) before deciding on a suitable 'coarse' grouping for analysis. One approach is to divide the sample into quartiles or quintiles with respect to the variable under study (that is, 4 or 5 groups of equal size). A slight disadvantage of this is that such groupings seem 'unnatural' as the cut-off points are 'odd' numbers (for example, monthly income US$53 to $87, instead of, say, US$50 to $99).

Even for categorical variables, recoding is often necessary. When analysing reasons for stopping breast feeding, for example, a number of distinct answers may be grouped under 'concern with milk quality', others under 'reduced milk output', and so forth. Such grouping increases the statistical power of the analysis and may make findings easier to understand.

After deciding if and how each variable should be categorized, the different categories should be assigned 'labels', and those saved in a file, which will eliminate the need to return to the questionnaires or code books during the analysis.

When recoding of a variable is undertaken it is advisable to allocate it a different name from the original variable so as to preserve the basic data. Thus the variable 'AGE' might be recoded and allocated to another variable given the name 'AGEGP' for information on the age group.

7.2 Computing new variables

It is often necessary to use two or more existing variables to create new variables, such as per capita income, number of persons per bedroom, or weight for age. Such new variables may be calculated either in a straightforward way (such as per capita income), or be obtained by comparison with a given standard (as in the case of weight for age). Special types of computed variables are those related to time, such as age, and duration of exposure to a risk factor. Depending on the characteristics of the variable and of the population under study, it may be preferable to record relevant dates on the questionnaires and to subtract them at the time of analysis to compute ages, etc. Most databases and statistical packages handle these calculations without difficulty. However, when computing age in full years or months, the usual convention is to truncate the variable (that is, round downwards), whereas statistical programs may round them, for example, to the nearest integer, unless programmed to truncate them.

After computing a composite variable, it is useful to check that the distribution of the new variable seems reasonable. It is also appropriate to check the range of the new variable as described above, as data errors may only show up at this stage. For example, negative ages or extreme weights-for-age may result from errors in the date of birth (or date of interview) in the questionnaire (though such errors should have been detected through consistency checks at an earlier stage).

If the field work lasts some time and inflation rates are high, currency variables, such as monthly incomes, may have to be adjusted for inflation. This may be done by expressing them in terms of an inflation-adjusted index (such as minimum wages or government bonds), or in some circumstances by converting them to a stable foreign currency using the exchange rate at the time of the interview.

7.3 Combining data from several files

The data required for a particular analysis may come from several files (for example, interview replies concerning morbidity may need to be linked to laboratory results). It will be necessary to produce extra data files in the computer, combining the necessary information from the original files. This may involve programming using the database package.

With hierarchical data an added complication arises. It is necessary to decide the 'unit of observation' for each analysis (for example, in morbidity surveillance, is the unit the child or the episode?). It may be necessary to combine data from several records, as averages or counts or proportions, to derive each value of a given variable for the analysis (in the example, the number of episodes or the number divided by the surveillance time may be needed).

REFERENCES

Byass, P., Hanlon, P.W., Hanlon, L.C.S., Marsh, V.M. and Greenwood, B.M. (1988). Microcomputer management of a vaccine trial. *Computers in Biology and Medicine*, **18**, 179–93.

Forster, D., Behrens, R.H., Campbell, H. and Byass, P. (1991). The evaluation of a computerized field data collection system for health. *Bulletin of the World Health Organization*, **69**, 107–11.

Forster, D. and Snow, R.W. (1995). An assessment of the use of hand-held computers during demographic surveys in developing countries. *Survey methodology*, **21**, 193–199.

Rowan, K.M., Byass, P. and Snow, R.W. (1987). On-line tropical epidemiology – a case-study from The Gambia. *Methods of Information in Medicine*, **26**, 73–6.

Stephens, J., Alonso, P.L., Byass, P. and Snow, R.W. (1989). Tropical epidemiology: a system for continuous demographic monitoring of a study population. *Methods of Information in Medicine*, **28**, 155–9.

14
Methods of analysis

1 Introduction

2 Basics of statistical inference
    2.1 Types of outcome measure
    2.2 Confidence intervals
    2.3 Significance tests

3 Analysis of proportions
    3.1 Confidence interval for a single proportion
    3.2 Difference between two proportions
    3.3 Ratio of two proportions
    3.4 Trend test for proportions

4 Analysis of mean values
    4.1 Confidence interval for a mean
    4.2 Difference between two means
    4.3 Analysis of more than two groups

5 Analysis of rates
    5.1 Risks, rates and person-time-at-risk
    5.2 Confidence interval for a rate
    5.3 Difference between two rates
    5.4 Ratio of two rates
    5.5 Trend test for rates

6 Controlling for confounding variables
    6.1 The nature of confounding variables
    6.2 Adjusting for confounding variables
    6.3 Adjusting risks
        6.3.1 Overall test of significance
        6.3.2 Pooled estimate of risk difference
        6.3.3 Pooled estimate of risk ratio
        6.3.4 Confidence intervals
    6.4 Adjusting rates
        6.4.1 Overall test of significance
        6.4.2 Pooled estimate of rate difference
        6.4.3 Pooled estimate of rate ratio
        6.4.4 Confidence intervals
    6.5 Adjusting means

1 INTRODUCTION

This chapter describes the principal statistical methods which are likely to be useful most frequently for the analysis of intervention trials. Reference to statistical or epidemiological texts, and probably also consultation with a statistician, will be necessary for more advanced analytical techniques. The choice of an appropriate method of analysis depends on the type of outcome measure which is of interest. The different types of outcome measure are discussed in Section 2, which also includes a brief review of the rationale behind confidence intervals and significance tests. In Sections 3, 4 and 5 methods are described which are appropriate for the analyses of data in the form of proportions, means, and rates, respectively. Randomized controlled trials have been recommended as the method of choice for determining the effects of an intervention because such trials avoid the problem of confounding. Where randomization is not feasible, any attempt to draw conclusions about the effects of an intervention must make allowance for possible confounding factors and, for completeness, simple methods for doing this are described in Section 6, even though randomized studies are the focus of this manual. The analysis of trials in which interventions are allocated to groups rather than individuals is discussed in Section 7. How the results of a trial may be used to assess the possible public health impact of an intervention is considered in Section 8.

A common mistake in the planning of a trial is to delay consideration of the analyses until the data become available. It is essential that the main analyses that will be undertaken are planned at the design stage, as this provides several major benefits. First, it encourages a clearer understanding of the basic questions to be answered, and thus assists with the formulation of clear and specific objectives. For example, in a vaccine trial, a simple comparison of the numbers of cases of the disease occurring over a five year period in the vaccinated and unvaccinated groups may answer the question of whether the vaccine has any protective effect. A comparison of the incidence rates of disease in vaccinated and unvaccinated individuals in the first, second, third, fourth and fifth years, answers a rather different question; namely, whether the protective effect is constant over the five year-period.

A second benefit of considering the analyses at the design stage is that it necessitates specification of which data need to be recorded. The investigator can check that arrangements have been made to measure and record all variables that will be needed in the analyses. Also, and perhaps as importantly, it may become clear that some variables will not be needed and these can then be omitted.

The process of planning the analyses may identify also the importance of subgroup analyses. In a vaccine trial, for example, it may reveal a need to assess the efficacy of the vaccine in children vaccinated at different ages. This may have major implications for the choice of sample size, as the need for age-specific estimates of efficacy requires a much larger sample in each age-group than would be needed if only an overall estimate of efficacy was wanted.

Finally, advanced planning of the analyses is desirable to ensure that adequate arrangements have been made for data handling, that the necessary computer software is available, and that sufficient time for data-cleaning and analysis has been allowed for in the study schedule.

Substantial developments have taken place in recent years in multivariate methods of analysis as applied to epidemiological studies. A discussion of these is beyond the scope of this manual. Generally, it is possible to elucidate the main findings of intervention trials without resort to these methods, but sometimes their use does aid interpretation. Detailed discussion of many of these methods is given in the two volumes by Breslow and Day (1980; 1987).

Prior to any formal statistical analyses of the kinds discussed from Section 2 onwards it is essential to perform simple tabulations of data and to construct simple diagrams to summarize the information that has been collected. The statistical 'package' programs described in Chapter 13 greatly facilitate doing this. The investigator should use these simple approaches to gain a good understanding of the data collected before embarking on more complex analyses. These simple analysis methods are not described further in this manual but they are discussed in most good textbooks on medical statistics (for example, Hill 1984; Armitage and Berry 1987).

2 BASICS OF STATISTICAL INFERENCE

2.1 Types of outcome measure

The appropriate method of statistical analysis depends on the type of outcome measure that is of interest. An outcome in an intervention study can usually be expressed as a proportion, as a mean, or as a rate. For example, in a trial of a new measles vaccine, an outcome measure of interest may be the *proportion* of vaccinated subjects who develop a high level of antibodies. In a trial of an anti-malarial intervention, it may be of interest to compare the *mean* packed cell volume (PCV) at the end of the malaria season in those in the intervention group and those in the comparison group. In a trial of multi-drug therapy for leprosy, the incidence *rates* of relapse following treatment may be compared in the different study groups under consideration.

2.2 Confidence intervals

An estimate of an outcome measure calculated in an intervention study is subject to *sampling error*, because it is based on only a sample of individuals and not on the whole population of interest. The term 'sampling error' does not mean that the sampling procedure or method of randomization was applied incorrectly, but that when random sampling is used to decide which individuals are in which group, there will be an element of random variation in the results. The methods of statistical inference allow the investigator to draw conclusions about the true value of the outcome measure on the basis of the information in the sample. In general, the observed value of the outcome measure gives the *best estimate* of the true value. In addition, it is useful to have some indication of the *precision* of this estimate, and this is done by attaching a *confidence interval* to the estimate. The confidence interval is a range of plausible values for the true value of the outcome measure based on the observations in the trial. It is conventional to quote the *95 per cent confidence interval* (also called *95 per cent confidence limits*). This is calculated in such a way that there is a 95 per cent probability that it includes the true value.

Suppose the true value of the outcome measure is ϕ, and that this is estimated from the sample data as $\hat{\phi}$. The 95 per cent confidence intervals to be presented here are generally of the form $\hat{\phi} \pm 1.96 \times SE(\hat{\phi})$, where $SE(\hat{\phi})$ denotes the *standard error* of the estimate. This is a measure of the amount of sampling error to which the estimate is susceptible. One of the factors influencing the magnitude of the standard error, and hence the width of the confidence interval, is the sample size. The larger the sample the narrower the confidence interval.

The multiplying factor 1.96, used when calculating the 95 per cent confidence interval, is derived from tables of the 'Normal' distribution. In this distribution 95 per cent of values are expected to fall within 1.96 standard deviations of the mean. In some circumstances, confidence intervals other than 95 per cent limits may be required and then different values of the multiplying factor are appropriate, as indicated in Table 14.1:

Table 14.1. Multiplying factors for calculating confidence intervals based on the Normal distribution

Confidence interval (%)	Multiplying factor
90	1.64
95	1.96
99	2.58
99.9	3.29

When analysing means, the multiplying factor sometimes has to be increased to allow for additional errors in estimating the standard error (see Section 4).

2.3 Significance tests

In some instances, as well as calculating a confidence interval to indicate a range of plausible values for the outcome measure of interest, it may be appropriate to test a specific *hypothesis* about the outcome measure. In the context of an intervention trial, this will often be the hypothesis that there is no true difference between the outcomes in the groups under comparison. (For this reason the hypothesis is often referred to as the *null hypothesis*.) The objective is thus to assess whether any observed difference in outcomes between the study groups may have occurred just by chance due to sampling error.

The method for testing the null hypothesis is known as a *significance test*. The sample data are used to calculate a quantity (called a *statistic*) which gives a measure of the difference between the groups with respect to the outcome(s) of interest. The details of how the statistic is calculated vary according to the type of outcome measure being examined, and are given in Sections 3–5. Once the statistic has been calculated, its value is referred to an appropriate set of statistical tables, in order to determine the *p-value* (probability value) or 'significance' of the results. The *p-value* measures the probability of obtaining a value for the statistic as extreme as the one actually observed if the null hypothesis were true.

For example, suppose a difference in mean PCV of 1.5 per cent is observed at the end of the malaria season between two groups of individuals, one of which was supplied with mosquito-nets. A *p*-value of 0.03 would indicate that, if nets had no true effect on PCV levels, there would only be a 3 per cent chance of obtaining an observed difference of 1.5 per cent or greater.

The smaller the *p*-value, the less plausible the null hypothesis seems as an explanation of the observed data. For example, a *p*-value of 0.001 means that the null hypothesis is highly implausible, and this can be interpreted as very strong evidence of a real difference between the groups. On the other hand, a *p*-value of 0.20 means that a difference of the observed magnitude could quite easily have occurred by chance, even if there were no real difference between the groups. Conventionally, *p*-values of 0.05 and below have been regarded as sufficiently low to be taken as reasonable evidence against the null hypothesis, and have been referred to as indicating a 'statistically significant difference‛, but it is preferable to specify the exact size of the *p*-value attained so that readers can draw their own conclusions about the strength of the evidence.

While a small *p*-value can be interpreted as evidence for a real difference between the groups, a larger 'non-significant' *p*-value must not be interpreted as indicating that there is no difference. It merely indicates that there is insufficient evidence to reject the null hypothesis, so that there *may* be no true difference between the groups.

Too much reliance should not be placed on the use of significance tests. Usually, it is more important to *estimate* the effect of the intervention, and to specify a confidence interval around the estimate to indicate the likely range of error, than it is to test a specific hypothesis. In any case, a null hypothesis of zero difference is often of no practical interest, as there may be strong grounds for believing the intervention has some effect, and the main objective should be to measure that effect.

The significance tests presented here are *two-sided* tests. This means that when the *p*-value is computed, it measures the probability (if the null hypothesis is true) of observing a difference as great as that actually observed *in either direction* (i.e. positive or negative). It is usual to assume that tests are two-sided unless otherwise stated, though not all authors adhere to this convention. A full discussion of the relative merits of one-sided and two-sided tests is given in Armitage and Berry (1987).

3 ANALYSIS OF PROPORTIONS

3.1 Confidence interval for a single proportion

Analysis of proportions is needed when the outcome of interest is a *binary* or yes/no variable (for example, the proportion of individuals who develop a disease). The standard error of a proportion p, calculated from a sample of n subjects, is estimated as $\sqrt{[p(1 - p)/n]}$. For example, if the prevalence of splenomegaly in a random sample of 200 children from a population is found to be 0.40 (40 per cent) (i.e. 80 had splenomegaly), the standard error (SE) is given by

$$SE(p) = \sqrt{(0.40 \times 0.60/200)} = 0.035 \ (3.5 \text{ per cent}).$$

The 95 per cent confidence interval for a proportion is given by $p \pm 1.96 \times SE(p)$. In the example, the 95 per cent confidence interval is $0.4 \pm 1.96 \times 0.035$, or $(0.33, 0.47)$, that is, 33–47 per cent. There is a 95 per cent chance that the true prevalence of splenomegaly in the population, from which the sample of 200 was taken, was between 33 per cent and 47 per cent.

3.2 Difference between two proportions

Suppose now that the objective is to compare the proportions observed in two groups of individuals; for example, an intervention and control group. The standard error of the *difference* between two proportions p_1 and p_2, based on n_1 and n_2 observations, respectively, is estimated, approximately, as $\surd\{\bar{p}(1 - \bar{p})[(1/n_1) + (1/n_2)]\}$ where $\bar{p} = (n_1 p_1 + n_2 p_2)/(n_1 + n_2)$. For example, if the proportions to be compared are 90/300 (30 per cent) and 135/300 (45 per cent), the observed difference between the two proportions is -0.150, $\bar{p} = 0.375$, and the standard error of the difference is given by $\surd\{0.375 \times 0.625[(1/300) + (1/300)]\} = 0.040$.

A 95 per cent confidence interval for the difference between the proportions is given by $(p_1 - p_2) \pm 1.96 \times$ SE. In the example, this gives $(-0.15) \pm 1.96(0.040)$, i.e. $(-0.23, -0.07)$, or -23 per cent to -7 per cent.

To test the null hypothesis that there is no true difference between the two proportions, the data are first arranged in a 2×2 table, as in Table 14.2.

In the table a is the number in group 1 who experience the outcome of interest. The expected value of a, $E(a)$, and the variance of a, $V(a)$, are calculated under the hypothesis of no difference between the two groups.

Table 14.2. Comparison of two proportions

Group	Outcome		Total	Proportion with outcome
	Yes	No		
1	a (90)	b (210)	n_1 (300)	$p_1 = a/n_1$ (0.30)
2	c (135)	d (165)	n_2 (300)	$p_2 = c/n_2$ (0.45)
Total	m_1 (225)	m_2 (375)	N (600)	

$$E(a) = m_1 n_1 / N \tag{14.1}$$

$$V(a) = n_1 n_2 m_1 m_2 / [N^2(N-1)] \tag{14.2}$$

The chi-squared (χ^2) statistic is then calculated. This gives a measure of the extent to which the observed data differ from those expected if the two proportions were equal.

$$\chi^2 = (|a - E(a)| - 0.5)^2 / V(a) \tag{14.3}$$

where $|a - E(a)|$ indicates the *absolute* value of $[a - E(a)]$. The calculated value of χ^2 is compared with tables of the chi-squared distribution with 1 degree of freedom (df). If it exceeds 3.84, then $p < 0.05$, indicating some evidence of a real difference in the proportions. If it exceeds 6.63, then $p < 0.01$, and there is strong evidence of a difference.

In the example, $a = 90$; $E(a) = (225)(300)/600 = 112.50$ and $V(a) = (300 \times 300 \times 225 \times 375)/(600 \times 600 \times 599) = 35.215$. Thus $\chi^2 = (|90 - 112.50| - 0.5)^2 / 35.215 = 13.74$. From tables of the chi-squared distribution the statistical significance of $p < 0.001$ may be obtained, indicating a difference as large as that observed would be very unlikely to arise by chance if there really was no difference between the two groups.

If any of the quantities $E(a)$, $E(b)$, $E(c)$ or $E(d)$ [for example, $E(b) = m_2 n_1 / N$] are less than 5.0 and N is less than 40, the χ^2 test is invalid, and a test called 'Fisher's exact test' should be used instead (see Armitage and Berry 1987).

3.3 Ratio of two proportions

The ratio of two proportions is sometimes referred to as the *relative risk* (R). To construct a confidence interval for a relative risk the natural logarithm of the estimate of the relative risk is computed:

$$\log_e(R) = \log_e(p_1/p_2) = \log_e[an_2/(cn_1)]$$

Its standard error is estimated by

$$SE[\log_e(R)] = \sqrt{\{[b/(an_1)] + [d/(cn_2)]\}} \tag{14.4}$$

The 95 per cent confidence interval for $\log_e(R)$ is then given by $\log_e(R) \pm 1.96$ SE, and the 95 per cent confidence interval for the relative risk is obtained by taking anti-logarithms.

In the example given in Table 14.2, the relative risk is estimated as $0.30/0.45 = 0.667$, and $\log_e(R) = -0.405$. The $\text{SE}[\log_e(R)]$ is estimated as $\sqrt{\{[210/(90 \times 300)] + [165/(135 \times 300)]\}} = 0.109$ and the 95 per cent confidence interval for $\log_e(R)$ is given by $-0.405 \pm 1.96(0.109)$, i.e. $(-0.619, -0.191)$. Taking antilogarithms, the 95 per cent confidence interval for the relative risk is $(0.538, 0.826)$.

3.4 Trend test for proportions

Sometimes it is of interest to examine whether there is a trend in a series of proportions associated with different levels of some underlying characteristic. For example, consider the proportion of leprosy patients who report regularly to collect their monthly drug supply from a clinic when the accessibility of the clinic is rated as very poor, poor, fair, or good (Table 14.3).

Table 14.3. Regularity of collection of drugs by leprosy patients according to accessibility of clinic

Accessibility of clinic	Collection of drugs		Total	'Score' x_i
	Regular	Not regular		
Very poor	a_1 (5)	$n_1 - a_1$ (20)	n_1 (25)	0
Poor	a_2 (12)	$n_2 - a_2$ (28)	n_2 (40)	1
Fair	a_3 (25)	$n_3 - a_3$ (25)	n_3 (50)	2
Good	a_4 (21)	$n_4 - a_4$ (14)	n_4 (35)	3
Total	A (63)	$N - A$ (87)	N (150)	

A 'score' (x_i) is assigned for each kind of clinic, whose value relates to the level of accessibility. For example, '0' has been assigned to those with 'very poor' accessibility and '3' to those with 'good' accessibility. A test for trend in the proportions a_1/n_1, a_2/n_2, a_3/n_3 and a_4/n_4 is provided by testing, as a chi-squared with 1 degree of freedom, the expression:

$$\chi^2 = N[(N\Sigma a_i x_i) - (A\Sigma n_i x_i)]^2 / \{A(N - A)[(N\Sigma n_i x_i^2) - (\Sigma n_i x_i)^2]\}$$

$$(14.5)$$

For example, suppose the proportions attending regularly are 5/25 (20 per cent), 12/40 (30 per cent), 25/50 (50 per cent), and 21/35 (60 per cent) in the four groups (as shown in Table 14.3). The value of χ^2 is $150[(150 \times 125) - (63 \times 245)]^2/\{63 \times 87[(150 \times 555) - 245^2]\} = 12.95$, which is highly significant ($p < 0.001$). It may be concluded, therefore, that there is strong evidence that the regularity of drug collection increases with the accessibility of the clinic.

4 ANALYSIS OF MEAN VALUES

4.1 Confidence interval for a mean

If the outcome measure is taken as the mean ($\bar{x}$) of a sample of n observations, for example, the weights of a sample of newborn infants, the standard error of the mean is given by $\sigma/\sqrt{n}$, where σ is the standard deviation of the variable measured (for example, weights of newborn infants) in the population from which the sample of n observations was taken. The 95 per cent confidence interval on the mean is given by $\bar{x} \pm 1.96(\sigma/\sqrt{n})$.

In general, σ (the standard deviation in the population) will not be known but must be *estimated*, based on the n observations in the sample. Thus, the estimate of σ is subject to sampling error also, and this must be taken into account in the computation of the confidence interval on the mean. This is done by using a multiplying factor in the confidence interval calculation taken from tables of the t-distribution rather than from tables of the 'Normal' distribution on which Table 14.1 was based. The value of the multiplying factor will depend on the size of the sample from which the standard deviation was estimated. For example, for 95 per cent confidence intervals, appropriate multiplying factors for sample sizes of 10, 20, 50, 100, are 2.26, 2.09, 2.01, and 1.98, respectively. (Note that in using the tables the values of t are given for different 'degrees of freedom'. In the situation considered here the degrees of freedom correspond to the sample size minus one, i.e. $n - 1$). If the sample size is around 30 or more, little error is introduced by using the value of 1.96 derived from the Normal distribution, rather than the appropriate t-value, when calculating 95 per cent confidence intervals.

If the estimate of the standard deviation based on the sample is

s, the 95 per cent confidence interval on the mean is given by $\bar{x} \pm t(s/\sqrt{n})$. For example, if the mean birthweight of 25 infants was 3.10 kg and the standard deviation of the weights in the sample was 0.90 kg, the 95 per cent confidence interval would be given by $3.10 \pm 2.06(0.90/\sqrt{25})$, i.e. 2.73–3.47 kg, where the multiplying factor 2.06 is taken from a table of the t-distribution corresponding to 24 degrees of freedom.

4.2 Difference between two means

In a trial it is very common to want to compare the means of observations in different groups; for example, to compare observations from an intervention group with those from a control group. Suppose that two groups are to be compared and the means are $\bar{x}_1$ and $\bar{x}_2$, respectively, and the corresponding standard deviations observed in the groups are s_1 and s_2. The standard error of the difference between the means is given by $\sqrt{\{s[(1/n_1) + (1/n_2)]\}}$, where s is the *pooled* estimate of the standard deviation based on the observations from the two groups. s is estimated as: $s = \sqrt{\{[(n_1 - 1)s_1^2 + (n_2 - 1)s_2^2]/(n_1 + n_2 - 2)\}}$.

The 95 per cent confidence interval for the difference between the means is given by $(\bar{x}_1 - \bar{x}_2) \pm ts\sqrt{[(1/n_1) + (1/n_2)]}$, where t is taken from a table of the t-distribution with $(n_1 + n_2 - 2)$ degrees of freedom.

For example, suppose erythrocyte sedimentation rates (ESRs) were measured in an intervention group and in a control group, as shown in Table 14.4.

The standard deviation s may be calculated as $\sqrt{\{[(9 \times 2.41^2) + (11 \times 2.54^2)]/(10 + 12 - 2)\}} = 2.48$, and the 95 per cent confidence interval on the difference is given by:

$$(9.7 - 6.5) \pm \{(2.09 \times 2.48)\sqrt{[(1/10) + (1/12)]}\} = 3.2 \pm 2.2$$
$$= 1.0\text{–}5.4.$$

To test the null hypothesis that there is no true difference in the mean ESRs between the two groups a test of statistical significance must be performed. A test statistic is calculated to assess the statistical significance of the difference. The difference of the means divided by the standard error of the difference gives a value of a test statistic that may be looked up in tables of the t-distribution with $(n_1 + n_2 - 2)$ degrees of freedom. For the

Table 14.4. Erythrocyte sedimentation rates (ESRs) in an intervention and in a control group

	Intervention group ($i = 1$)	Control group ($i = 2$)
No. of subjects (n_i)	10	12
Mean ESR ($\bar{x}_i$)	9.7	6.5
Standard deviation (s_i)	2.41	2.54

example above the test statistic $= (\bar{x}_1 - \bar{x}_2)/\{s\sqrt{[(1/n_1) + (1/n_2)]}\} = 3.01$. As this value is higher than the tabulated critical value of t at 1 per cent (with 20 degrees of freedom) of 2.85, it may be concluded that the mean ESR in the intervention group is significantly higher than that in the control group at the 1 per cent level of significance ($p < 0.01$); i.e. if there really is no effect of the intervention on ESRs the chance of observing a difference in means as large or larger than that in the study is less than 1 per cent (i.e. not impossible, but rather unlikely!).

4.3 Analysis of more than two groups

If a study involves the comparison of observations in more than two groups it is necessary to generalize the methods given in Section 4.2. This is straightforward, but is beyond the scope of this manual and the reader is referred to standard statistical texts, such as that by Armitage and Berry (1987), for details. The relevant sections to which to refer are those on 'one-way analysis of variance'.

Of course, it is always possible to use the methods given in Section 4.2 to compare groups just two at a time. This is a reasonable approach but some caution must be exercised when interpreting the findings as the chances of finding at least one pair to be significantly different may be substantial even if there are, in truth, no differences between the groups. To illustrate this, suppose 6 groups are being compared. In an analysis of variance, the question is asked: 'considered as a whole, is the variation between the means observed in the six groups more than might be expected to arise by chance if there were no differences in the true means?'. This question may be answered with one statistical test in an analysis of variance and the null hypothesis may, or may not, be rejected on the basis of this one test. Suppose, however, it was decided to examine all possible pairs of comparisons of the groups. There are 15 possible pairs and if a *t*-test was done on each pair there is a reasonable chance that at least one comparison would be found to be 'statistically significant' by chance alone, because of the number of different tests that had been performed. There are ways of adjusting the significance levels to allow for this effect and the reader is referred to standard texts again for a discussion of 'the multiple comparison problem'.

5 ANALYSIS OF RATES

5.1 Risks, rates and person-time-at-risk

The terms 'risk' and 'rate' are often used rather loosely and interchangeably to describe the frequencies of events in epidemiological studies. Usually this is of no great consequence, but in some circumstances the distinction is important and, in particular, may affect the way in which a study is analysed. A *risk* is essentially a proportion or, equivalently, a probability. The numerator consists of the number of individuals who experience the event of interest (say, develop disease) in a defined period. The denominator consists of the total number of individuals who were followed for the defined period, some of whom experienced the event of interest (for example, developed the disease) and the remainder of whom did not (ignoring for the moment complications that might arise if some individuals are lost to follow-up). A *rate* takes into account both the number of persons at risk and also the duration of observation for each person. In the simplest case, the numerator is the number of individuals who experience the event of interest during the study period (i.e. the same as the numerator for a risk) but the denominator is expressed as the number of person-years (or person-months, and so on) at risk for the individuals in the study. For example, if 120 persons are observed for 3 years and 40 of them die at some time during the period, the *risk* of death over the three years is estimated as $40/120 = 0.33$, whereas the death *rate* is estimated as $40/$(the number of person-years-at-risk). The denominator for the rate calculation is $(80 \times 3) + (40 \times 1.5) = 300$

years, as 80 persons were 'at risk' for the full 3-year period and 40 were at risk until they died (which, on average, is likely to have been about half way through the follow-up period if deaths occurred uniformly over the period). Thus, the death rate is $40/300 = 0.133$ per person-year-at-risk (which is not the same as the risk of death during the three years of 0.33 divided by 3).

Mathematically, it is straightforward to convert rates to risks and vice versa, if it may be assumed that the rates are constant over time (see, for example, Breslow and Day 1980). The reason for discussing the distinction in this chapter is that different methods of statistical analysis are appropriate for risks and rates. As mentioned above, risks are proportions and thus the methods described in Section 3 are applicable. Modifications of these methods for the analysis of rates are discussed below.

Rates are useful if different individuals in a study have been followed for different periods. This may arise if recruitment to the study population is staggered over time but follow-up is to a common date, or if individuals are lost to follow-up at different times (for example, because of death, migration, or non-cooperation).

An example of the computation of person-years-at-risk in a large study is given in Table 14.5. In this study a census was done of the study population on the 1st November each year and the number of persons remaining at risk was ascertained.

Alternatively, the exact period of follow-up may be known for each subject in the study (if the dates of entry and exit are available for each person); in which case these periods would be summed to derive the total person-years-at-risk.

Another situation in which rates, rather than risks, may be more appropriate is when each individual may be at risk of experiencing the event of interest more than once during the study period (for example, an episode of diarrhoea). The incidence rate in the study population would be calculated as the total number of events (for example, episodes of diarrhoea) for those in the study divided by the total person-years-at-risk (which, in this case, would not end at the first episode). Responses such as this can always be converted to a risk by expressing the outcome as the proportion of individuals who experience more than a specified number of events (for example, one or more episodes of diarrhoea), but in doing this some information may be lost, with a consequent reduction in the power of the study to detect a difference between groups being

Table 14.5. Example of the computation of person-years-at-risk in a large study

	Date (a)	No. of persons under observation (b)	Average of successive numbers (c)	Years of observation (d)	Person-years (c × d)
Start date	1.11.1984	10140			
	1.11.1985	9145	9642.5*	1	9642.5
	1.11.1986	8232	8688.5	1	8688.5
	1.11.1987	7389	7810.5	1	7810.5
	1.11.1988	6281	6835.0	1	6835.0
End date	1. 4.1989	5779	6030.0	5/12	2512.5
				Total	35489.0

* If 10140 persons were alive on 1.11.84 and 9145 of them were known to be alive on 1.11.85 and if losses to follow-up occurred evenly throughout the year, there would have been, on average, (10140 + 9145)/2 = 9642.5 persons at risk on each day during the first year, hence a total of 9642.5 person-years.

compared. The analysis of rate data of this kind is not straightforward as the approach depends upon whether it is reasonable to assume that once an individual has experienced one event he or she is no more or less likely to experience another event than anyone else in the same intervention group (say, of the same age and sex). Usually it is not reasonable to make this assumption as it is frequently found that susceptibility to disease varies considerably between individuals in ways that cannot be predicted. A simple way out of the analytical problem is to use the approach suggested above, and to classify individuals according to whether or not they experienced any events or not. If this is done, the data can either be analysed as a proportion (using the methods given in Section 3) or the individual can be excluded from follow-up, for purposes of analysis, from the time the *first* event occurs (i.e. they are not counted as 'at risk' after the first event) and the methods given below can be used.

5.2 Confidence interval for a rate

Suppose e is the number of events that occurred during the study period and the total person-years-at-risk during the period was y.

(Note that the period does not have to be measured in 'years'; it could be in, for example, days, weeks, or months.) The event rate (r) is estimated by e/y. For example, suppose 5000 patients who have received a new anti-leprosy vaccine have been followed for 5 years, but due to losses in follow-up, the total person-years-at-risk is 20 000 [instead of the nearly 25 000 that would have been appropriate if every patient (except the cases, whose follow-up period would be counted up to the time they developed leprosy) had been followed up throughout the 5 years]. If the number of new cases of leprosy that were detected during the follow-up was 80, the estimated incidence rate of leprosy would be $80/20\,000 = 0.0040$/person-year i.e. 4 per thousand person-years.

The standard error of a rate (r) is $\sqrt{(r/y)}$ and the approximate 95 per cent confidence interval for the rate is given by $r \pm 1.96\sqrt{(r/y)}$. Thus, in the example given above, the 95 per cent confidence interval for the leprosy incidence rate is $0.0040 \pm 1.96\sqrt{(0.0040/20\,000)} = 0.0040 \pm 0.0009$ i.e. 3.1–4.9 per thousand person-years.

5.3 Difference between two rates

Suppose it is required to compare event rates in two groups and the numbers of events and the person-years-at-risk in the two groups are as in Table 14.6.

The standard error of the difference between two rates is given by: $\sqrt{[(r_1/y_1 + r_2/y_2)]}$ and the 95 per cent confidence interval on the difference is given by: $(r_1 - r_2) \pm 1.96\sqrt{(r_1/y_1 + r_2/y_2)}$.

Thus, for the example, the 95 per cent confidence interval on the rate difference is: $(0.0041 - 0.0084) \pm 1.96\sqrt{[(0.0041/19470) +}$

Table 14.6. Leprosy incidence rates in vaccinated and unvaccinated groups

	No. of events (new leprosy cases)	Person-years at-risk (pyar)	Event rate (leprosy cases per 1000 pyar)
Vaccinated	e_1 (80)	y_1 (19 470)	r_1 (4.1)
Not vaccinated	e_2 (160)	y_2 (19 030)	r_2 (8.4)
Total	e (240)	y (38 500)	r

$(0.0084/19030)] = -0.0043 \pm 0.0016 = -0.0059$ to -0.0027 i.e.
-5.9 to $-2.7/1000$/year

To determine the level of statistical significance it is necessary to calculate a test statistic, which may be done along similar lines to those described in Section 3.2. If e_1 is the observed number of events among those in group 1, then:

$$\text{Expected value of } e_1 = E(e_1) = ey_1/y \qquad (14.7)$$

$$\text{Variance of } e_1 = V(e_1) = ey_1y_2/y^2 \qquad (14.8)$$

$$\text{Then } \chi^2 = (|e_1 - E(e_1)| - 0.5)^2/V(e_1) \qquad (14.9)$$

and the value of chi-squared is looked up in tables of the chi-squared distribution, with one degree of freedom, to assess the statistical significance.

In the example shown in Table 14.6 $e_1 = 80$; $E(e_1) = 240 \times 19470/38500 = 121.37$, and $V(e_1) = (240 \times 19470 \times 19030)/(38500 \times 38500) = 59.99$.

Thus, $\chi^2 = (|80 - 121.37| - 0.5)^2/59.99 = 27.84$ and $p < 0.000001$; a very highly significant difference.

5.4 Ratio of two rates

In some situations, the *ratio* of two rates will be of greater interest than their *difference*. For example, vaccine efficacy is usually calculated from a ratio. The test of the null hypothesis is identical in the two situations (i.e. that the difference is zero or that the ratio is unity), but the confidence intervals are calculated in a different way.

The ratio of two rates, sometimes called the relative risk, but more correctly called the relative rate, is $(e_1/y_1)/(e_2/y_2)$ and the standard error of the logarithm of this ratio is approximated by $\sqrt{[(1/e_1) + (1/e_2)]}$. In the example given in Table 14.6 the ratio of the rates is 0.489 and the standard error of the logarithm of the ratio is $\sqrt{[(1/80) + (1/160)]} = 0.1369$. The 95 per cent confidence interval of the logarithm of the ratio is given by $-0.715 \pm 1.96(0.1369)$, i.e. -0.983 to -0.447. Thus, the 95 per cent confidence interval for the ratio of the two rates is 0.37–0.64 [or the 95 per cent confidence interval on the estimate of vaccine efficacy is from 36 per cent to 63 per cent, i.e. $100(1 - 0.64)$ to $100(1 - 0.37)$].

5.5 Trend test for rates

Directly analogous to the trend test for proportions described in Section 3.4, a similar test exists to test for a trend in rates. Suppose data have been collected on the time since the start of a study to the first attack of malaria among children of different ages, and it is of interest to test whether the attack rate declines with age. The data may be summarized as in Table 14.7.

Table 14.7. Malaria attack rates in children of different ages

Age of children (years)	'Score' x_i	No. with malaria attack	Child-weeks-at-risk	Attack rate e_i/y_i
1–2	x_1 ($= 2.0$)	e_1 (30)	y_1 (200)	0.150
3–4	x_2 ($= 4.0$)	e_2 (20)	y_2 (150)	0.133
5–7	x_3 ($= 6.5$)	e_3 (10)	y_3 (150)	0.067
Total		e (60)	y (500)	0.120

A 'score' has been assigned to each group. In the example the scores have been taken as the mid-points of the different age groups (for example, those aged 1 to 2 years range in age from 1.00 to 2.99 years).

A test for trend in the attack rates in the three age groups e_1/y_1, e_2/y_2 and e_3/y_3 is provided by testing, as chi-squared with 1 degree of freedom, the expression:

$$\chi^2 = \{[\Sigma e_i x_i - [(e/y)\Sigma y_i x_i]\}^2 / \{(e/y^2)[y\Sigma y_i x_i^2 - (\Sigma y_i x_i)^2]\}} \tag{14.10}$$

For example, suppose the malaria attack rates (attacks/weeks-at-risk) were 30/200, 20/150 and 10/150 in the three age groups, respectively, as in Table 14.7, then the value of χ^2 is $\{205 - [(60/500)1975]\}^2 / \{(60/500^2)[(500 \times 9537.5) - 1975^2]\} = 4.91$, which is significant at the 5 per cent level ($p < 0.05$) and thus there are grounds for believing that in the study area the risk of a malaria attack declined with increasing age.

6 CONTROLLING FOR CONFOUNDING VARIABLES

6.1 The nature of confounding variables

A risk factor for the disease under study that is differentially distributed among the groups receiving different interventions in which disease incidence is being compared is called a *confounding* factor. Unless the trial is very small, confounding factors are not likely to bias the comparisons between intervention and control groups in randomized trials as the process of randomization ensures that any such factors, whether known or unknown, will be equally distributed in the different groups (apart from random variation). In studies in which those in the different groups have not been allocated at random, the control of confounding factors is a critical component in the analysis. For example, consider a comparative study of tuberculosis incidence in persons who received BCG in a routine vaccination programme and those who were not vaccinated. BCG coverage is often higher in urban areas and, independently of any effect of BCG, those living in urban areas also tend to have a higher incidence of tuberculosis (TB) because of over-crowding and other environmental factors. In this instance, residential status (rural/urban) could be a confounding factor and, if it is not taken into account in the analyses, any protective effect of BCG against TB might be underestimated. Consider the hypothetical situation depicted in the Table 14.8, which shows the incidence of TB over a ten-year period in BCG-vaccinated and unvaccinated individuals in urban and rural areas.

BCG coverage is appreciably higher in the urban population (80 per cent) than in the rural population (50 per cent). Also, in unvaccinated persons, the incidence of TB is higher in the urban population (20 per thousand over 10 years) than in the rural population (10 per thousand). In consequence, although BCG vaccine efficacy is 50 per cent in both urban and rural areas, the estimate obtained from a comparative study in which place of residence is ignored is only 41 per cent. This difference is due to the confounding effect of place of residence on the estimate of efficacy (place of residence being related to both disease incidence and, independently, to the prevalence of vaccination).

Table 14.8. Tuberculosis incidence rates by BCG vaccination status and urban or rural residence

BCG vaccination status	Urban			Rural			Both groups		
	Total Popn.	TB cases* No.	/1000	Total Popn.	TB cases* No.	/1000	Total Popn.	TB cases* No.	/1000
Vaccinated	16 000	160	10	40 000	200	5	56 000	360	6.4
Unvaccinated	4000	80	20	40 000	400	10	44 000	480	10.9
Vaccine efficacy		50%			50%				41%

* over a period of 10 years.

6.2 Adjusting for confounding variables

A powerful way of removing the effect of a confounding variable is to restrict comparative analyses to individuals who share a common level of the confounding variable and then to combine the results across the different levels in such a way so as to avoid bias. Thus, in the example above, if the vaccine efficacy was first estimated separately for rural and urban dwellers and then the two estimates were to be combined, the estimate of efficacy obtained (50 per cent) would be free of the confounding bias of place of residence. In general, the study population is divided into a number of *strata*. Within each stratum individuals share a common level of the confounding variable. Estimates of risk, mean or rate differences, or ratios, are made within each stratum and the resulting estimates are then *pooled* in some way across strata in order to obtain an overall measure of effect which is free of any confounding due to the variable on which the stratification was made. Such stratification may be carried out on several confounding variables simultaneously (for example, age and sex).

If it is known when a study is planned that it will be necessary to allow for confounding variables in the analysis, it is desirable to give consideration to this at the design stage, both in terms of the information which must be collected and because it will require an increase in the required sample sizes (to achieve the desired statistical power, see Chapter 3). Usually the necessary increase in sample size to allow for confounding variables is not great (for example, less than 20 per cent) and often the information needed for these sample size calculations is not available before the study starts anyway. Formal methods for calculating sample sizes, allowing for adjustment for confounding variables, are given in Breslow and Day (1987).

6.3 Adjusting risks

6.3.1 Overall test of significance

After stratifying on the basis of the confounding variable(s), the analysis is conducted one stratum at a time and then the results are pooled. In the ith stratum the data may be depicted as shown in Table 14.9.

Table 14.9. Comparison of proportions developing disease in two intervention groups for individuals in ith stratum

Intervention Group	Developed disease	Did not develop disease	Total
1	a_i	b_i	$a_i + b_i = n_{1i}$
2	c_i	d_i	$c_i + d_i = n_{2i}$
Total	$a_i + c_i = m_{1i}$	$b_i + d_i = m_{2i}$	N_i

To test the hypothesis that the relative risk is 1 in all strata or, equivalently, that the risk difference is zero in each stratum, a generalization of the method given in Section 3.2 may be used. The statistical test is known as the Mantel–Haenszel test.

In the ith stratum:

Expected value of $a_i = E(a_i) = m_{1i}n_{1i}/N_i$ $\quad\quad\quad$ (14.11)

Variance of $a_i = V(a_i) = n_{1i}n_{2i}m_{1i}m_{2i}/[N_i^2(N_i - 1)]$ $\quad\quad$ (14.12)

An overall test of the null hypothesis that the relative risk is unity is given by calculating $\chi^2 = (|\Sigma a_i - \Sigma E(a_i)| - 0.5)^2/\Sigma V(a_i)$, where the summation is over all strata, which may be tested for statistical significance using tables of the chi-squared distribution with one degree of freedom.

The calculations are illustrated in Table 14.10 with data on

Table 14.10. Disease incidence rates in urban, semi-urban, and rural areas according to vaccination status

Area (i)	Vaccinated			Unvaccinated			Grand total (N_i)	$E(a_i)$	$V(a_i)$
	Cases (a_i)	Non-cases (b_i)	Total (n_{1i})	Cases (c_i)	Non-cases (d_i)	Total (n_{2i})			
1. (Urban)	160	15 840	16 000	80	3 920	4 000	20 000	192	37.94
2. (Semi-urban)	170	23 830	24 000	240	15 760	16 000	40 000	246	97.39
3. (Rural)	200	39 800	40 000	400	39 600	40 000	80 000	300	148.88
Total	530	79 470	80 000	720	59 280	60 000	140 000	738	284.21

disease incidence rates in vaccinated and unvaccinated individuals in 3 areas; urban, semi-urban, and rural.

$\Sigma a_i = 530$; $\Sigma E(a_i) = 738$; $\Sigma V(a_i) = 284.21$;
Thus, $\chi^2 = (|530 - 738| - 0.5)^2/284.21 = 151.49$

Thus, there is very strong evidence against the null hypothesis as $p < 0.000001$ (from tables of the chi-squared distribution).

6.3.2 Pooled estimate of risk difference

If it is considered that the risk *difference* (rather than the risk ratio) is likely to be constant across different strata, a pooled estimate of the common risk difference may be required. This may be obtained by taking a weighted average of the risk differences in each stratum, weighting each by the inverse of its variance (as this may be shown to give the 'best' estimate of the common risk difference).

In the ith stratum the risk difference is

$d_i = p_{1i} - p_{2i} = (a_i/n_{1i}) - (c_i/n_{2i})$

and the variance of the risk difference is

$V(d_i) = \{p_i(1 - p_i)[(1/n_{1i}) + (1/n_{2i})]\}$ (as given also in Section 3.2), where
$p_i = [n_{1i}p_{1i} + n_{2i}p_{2i}]/(n_{1i} + n_{2i}) = (a_i + c_i)/(n_{1i} + n_{2i})$.

Now, let $w_i = 1/V(d_i)$

The pooled estimate of the common risk difference is given by $d = \Sigma w_i d_i/\Sigma w_i$. For the data in the example given in Table 14.10 the computations for the common risk difference are shown in Table 14.11.

Table 14.11. Computation of the common risk difference for the data in Table 14.10

Area	p_{1i}	p_{2i}	d_i	$V(d_i)$	w_i
Urban	0.0100	0.0200	−0.0100	3.705×10^{-6}	270×10^3
Semi-urban	0.0071	0.0150	−0.0079	1.057×10^{-6}	946×10^3
Rural	0.0050	0.0100	−0.0050	37.219×10^{-6}	27×10^3

$d = \Sigma w_i d_i/\Sigma w_i = -0.0083$

6.3.3 Pooled estimate of risk ratio

A pooled estimate of the common risk ratio, R, across strata, may be obtained using the following formulae.

In the ith stratum the risk ratio is given by

$$R_i = (a_i/n_{1i})/(c_i/n_{2i}) = a_i n_{2i}/(c_i n_{1i}). \qquad (14.13)$$

A pooled estimate across all strata is given by

$$R = \Sigma(a_i n_{2i}/N_i)/[\Sigma(c_i n_{1i}/N_i)]$$

Thus, for the example in Table 14.10

$$R = \frac{[(160)(4000)/20000] + [(170)(16000)/40000] + [(200)(40000)/80000]}{[(80)(16000)/20000] + [(240)(24000)/40000] + [(400)(40000)/80000]}$$

$$= 200/408 = 0.49$$

6.3.4 Confidence Intervals

The easiest way of obtaining confidence intervals on the estimates of the common risk difference or the common relative risk is to use the 'test based' method (Miettinen 1976).

The approximate 95 per cent confidence interval on the risk difference is given by

$$d\,(1 \pm 1.96/\sqrt{\chi^2}) \qquad (14.15)$$

Thus, in the example in Tables 14.10 and 14.11 the confidence limits are

$$-0.0083(1 \pm 1.96/\sqrt{151.49}) = -0.0096 \text{ to } -0.0070.$$

The 95 per cent confidence interval on the logarithm of the relative risk is given by

$$\log_e R\,(1 \pm 1.96/\sqrt{\chi^2}) \qquad (14.16)$$

In the example, the confidence limits are

$$\log_e(0.49)\,(1 \pm 1.96/\sqrt{151.49}) = -0.8269 \text{ to } -0.5998$$

and thus the confidence limits on the relative risk are 0.44 to 0.55.

6.4 Adjusting rates

The computations for adjusting rates are very similar to those for adjusting risks and involve only some changes to the formulae given in Section 6.3.

Suppose the results observed in the ith stratum are as shown in Table 14.12.

Table 14.12. Disease rates in two intervention groups for individuals in the i th stratum

Intervention group	Developed disease	Person-years-at-risk
1	e_{1i}	y_{1i}
2	e_{2i}	y_{2i}
Total	e_i	y_i

6.4.1 Overall test of significance

In the ith stratum e_{1i} is the number of individuals who developed disease in group 1.

$$\text{Expected value of } e_{1i} = E(e_{1i}) = e_i y_{1i}/y_i \tag{14.17}$$

$$\text{Variance of } e_{1i} = V(e_{1i}) = e_i y_{1i} y_{2i}/y_i^2 \tag{14.18}$$

An overall test of significance (that the common rate ratio is unity, or the common rate difference is zero) is given by:

$$\chi^2 = (|\Sigma e_{1i} - \Sigma E(e_{1i})| - 0.5)^2/\Sigma V(e_{1i}) \tag{14.19}$$

where the summation is over all strata. The value calculated should be looked up in tables of the chi-squared distribution with one degree of freedom.

6.4.2 Pooled estimate of rate difference

In the ith stratum the rate difference is

$$d_i = r_{1i} - r_{2i} = (e_{1i}/y_{1i}) - (e_{2i}/y_{2i})$$

and its estimated variance, $V(d_i)$, is $(r_{1i}/y_{1i} + r_{2i}/y_{2i})$. Let $w_i = 1/V(d_i)$, then the estimate of the common rate difference across all strata is given by: $d = \Sigma w_i d_i / \Sigma w_i$

6.4.3 Pooled estimate of rate ratio

In the ith stratum the rate ratio is

$$R_i = r_{1i}/r_{2i} = (e_{1i}/y_{1i})/(e_{2i}/y_{2i})$$
$$= e_{1i}y_{2i}/e_{2i}y_{1i}$$

and a pooled estimate of the common rate ratio is given by:

$$R = \Sigma(e_{1i}y_{2i}/y_i)/\Sigma(e_{2i}y_{1i}/y_i) \tag{14.20}$$

6.4.4 Confidence intervals

The 95 per cent confidence interval on the common rate difference is given by:

$$d(1 \pm 1.96/\sqrt{\chi^2}) \tag{14.21}$$

and, on the logarithm of the common rate ratio, is given by:

$$\log_e(R)(1 \pm 1.96/\sqrt{\chi^2}) \tag{14.22}$$

Example: In Table 14.13 the numerical computations are illustrated, as before, with data on disease incidence in vaccinated and unvaccinated individuals in 3 areas; urban, semi-urban, and rural.

Overall test of significance:

$$\chi^2 = (|\Sigma e_{1i} - \Sigma E(e_{1i})| - 0.5)^2/\Sigma V(e_{1i}) \tag{14.23}$$
$$= (|245 - 359| - 0.5)^2/138.40 = 93.08 \; (p < 0.000001)$$

The estimation of the common rate difference is shown in Table 14.14.

95 per cent confidence interval on the common rate difference

$$= d(1 \pm 1.96/\sqrt{\chi^2})$$
$$= -0.0066(1 \pm 1.96/\sqrt{93.08}) \tag{14.24}$$
$$= -0.0079 \text{ to } -0.0053$$

Estimate of common rate ratio

$$R = \Sigma(e_{1i}y_{2i}/y_i)/\Sigma(e_{2i}y_{1i}/y_i)$$
$$= \frac{[(80)(2000)/10000] + [(85)(8000)/20000] + [(80)(20000)/40000]}{[(40)(8000)/10000] + [(120)(12000)/20000] + [(200)(20000)/40000]}$$
$$= 90/204 = 0.44$$

Table 14.13. Disease incidence rates in urban, semi-urban, and rural areas according to vaccination status

Area (i)	Vaccinated		Unvaccinated		Both groups			
	Cases (e_{1i})	Person-years (y_{1i})	Cases (e_{2i})	Person-years (y_{2i})	Cases (e_i)	Person-years (y_i)	$E(e_{1i})$	$V(e_{1i})$
1 (Urban)	80	8 000	40	2 000	120	10 000	96	19.2
2 (Semi-urban)	85	12 000	120	8 000	205	20 000	123	49.2
3 (Rural)	80	20 000	200	20 000	280	40 000	140	70.0
Total	245	40 000	360	30 000	605	70 000	359	138.4

Table 14.14. Computation of the common rate difference for the data in Table 14.13

Area	r_{1i}	r_{2i}	difference d_i	$V(d_i)$	$w_i = 1/V(d_i)$
1 (Urban)	0.0100	0.0200	-0.0100	11.250×10^{-6}	89×10^3
2 (Semi-urban)	0.0071	0.0150	-0.0079	2.465×10^{-6}	406×10^3
3 (Rural)	0.0040	0.0100	-0.0060	0.700×10^{-6}	1429×10^3

$d = \Sigma w_i d_i / \Sigma w_i = -0.0066$

95 per cent confidence limits on the logarithm of the common rate ratio

$$= \log_e(R)(1 \pm 1.96/\sqrt{\chi^2}) = \log_e(0.44)(1 \pm 1.96/\sqrt{93.08})$$

$$= -0.988 \text{ to } -0.654$$

and, taking antilogarithm, 95 per cent confidence limits on the common rate ratio are 0.37 to 0.52.

6.5 Adjusting means

If the outcome variable is a quantitative measure other than a risk or a rate, adjustment for the effects of a confounding variable involves performing a stratified t-test.

A numerical example is given in Table 14.15, where the comparison is between subjects using mosquito nets (intervention group) and those not using them (control group), and the outcome measure (x) is the number of episodes of malaria over a period of one year. In this example, age is considered as the confounding variable and the stratification has been made by dividing the study subjects into 3 age-groups. The size of each subgroup has been made small to simplify the computations for illustrative purposes.

The data may be represented, algebraically, for those in the ith stratum as shown in Table 14.16.

An estimate of the common difference in response between the intervention and control group is obtained calculating a weighed average of the differences within each stratum: by $d = \Sigma w_i d_i / \Sigma w_i$, where $w_i = [n_{1i} n_{2i}/(n_{1i} + n_{2i})]$.

Table 14.15. Attacks of malaria in children of different ages in those using (intervention) and not using (control) mosquito nets

(Stratum) Age group		Attacks of malaria/child (x)	No. of children n	Mean $\bar{x}$	Standard deviation s
(1) <2y	I*	1,0,2,3,1,2,1,0	8	1.25	1.0351
	C	2,3,1,2	4	2.00	0.8165
(2) 2–3y	I	0,1,1,2,1,1,0,2,2,1,1,0	12	1.00	0.7385
	C	2,2,1,1,1,2,1,1,2,2,1	11	1.45	0.5222
(3) 4–5y	I	1,0,1,1,1	5	0.80	0.4472
	C	1,1,2,0,1,1,0,2,1,1	10	1.00	0.6667

* I = intervention group, C = control group

Table 14.16. Algebraic representation of data in Table 14.15 for those in the ith stratum

Intervention group	No. in group	Mean	Standard deviation
1 (I)	n_{1i}	$\bar{x}_{1i}$	s_{1i}
2(C)	n_{2i}	$\bar{x}_{2i}$	s_{2i}

Difference $d_i = \bar{x}_{1i} - \bar{x}_{2i}$

Thus, in the example:

$$d = \frac{[(-0.75)32/12] + [(-0.45)132/23] + [(-0.20)50/15]}{(32/12) + (132/23) + (50/15)}$$

$$= -5.25/11.74 = -0.45$$

An overall test of significance is obtained by calculating a test statistic $= \Sigma w_i d_i/[s\sqrt{\Sigma(w_i)}]$
where $s = \sqrt{\{[\Sigma(n_{1i} - 1)s_{1i}^2 + \Sigma(n_{2i} - 1)s_{2i}^2]/\Sigma(n_{1i} + n_{2i} - 2)\}}$
and the value of the test statistic can be compared with tables of the t-distribution with $\Sigma(n_{1i} + n_{2i} - 2)$ degrees of freedom.

In the example, $s = \sqrt{(23.0265/44)} = 0.7234$
The test statistic (44df) $= -5.25/[0.7234 \times \sqrt{(11.74)}]$
$= -2.12$

The absolute value is larger than 2.02, which is the tabulated 5 per cent value for t with 44 degrees of freedom. Thus, there is statistically significant evidence regarding the efficacy of intervention; the reduction in the average number of episodes of malaria is estimated as 0.45 per child per year. 95 per cent confidence limits on the difference are given by:

$$(\Sigma w_i d_i / \Sigma w_i) \pm ts / \sqrt{\Sigma w_i} \qquad (14.26)$$

where t is taken from tables of the t distribution for 95 per cent confidence limits with $\Sigma(n_{1i} + n_{2i} - 2)$ df.

Thus 95 per cent confidence limits are: $-0.45 \pm 2.02\,(0.7234)/\sqrt{(11.74)}$

$$= -0.88 \text{ to } -0.02 \text{ episodes/year/child.}$$

If it is thought that the intervention is likely to affect the response measured in a *relative* rather than an *absolute* fashion (i.e. a constant percentage reduction in the number of malaria attacks rather than a constant absolute reduction in the number of malaria attacks) then it would be appropriate to *transform* the data initially by taking logarithms of the number of attacks [or, say, $\log_e$ (number of attacks + 0.1) to avoid zero numbers] and to perform the calculation detailed above on the transformed values.

7 ANALYSES WHEN COMMUNITIES HAVE BEEN RANDOMIZED

In some intervention studies, communities rather than individuals are used as the unit of randomization. If this has been done it is inappropriate to base analyses on responses of individuals, ignoring the fact that randomization was over larger units.

The appropriate method of analysis would be to summarize the response in each sampling unit by a single value, and analyse these summary values as though they were individual values; i.e. the statistical test should be based on the variation between the community summary values, and not on the variation between individuals.

7.1 Calculation of standardized responses

Often, trials in which communities have been randomized suffer

problems with confounding variables. If the number of units randomized is large, confounding variables are likely to balance out
between groups, but if the number of units is small (as may be the
case when communities have been randomized, even though the
number of individuals in each community is large), confounding
may be a potentially serious problem and some adjustment should
be made in the analysis. One method of doing this is by *standardization*.

Within each community, the sampled population is divided into
strata on the basis of the confounding variable(s) (for example,
age and sex groups). The average value of the outcome measure is
computed for those in each stratum (for example, a disease incidence rate). A weighted average of the rates in the different strata
is then computed to give a single 'standardized' measure for the
community; the weights being based on some 'standard' population. The same standard population is used for each community
and thus the standardized measures for each community are not
biased by the differential composition of each community with
respect to the confounding variable that is being standardized for.

The method outlined above is called the 'direct' method of
standardization. If the number of individuals in some strata is
small it may be better to use the 'indirect' method and details of
both are given below—see Armitage and Berry (1987) for a more
detailed discussion of these methods.

Consider a community in which disease risks, p_i, have been
measured for individuals in k strata (for example, age groups).
This may be represented in Table 14.17. Also shown are the
corresponding data for a 'standard' population. For example, this
might be chosen as the combined data for all communities in the
study.

The *directly standardized* disease risk for the community (standardized to the standard population) is given by: $(\Sigma p_i N_i)/\Sigma N_i$

The *indirectly standardized* disease risk for the community is
given by: $[\Sigma a_i/(\Sigma n_i P_i)](A/N)$

Having calculated standardized values for each community the
means of the standardized values for the intervention communities
may be compared with those for the control communities using a
simple t-test (Section 4.2).

It is usually safer, however, to perform a non-parametric test if
the assumptions underlying the t-test are in any doubt (see Armi-

Table 14.17. Disease risks in study community and in standard
population in each of k strata

Stratum	Study community			Standard population		
	Total	Cases		Total	Cases	
		No.	Risk		No.	Risk
1	n_1	a_1	p_1	N_1	A_1	P_1
2	n_2	a_2	p_2	N_2	A_2	P_2
i	n_i	a_i	p_i	N_i	A_i	P_i
.						
.						
k	n_k	a_k	p_k	N_k	A_k	P_k
Total	n	a	p	N	A	P

tage and Berry 1987), as it may be impossible to verify the
assumptions if the study involves a small number of communities.

7.2 Non-parametric rank sum test

Suppose there are n_1 communities in one group and n_2 in the other
($n_1 \leq n_2$) and a summary response has been derived for each community. To perform a non-parametric test, consider all the ($n_1 +
n_2$) observations together, and rank them, giving a rank of 1 to the
smallest value and ($n_1 + n_2$) to the highest. Tied ranks are allotted
the mid-rank of the group. Let T_1 = sum of the ranks in group 1
with n_1 observations. Under the null hypothesis the expectation
of $T_1 = n_1(n_1 + n_2 + 1)/2$. Then calculate:

$T^1 = T_1$; if T_1 is less than or equal to the expected value
  $= n_1(n_1 + n_2 + 1) - T_1$; if T_1 is more than its expected value.

T^1 may be compared with tabulated critical values (see Table A8
of Armitage and Berry 1987) to determine statistical significance.

Consider the example shown in Table 14.18 in which age-
standardized leprosy prevalence rates are compared in 12 'intervention' villages and 10 'control' villages.

The expected value of $T_1 = n_1(n_1 + n_2 + 1)/2 = 10(10 + 12 + 1)/
2 = 115$. As T_1 is greater than its expectation, T^1 is

Table 14.18. Age-standardized leprosy prevalence rates and ranks in 12 'intervention' and 10 'control' villages

Intervention villages		Control villages	
Prevalence rate/1000	Rank	Prevalence rate/1000	Rank
3	1.5	10	18.5
9	15.5	13	22
8	12.5	6	7.5
6	7.5	11	21
5	5	10	18.5
5	5	7	9.5
7	9.5	8	12.5
3	1.5	8	12.5
10	18.5	5	5
8	12.5	9	15.5
10	18.5		
4	3		
Sum of ranks $T_2 = 110.5$		$T_1 = 142.5$	

$10(10 + 12 + 1) - 142.5 = 87.5$. The critical value of T^1 at the 5 per cent level of significance is 84 (from tables in Armitage and Berry 1987). As T^1 is greater than the critical value, it is concluded that the intervention has not had a statistically significant effect (the average prevalence was 6.5 per thousand in intervention villages and 8.7 per thousand in control villages).

7.3 Tests on paired data

In some study designs, communities may be 'paired' on the basis of similarity with respect to confounding variables and baseline disease prevalence or incidence rates. Within each pair of communities, one receives the intervention and the other serves as the control. If this has been done, the analysis should take the pairing into account.

First, standardized response rates are computed for each community (as discussed in Section 7.1) and then the standardized response rates are compared using a paired t-test (Armitage and Berry 1987) or a non-parametric test.

To perform a paired t-test for n pairs of communities, suppose d_i is the difference in outcome measured between the intervention and control unit for the ith pair. Calculate a test statistic $= (\Sigma d_i/n)/(s/\sqrt{n})$ where s is the standard deviation of the n differences. This value of the test statistic may be compared to tabulated values of the t-distribution with $(n-1)$ degrees of freedom.

Consider the data shown in Table 14.19, which shows leprosy prevalence rates in 10 pairs of communities.

Table 14.19. Leprosy prevalence rates in ten pairs of communities

Village pair no.	Prevalence of leprosy (per thousand)		Difference (d_i)	Rank (ignoring sign)
	Intervention	No Intervention		
1	6	10	− 4	8
2	9	13	− 4	8
3	3	6	− 3	5
4	12	11	+1	1.5
5	10	10	0	
6	4	7	− 3	5
7	7	8	− 1	1.5
8	5	8	− 3	5
9	7	5	+2	3
10	5	9	− 4	8

The mean difference $d = -19/10 = -1.9$ and the standard deviation of the difference (s) is 2.23. Thus the test statistic $= -1.9/(2.23/\sqrt{10}) = -2.69$ with 9 degrees of freedom. From tables of the t-distribution, $p < 0.05$ and it may be concluded that the prevalence of leprosy is significantly lower in the intervention villages.

Alternatively, a non-parametric test may be preferred. In this instance the appropriate such test is Wilcoxon's signed rank test.

The differences between each pair of villages are arranged in ascending order of magnitude of the absolute value of the differences (i.e. ignoring the sign) and given ranks 1 to n; zero values are excluded from analysis. Any group of tied ranks is allotted the mid rank of the group. Let:

T_+ = sum of ranks of positive differences,
T_- = sum of ranks of negative differences.

The smaller of the two, T_+ and T_-, is compared with tabulated critical value (see Table A9 of Armitage and Berry 1987). If it is lower than the tabulated value, it is concluded that there is a significant difference. For the data in the table, $T_+ = 4.5$ and $T_- = 40.5$; $n = 9$ (excluding one zero difference). The tabulated critical 5 per cent value is 5. Since $T_+ = 4.5$ is less than 5, it is concluded that the difference is significant at the 5 per cent level.

8 PREVENTED FRACTION OF DISEASE

The objective of most field trials is to measure the effect of an intervention in reducing disease rates. The results of such studies may be used to estimate the impact that an intervention might have on disease rates if it was introduced into a public health programme. In such circumstances, the overall effect is much influenced by the *coverage* achieved by the programme.

The *prevented fraction* among individuals exposed to an intervention measure is defined as the percentage of the disease incidence in such individuals that has been prevented due to having received the intervention. For example, if the efficacy of BCG vaccination against TB is 60 per cent, among persons who receive BCG vaccination, 60 per cent of the tuberculosis cases that would have developed otherwise have been prevented by the vaccination. For vaccine studies the prevented fraction is directly equivalent to the *vaccine efficacy*, but the former term may be used for interventions other than vaccines.

The prevented fraction is computed by subtracting the disease risk in individuals with the intervention measure (for example, an anti-leprosy vaccine) from the disease risk in individuals without the intervention, and expressing the difference as a proportion of the latter. For example, if the annual incidence of leprosy is 2.8 per thousand in the vaccinated and 4.2 in the unvaccinated, the prevented fraction is equal to $[(4.2 - 2.8)/4.2] = 0.33$ (or 33 per cent).

If the relative risk (R) (of disease in those who receive the intervention compared to those who do not) is known, the prevented fraction may be obtained by calculating ($1 - R$). For example, if the relative risk of developing malaria in homes where mosquito nets are used is a quarter of that in homes where they are not used, the prevented fraction is equal to $1 - 0.25$, i.e. 75 per cent.

The *population prevented fraction* is defined as the proportion of cases of the disease in the *total population* that have been prevented by the intervention. If the relative risk (R) and the proportion of individuals in the population who receive the intervention measure (P) are known, the population prevented fraction is obtained by calculating $P(1 - R)$. Thus, the extent of reduction possible in disease incidence in the total population, if all individuals were to receive the intervention measure ($P = 1$), is $(1 - R)$.

Consider a situation in which the annual incidence of tuberculosis is 2.0 per thousand in those who do not receive BCG vaccination and 0.8 per thousand in those who do, i.e. the relative risk in those vaccinated is $0.8/2.0 = 0.4$. Table 14.20 shows the fraction of all cases prevented by the intervention according to the disease incidence in the total population and the vaccination coverage.

Table 14.20. Population prevented fraction according to vaccination coverage and disease incidence rate

Vaccination coverage (%) ($P \times 100$)	Disease incidence in total population (per thousand) $[0.8P + 2.0(1-P)]$	Population prevented fraction (%) $[P(1-R)\times100]$
0	2.00	0
20	1.76	12
40	1.52	24
60	1.28	36
80	1.04	48
100	0.80	60

REFERENCES

Armitage, P. and Berry, G. (1987). *Statistical methods in medical research*, (2nd edn), Blackwell, London.

Breslow, N. E., and Day, N. E (1980). *Statistical methods in cancer research. Volume 1: the analysis of case-control studies*. Scientific Publication No. 32. International Agency for Research on Cancer, Lyon, France.

Breslow, N. E. and Day, N. E. (1987). *Statistical methods in cancer research. Volume 2: the design and analysis of cohort studies*. Scientific Publication No. 82. International Agency for Research on Cancer, Lyon, France.

Hill, A. B. (1984). *A short textbook of medical statistics*, 11th edition. Hodder and Stoughton, London.

Miettinen, O. S. (1976). Estimability and estimation in case-referent studies. *American Journal of Epidemiology*, **103**, 498–502.

15
Preparing grant applications

·1 INTRODUCTION

All intervention trials cost money. Sometimes the amount required is small and it may not be necessary to seek additional support to conduct the investigation. Often, however, extra human and material resources are essential to ensure that a trial is carried out properly, and for some the amounts required may be considerable. In these circumstances, investigators must estimate the resources required and know where and how to submit an application for support to an appropriate grant awarding agency, which may be local, national or international.

In this chapter we outline the grant awarding requirements and procedures used by many agencies. The orientation will be towards the general steps to be followed in seeking grants from international agencies, but the procedures and requirements are likely to be similar in broad outline, no matter what source of funding is pursued.

2 INTERNATIONAL GRANT AWARDING AGENCIES

The international agencies that may provide funding for field trials in developing countries fall into three groups: international multilateral agencies, such as the World Health Organization (WHO), the United Nations Children's Fund (UNICEF) and the World Bank; bilateral agencies, such as the British Overseas Development Administration (ODA), the United States Agency for International Development (USAID), the European Community (EC), the Japanese International Co-operation Agency (JICA) and the Swedish Agency for Research Co-operation with Developing Countries (SAREC); and private foundations and non-governmental organizations (NGOs) such as the Rockefeller Foundation, the Ford Foundation, the Carnegie Corporation, the African Medical and Research Foundation (AMREF) and the Helen Keller Foundation. Sometimes agencies which are major funders of domestic research, such as the United States National Institute of Health and the British Medical Research Council, also support some kinds of research in developing countries. Each agency has been established for a particular purpose and each has its own set of operating rules. Many have a defined research agenda with a written plan of research questions for which they are interested in receiving proposals. Generally they will provide application forms with instructions that detail the information, procedures, and timetable for submitting grant proposals. These may guide potential applicants in the formulation of research questions or may help an applicant chose the agency to which to submit a proposal for a particular piece of research. The first step is to find out which agencies might support the research you wish to conduct and to write to obtain all relevant grant information from them. Once it has been decided to which agency a proposal will be submitted, it will be worthwhile to obtain one or more applications that have been successfully submitted to that agency to get an idea of what is expected in the application.

It is important both to read the information sent by the agency and to follow their instructions with care. Pay particular attention to date deadlines and to the length of the various sections of information requested. Note that the deadline is usually based on when the application is to be received by the grant agency rather than when it should be posted! In countries where the mail service is unreliable, it may be worth sending the application by a special courier. If not done automatically, the grant agency should be asked to confirm receipt of the application.

Also, to plan the timing of the study, applicants should find out what the interval is likely to be between the approval of a grant at a review committee meeting and the arrival of research funds into a bank account. In some circumstances, it may be possible to subsidize a study from another account until the money arrives, but in many cases this cannot be done. It is frustrating to have planned to start a study by a particular date, say before the start of the rains, only to find that the funding is delayed. There are many steps to be taken even after the agency has completed the review process and agreed to fund the proposal. These include steps internal to the agency, particularly the financial management and the assurance of ethical clearances, then transfer of funds to the appropriate department of the agency's bank, the subsequent transfer to the investigator's banking system often requiring lengthy foreign exchange arrangements and then to the investigator's institution and to the investigator's account. It is vital to understand fully the many steps and to do as much advance preparation as possible, in anticipation of possible problems. Grant agencies tend to be optimists about the time lags that commonly occur; so try to obtain realistic information from others who have received funding from the same source. Unfortunately, with some agencies, not only is the mean interval many months, but the variation is also large.

Proposals for research may be sent to the grant agency as an 'unsolicited' investigator initiated proposal, or may be submitted in response to a call for proposals to address a particular topic that has been put out for bidding by the agency (commonly known by the letters RFP – 'request for proposal').

Contrary to the impression that many of us sometimes gain, funding agencies really do want to spend their money and to sponsor research! It is almost always worthwhile making a preliminary approach to the funding agency before submitting a full application. The staff of the agency often give considerable help and assistance before a full proposal is submitted to the agency, so as to increase the chances of funding or to warn, at an early stage, that an application for a particular type of research is unlikely to be successful. Potential applicants should send a brief description of the proposed study to the agency, perhaps in the form of a one or two page letter, together with an enquiry as to whether the agency would be interested in having a full proposal developed. The response may be a straight 'no' thus saving the potential applicant a great deal of fruitless effort. Alternatively, the agency may respond that it would be more interested in funding a proposal if it were changed in certain ways. This does not guarantee, of course, that they will fund the modified proposal, but it does usually increase the chances of a successful application. The secretariat of the granting agency will also be able to advise on the normal size of awards they make, so an applicant can judge if the proposal is likely to be in the right range.

Most international funding agencies appreciate that investigators in developing countries may face severe difficulties in conducting research and many have a genuine interest in strengthening research competencies in these countries' institutions. Further, many of the most important disease problems, as well as a wealth of opportunities for important and innovative public health research, are in these countries. Thus there is a considerable desire to fund good research proposals submitted by applicants from developing countries and to assist in every way possible. The World Health Organization and several of its special programs (notably the WHO Tropical Diseases Research Programme (TDR)) are especially concerned with building capacity for research in developing countries and make extra efforts to assist investigators in the development of their research. Sometimes a member of the secretariat of the grant agency or a committee member may be prepared to do considerable work with an applicant to get a proposal into a fundable form. If this kind of assistance is offered, it is usually wise to accept it.

3 THE GRANT AWARDING PROCESS

Most grant awarding agencies select the projects they will fund competitively, using a 'peer-review' procedure for which a committee of experts in relevant scientific areas is convened once or twice a year to review proposals. The committee is charged to judge each proposal on the basis of several specific factors, such as relevance, scientific merit, adequacy of study design, feasibility and cost. Usually there are specific criteria for scoring and the proposals are ranked by score to determine which are to receive funding.

Typically a grant review committee will judge 20 or more (even up to 60) applications in a day. Often committee members receive the applications only a few days or a week or two before the review meeting and, consequently, may not have had time to read them all in detail. Commonly one or two members with expertise pertinent to the research topic are designated to review a particular proposal in detail and introduce it to the committee pointing out its strengths and weaknesses. The views of these committee members are likely to carry great weight.

In addition to the review committee, it is common practice for the granting agency to send proposals to several external reviewers with special expertise in the topic of the research application. Applications for substantial funding may be sent to six or even more reviewers. Each external reviewer submits a written review of the proposal and often is asked to rate particular aspects of the proposal on a quantitative scale. Reviewers are usually asked to conclude their review by giving the proposal an overall score (on a scale ranging from very good to very bad) and to give their opinion on whether or not the grant should be funded. They will also be asked to give their opinion as to whether the amount of funding requested is appropriate for the studies proposed.

The reports of the external reviewers will usually be circulated to all members of the review committee. The salient points in the reviews and the opinions of the reviewers regarding each proposal will often be summarized by the members charged with presenting the proposal to the committee. Opinions of external reviewers carry substantial weight with the committee, but generally the members presenting the proposal are likely to have most influence with the other committee members.

Some agencies provide applicants with the written comments of the external reviewers, usually anonymously, and sometimes the secretariat provides suggestions for improvement and an opportunity for clarification. This is a good system, as it gives the applicant a chance to correct misunderstandings or to modify the proposal in the light of criticisms, but few grant awarding bodies have adopted this way of working as it takes up too much time and requires that reviewers submit their review in good time, which many do not!

More commonly, edited versions of the reviewers' comments are given to applicants at the time the decision about the award is communicated. Unsuccessful applicants may be invited to modify their proposals in the light of specific comments and to resubmit the proposal, though normally with no commitment concerning funding for a resubmission which again would have to compete with the next round of applications. A successful award may be made conditional on the incorporation of changes suggested by referees or by members of the review committee.

Most grant awarding bodies have many more grant applications than they can fund and it is not possible for committees to spend much time discussing the pros and cons of each grant. Each application has a relatively small amount of time allocated to it at a meeting (certainly small in relation to the time that it is likely to have taken to prepare the proposal!) and it is important therefore that the grant is written in such a way that anyone reading it, either by skimming it or by examining it in detail, comprehends that an important research question is being addressed with an appropriate research design and that the applicants are highly competent people to address the question. Particularly for those without a track record of successful research behind them, the application is the document by which the review committee is going to judge the competence of the applicants.

Funding agencies generally like to support persons they have supported before, especially if the previous research was successfully completed. Young investigators are more likely to win a grant award if they have been a member of a proven research team. Investigators are also more likely to be successful in obtaining a grant for a large study if they have previously been successful in gaining support for a smaller study. Many intervention trials are relatively large undertakings and, if possible and time allows, a good strategy for relatively inexperienced investigators is to seek support for a small pilot study to investigate the feasibility of the main trial. If the pilot study is conducted well and the study is properly written up for the funding agency, the chances of obtaining funding for the main study may be greatly enhanced.

4 PREPARING A GRANT APPLICATION

4.1 The research plan

In reviewing a grant application, reviewers will be looking for the answers to some key questions:

1. What are the research questions that will be addressed by the proposed study?
2. Why is it important that this research be carried out? How will the study contribute, directly or indirectly, to the advancement of public health?
3. Are the applicants familiar with previous work in the area of the research and does the study proposed build on and complement that work. Have the applicants done pilot studies that demonstrate the feasibility of the proposed research?
4. What is the research design and how will it be carried out? Is the design appropriate? Is the size of the study correct? Is the time schedule for the work appropriate?
5. How much will the research cost? Are the costs justified in terms of different components of the research, for example staffing levels, equipment costs?
6. Have the applicants considered the possible obstacles they might encounter in conducting the research and devised ways of overcoming these?
7. Have the applicants assembled the right team to do the research? What is their track record in research of this kind? Is their training and experience appropriate?

Usually, grant agencies are fairly specific with respect to the form in which they are prepared to receive applications for support and many have their own specially printed forms for this purpose. The forms will usually come with guidelines as to what aspects of the research should be discussed under different headings. Guidelines may also be given on the maximum length of the overall proposal or on specific sections. These guidelines should be followed carefully.

Box 15.1 shows the instructions that are given to new applicants for grants from the United States Public Health Service (PHS). They are shown as an example only, and other agencies will have different requirements. In particular, many agencies restrict the maximum number of pages to around six, rather than the 20 specified in the Box. However, most agencies require most of the information requested on the PHS form.

Box 15.1. Instructions for the completion of grant applications based on those given by the United States Public Health Service

Research plan. Organize Sections A–D of the Research Plan to answer these questions: (A) What do you intend to do? (B) Why is the work important? (C) What has already been done? (D) How are you going to do the work? **Do not exceed 20 pages for Sections A–D**. You may use any page distribution within this overall limitation; however, the PHS recommends the following format and distribution:

A. *Specific aims*. State the broad, long-term objectives and describe concisely and realistically what the specific research described in this application is intended to accomplish and any hypothesis to be tested. **One page is recommended.**

B. *Background and significance*. Briefly sketch the background to the present proposal, critically evaluate existing knowledge, and specifically identify the gaps which the project is intended to fill. State concisely the importance of the research described in this application by relating the specific aims to the broad long-term objectives. **Two to three pages are recommended**.

C. *Preliminary Studies*. For NEW applications a report of the principal investigator/program director's preliminary studies is useful but optional.

Applicants may use this section to provide an account of the principal investigator/program director's preliminary studies pertinent to the application and/or any other information that will help establish the experience and competence of the investigator to pursue the proposed project. The titles and complete references to appropriate publications and manuscripts **accepted** for publication may be listed, and six collated sets of **no more than ten** such items of background material may be submitted as an Appendix. **Six to eight pages are recommended for the narrative portion of the Preliminary Studies**.

> **Box 15.1.** Continued
>
> D. *Experimental design and methods.* Outline the experimental design and the procedures to be used to accomplish the specific aims of the project. Include the means by which the data will be collected, analysed and interpreted. Describe any new methodology and its advantage over existing methodologies. Discuss the potential difficulties and limitations of the proposed procedures and alternative approached to achieve the aims. Provide a tentative sequence or timetable for the investigation. Point out any procedures, situations, or materials that may be hazardous to personnel and the precautions to be exercised. **Although no specific number of pages is recommended for this section of the application, the total for Sections A to D may not exceed 20 pages.**

4.2 Aims of the research

The information included in describing the aims of the research should be as outlined in Chapter 2, Sections 2.2 to 2.4. The aims include the overall purpose of the research, that is the wider public health goals, together with the specific objectives, which should be as precise as possible and should include specification of the nature and size of the effects sought for the interventions under test.

Questions which are subsidiary to the main objectives, but which might be answered by the research proposed, should be clearly distinguished from the main objectives. In general, reviewers will be more impressed by a study that is designed to provide a clear answer to a single question, than by one diffusely spread over a range of different questions.

4.3 Background to the research

Having stated what questions the research will address, the application should then include a discussion of why these are important questions and how the answers to these questions will add to existing knowledge. Reviewers will expect the applicants to put the specific aims into a broader public health perspective. If a trial of a malaria vaccine is proposed, there should be a *brief* description of why there is a need for such a vaccine to control malaria (for example, the inadequacy of existing control measures in the area in which the trial will be conducted). Usually, in the context of intervention trials, this broader public health perspective will be fairly obvious and this section of the proposal should be brief. However, where the public health implications are not so obvious, more justification may be required. For example, a longer discussion of the public health issues would be required for a study to evaluate whether periodic mass treatment of a population in a developing country with an expensive antibiotic will control sexually transmitted diseases and inhibit HIV transmission.

Applicants should demonstrate their familiarity with all previous work directly relevant to the proposed research. The most important papers/studies should be identified and reference made to these and to appropriate review papers. What is not expected is an exhaustive list of all the papers that have ever been published on the subject, nor should material be included that is not directly relevant to the proposal. Making this section unnecessarily long may suggest to reviewers that the applicants have not adequately sorted the 'wheat from the chaff' in considering previous work; also it will use up valuable space in the application that could otherwise be used to describe the study procedures in more detail, which is generally the part that reviewers will focus their attention on.

4.4 Pilot studies

Success in seeking support for a large or innovative field research project will be enhanced if the applicants can give evidence, based on pilot studies, that the study is feasible. If pilot studies have been done, they should be described in the grant application. For example, if a trial of an HIV vaccine is planned, prior studies could be conducted to assess what proportion of the target population for the trial would be likely to agree to participate in a trial. Sometimes such pilot studies can be conducted prior to a grant application without need for additional financial support, but often the first application to an agency may be for a modest amount to enable pilot investigations to be undertaken, which, if successful, will strengthen the case for supporting the main study.

4.5 Experimental design and methods

The material to be included under this heading is described in Sections 3–10 of Chapter 2. The study design should be described and reasons given why this design was chosen instead of alternative ones. The study population, the interventions and the outcome measures should be fully described. The size of the study must be justified, using realistic assumptions and appropriate statistical procedures. Precise definitions should be given of measurement techniques to be employed and, if questionnaires are to be used, drafts of these should be included as an appendix. If novel methods are to be used, their advantage over existing methods should be given. The means by which information will be recorded, stored and analysed should be specified, as should the measures that will be taken to monitor and ensure the quality of field and laboratory procedures.

If the study design is complicated, it may help to include a diagram which shows, for example, the different treatment schedules and the different points in the trial at which blood or other samples will be taken. A diagram may also be useful to map out the timetable of the trial, indicating the time periods during which patients will be recruited and followed up and when interim and final analyses will be conducted (see Fig. 11.1). Certainly, reviewers will require evidence that the applicants have planned the trial in sufficient detail that it will be completed according to the time schedule given in the proposal.

An important section of the experimental design and methods section is that which discusses the aspects of the study that may give rise to problems and to how these problems will be handled. The proposal should include a discussion of potential problems which might jeopardize the achievement of the objectives of the trial and of approaches to their solution. The consequences of equipment and vehicle failures should be anticipated and evidence of contingency plans presented. For example, if continuous refrigeration of specimens is required and the power supply in the study area is unreliable, adequate provision must be made for the use of generators or other measures as appropriate.

4.6 The budget

The costing of research is often the aspect that gives investigators the most difficulty and getting it wrong can have serious consequences. Overestimating the required budget may be viewed poorly by the reviewers and the funding agency, while under-budgeting may result in resources being exhausted before a study is finished. Some funding agencies *may* be sympathetic to requests for supplementary funding, if there are good reasons, for example greater than expected inflation or a devaluation, but are less sympathetic when investigators have not properly anticipated costs while preparing the original proposal.

The essential characteristics of budgets are that they should be:

1. *Reasonable.* The costs shown should be appropriate for the purposes for which they will be used. Investigators should avoid 'padding' proposals and also avoid quoting unrealistically low costs.
2. *Well-researched.* Actual costs in the past provide a good guide for anticipating future costs for the same or similar procedures. Several independent quotes should be obtained for major items of equipment, to ensure that the costs quoted represent the best value for money.
3. *Detailed.* All significant costs should be given in detail. 'Petrol and servicing of vehicles $10,000' is inadequate! The anticipated mileage and evidence of past servicing costs should be given.
4. *Well-justified and explained.* The necessity for each cost should be given, including an indication of the consequences for the research of *not* having the particular piece of equipment or staff member, etc. A good general rule is to justify *everything*!

Most sponsors of research have specific forms for the budget and they will usually specify what kinds of costs they will and will not cover. For example, some sponsors expect the institution in which the applicants are based to cover local telephone and postage costs and office accommodation and supplies. Only in exceptional circumstances will they meet such costs and, if such expenses are requested, they should be justified in terms of the specific needs of the project.

Cost estimates will usually be divided into different categories of expenditure as given below.

4.6.1 Personnel

Give details of the names, positions and roles of personnel to be engaged on the proposed project. Indicate the percentage of their time that each person, including the principal investigator, will devote to the project and calculate their salary cost on a *pro rata* basis. Estimates should be made separately for each financial year of the study (usually based on the financial year of the grant agency) and should include provision for annual increases in salary, where appropriate. Some grant agencies will not contribute to the salary of the principal investigator, but will still expect to know what percentage of their time will be spent on the project. Appropriate amounts should be added to cover benefits, such as superannuation and health insurance costs, that may be part of the full salary cost (often 25 per cent or more of salary cost).

4.6.2 Consultant costs

The funding agency may have guidelines for the rates of remuneration of consultants to a project. In any case, rates should be agreed with the consultants at the time their participation in the project is sought. The grant application should specify the number of days that will be spent on the project by each consultant, together with their rate of remuneration and any associated costs, such as travel and per diem costs. The contribution that any consultant will make to the project must be specified.

4.6.3 Equipment

List each item of equipment separately and justify the need for each piece. For expensive equipment the agency might want to know if you or other investigators in the institution have similar equipment and if so, whether a sharing arrangement might be worked out. Estimates for the cost of equipment should be obtained from manufacturers or suppliers and should include shipping (and associated insurance) costs. Maintenance agreement costs should be included under 'other expenses'. Depreciation of equipment must be allowed for, but there are wide variations in what is permitted. Vehicles pose special problems in virtually all developing countries. If a vehicle is requested, reasons should be given why any existing vehicles cannot be used, with an appropriate kilometre charge (to cover depreciation, servicing and fuel costs). If the mileage to be covered in a project is considerable, it may be cheaper to buy a vehicle than to budget by the kilometre (for example 40 000 kilometres at 50 cents a kilometre may be more than the cost of a vehicle and fuel for that distance). If a new vehicle is bought for a project there will be servicing costs to add and maintenance costs in the years after the first year.

4.6.4 Supplies

Supplies should be itemized in separate categories (for example, chemicals, glassware, test kits) and should be justified in terms of the needs of the project (for example, number of tests to be performed). If a project requires experimental animals, the specification should include the species, number, unit purchase cost, unit care cost and number of care days. Most agencies will also require reassurance, on ethical grounds, that the animals are essential for the project and that the number requested is the minimum number necessary for the conduct of the research; increasingly, certification of animal care is required.

4.6.5 Travel

Specify the destination of each trip, the number of persons, the mode of transport and the basis for the costs (most agencies will pay only economy air fares). Justification should be given for the necessity for all travel in terms of achieving the goals of the project. Agencies have different rules about travel to conferences (some allow none, some allow one per year).

Per diem costs may be a significant proportion of the budget in field research projects and the rates paid should be based on existing practice in the institution in which the research is based. These costs should be justified for each member of the project staff to whom they will be paid, in terms of the necessity for spending the specified number of days away from the home institution.

4.6.6 Patient care costs

These are costs that may be incurred in a research project which are not directly related to the research objectives. A frequent concern in field studies in developing countries in which health care services are inadequate is provision of normal health care to those in the study. In principle, such costs should be borne in whatever manner health care costs are normally paid, but that is not always possible. In large or prolonged trials, arrangements should be worked out with the health authorities responsible for health care in the population to ensure that care is provided on a regular basis during and after the trial. In poor countries, however, where health care is generally inadequate, some kind of interim arrangements may have to be made. See Chapter 4 on ethical considerations concerning obligations of investigators.

Reimbursement to participants in a trial for travel or loss of earnings should be listed under 'other expenses'.

4.6.7 Alterations and renovations

If alteration or renovation of buildings is essential for the conduct of a research project, then the cost of these should be claimed. However, some agencies may argue that changes in the investigator's institution should be borne by that institution. In some circumstances it may be necessary to rent space for project activities. This may require special justification and should be included under 'other expenses'.

4.6.8 Other expenses

This section should contain items such as: rentals and leases, equipment maintenance (service contracts, repairs), computer charges (if there is not a separate claim for computers under 'equipment'), publication costs, fees for services related to the project (for example, library searches), office supplies, postage and telecommunication charges (telephone, telex, fax, e-mail).

Not all costs listed above may be allowed by a grant agency, but if in doubt it is better to include them in the application (and let the agency cross them out!).

4.6.9 Overhead (indirect) charges

There are 'hidden' costs associated with all research. Someone must pay the principal investigator's salary and must administer the grant, pay salaries, order supplies, supply heat or air conditioning and light to offices, supply the offices themselves, have them cleaned and maintained, etc. These costs, called 'institutional overheads' may be substantial and amount to a considerable portion of the project costs. In Europe and North America, such costs may amount to between 30 per cent and 90 per cent or more in different institutions. These costs are added on to the budgeted cost of the research when a grant is submitted to a funding agency. Some funding agencies refuse payment of overheads (for example, WHO and many charitable foundations), others will pay them in their own country but not outside (for example, US Public Health Service). Sometimes it is possible to directly budget for many of these items (to be listed as rental of space, cost of utilities, administration salary proportion, etc., but there must be justification and charges pro-rated in accordance of actual project use) and it is usually advantageous to do so. Institutions in developing countries have been more lax about claiming such costs than have those in developed countries with the result that, in some instances, institutions in the former countries have been subsidizing the costs of research projects. It is important to ascertain whether or not an agency will pay overhead costs. If it will not, the applicant should determine what costs might reasonably be put on a grant. For example, agencies which pay overheads may consider that local telephone costs should be borne by the institution (that is, they are included in the overhead costs). If the agency does not pay overheads, it may be appropriate to budget for total telephone costs, including their installation if necessary.

It is hard to give firm guidelines of what may or may not be included in the budget. The important points to bear in mind are, firstly, that all costs should be justified in terms of project needs and, secondly, if you do not ask for it, you are unlikely to get it!

4.7 General considerations

Those reviewing proposals submitted to funding agencies will examine each research proposal to be considered at a particular meeting, to look for evidence that the investigator has defined clearly an interesting and important research question, has demonstrated adequate familiarity with previous work in the area, has put forward an appropriate and efficient study design to answer the question(s) posed and has the capability of successfully completing the research at an appropriate cost and in an appropriate time-span. The reviewers will often have to assimilate a large number of proposals in a relatively short period of time and thus it is important that grant applications are written clearly and unambiguously to facilitate rapid understanding. Factors which some investigators might consider unimportant may carry more weight than they would expect in this process.

First, *brevity* has great merit! The length of the grant application should be the minimum necessary to demonstrate the competence of the investigator and of the appropriateness and importance of the study proposed. Reviewers are generally experts in the field and will be annoyed rather than impressed with information, however erudite, not relevant to the research question.

Second, read the instructions carefully and fill in the forms as directed. It is amazing how many applicants ignore this rule, and suffer as a consequence. Many funding bodies provide specific instructions as to how they would like to receive proposals. They may specify the maximum length for specific sections of the proposal. If the instructions specify no more than 6 pages, write no more than 6 pages. Also, in order to stay within the specified limit, do not use the facility on printers that allows the size of the script to be reduced so that it is barely legible without a magnifying glass! Instructions vary considerably from agency to agency and if a grant is rejected by one, do not send it in the same form to another agency, ignoring their different requirements.

Third, proof-read the application carefully to eliminate, as far as possible, all errors. Typographical errors create the impression, rightly or wrongly, that the applicant does not pay attention to detail, an important requirement for almost all research. Use the spell checker, but do not rely upon this to detect all typing errors!

Fourth, try to make the finished document as professional as possible. This may be a particular challenge to applicants from developing countries, who may have problems accessing suitable and functioning equipment. If possible use a laser printer to type the application, even if this means borrowing someone else's for the application. Try to avoid using a dot-matrix printer, but if there is no alternative, make sure the ribbon is fairly new. If the grant agency requires more than one copy of an application, find a photocopier that produces good copies and check all of the final documents to be sure that pages have not been missed out or collated in the wrong order. Before submitting an application, ask colleagues to read it who have not been involved in its generation. They should be able to understand it without difficulty and they may detect errors that you can no longer see, even though it has been through many drafts.

Finally, if an application is turned down by a funding body, reviewers comments will often be given to the applicant at that stage. If submission for the same research project is then made to another agency, it is wise to take account of the reviewers' comments in reformulating the proposal. Bear in mind that the application will often be sent to the same external reviewer by different agencies and few reviewers are impressed to see a rejected proposal resubmitted without change to a different agency!

5 COMMON PROBLEMS IN GRANT APPLICATIONS

Below is a list of common problems with grant applications, based on the experience of the authors in reviewing proposals:

(1) poorly formulated objectives;
(2) poor budget and budget justification;
(3) poor research design: inadequate attention to what specific research question is being addressed by the research. Why is it

important to answer this question? What impact may it have on public health practice?

(4) analysis not planned in relation to the main objectives with inadequate dummy tables, if at all;

(5) inadequate description of the study design and procedures: derivation of sample size is often done poorly. Inadequate description as to who is doing what and when. Few applications contain a detailed timetable for the research;

(6) too ambitious: trying to address too many questions in one study;

(7) not sufficient attention to previous literature on the research question;

(8) no pilot studies to investigate feasibility of proposed approach;

(9) insufficient attention to quality and quality control;

(10) inadequate allowance for data entry and analysis: often arrangements for analysis of data are not addressed at all in a proposal, other than that it will all go into a computer!

16
Reporting and using results

1 Reporting findings

2 From research to public health action
2.1 Policy makers and researchers
2.2 Introduction into operational control programmes
2.3 Managing the implementation
2.4 Costs

1 REPORTING FINDINGS

Whatever the outcome of the trial, a number of documents must be prepared. For all studies it is highly recommended that a comprehensive document be prepared detailing all the trial procedures and the full results. This document serves as a permanent record for the study team and will be a reference for anyone who wants to know exactly what was done in the investigation. It will also be invaluable for the conduct of any resurvey of the trial population, and may provide legal documentation with respect to registration of a new product or if questions about the study arise for any reason in the future. If the results of a trial may be used as part of the registration procedures for a new product, it is important to liaise with the regulatory authorities at an early stage in the planning of the trial so that the appropriate records are kept and the proper recording procedures are used.

In addition to the full report on the study, the investigators have the responsibility of making the findings available in the most appropriate format to several different audiences.

Firstly, it is the responsibility of the investigators to report back the results to those whose participation made the trial possible, that is, those in the study communities. As emphasized in Chapters 4 and 5, the investigating team should be in regular communication with the participants and their communities throughout the trial, but there is a special responsibility to review and discuss comprehensively both the findings at the end of the trial and also the public health actions that may be taken on the basis of the trial results. Should they wish to see them, copies of all written reports which do not contain confidential information (for example, names of patients) should be made available to the participants in the trial and to members of their communities. However, usually such documents are produced for technical audiences and it may also be important to convey the findings to the participants in a document written in such a way as to be readily comprehensible to a lay audience. Alternatively, or in addition, it may be appropriate to hold a meeting to explain and discuss the findings with community leaders and district or local officials and to have an open public meeting with community members to answer any questions they may have regarding the study and to consider the implications of the findings in the local setting. Such meetings must be discussed with all appropriate health officials, and it may be useful to have the meetings opened by the Minister of Health or the Director of Medical Services, or their representatives.

Secondly, the findings should be reported formally to the local and national health policy and decision makers. As well as reporting the results in full, the implications that the findings have for disease control programmes should be reviewed with all appropriate health authorities, both governmental and non-governmental. It is important that a clearly written summary of the main results be included, usually at the front of the report, as many of those to whom the results may be relevant will not have the time or inclination to study all the fine details.

Thirdly, papers must be prepared for national or international peer-reviewed journals. These papers will generally be much shorter than the comprehensive reference document discussed above. Guidance on the form these should take is generally detailed by the particular journal selected. Since different journals have different target audiences, it may be important to publish different aspects of the study in different journals in order to ensure dissemination of specific findings to the most relevant groups.

The funding agency will also require a final report on the outcome of the study. Sometimes it is sufficient to send drafts of papers that are to be published, but the different agencies will specify the information they require.

Preparation of all these reports, particularly those for peer-reviewed journals, are major undertakings in themselves, but they must be considered an integral part of the conduct of the study and a major responsibility of the investigators. Research that is not appropriately disseminated is likely to fail to achieve its proper impact.

2 FROM RESEARCH TO PUBLIC HEALTH ACTION

2.1 Policy makers and researchers

Final analyses and the publication of results are important tasks that must be completed at the end of a trial, but an important further responsibility of researchers is to review the findings with the relevant disease control authorities and to explore implications for the overall health policy of the country and for the design of specific disease control strategies. From the beginning of the planning of a trial directed towards an important public health problem, the appropriate policy and planning (as well as disease control) arms of the Ministry of Health should be involved. Even when the Ministry does not have direct responsibility for the actual conduct of the trial, formulation of conclusions from the analysis of trial results requires their input and participation, as they are usually responsible for changes to health programmes that may be necessary because of the results of the trial.

There is no point in conducting an intervention trial if the results of the study are not translated into specific public health actions. Policy makers and researchers share the responsibility for ensuring that research findings are put to their proper use. Unfortunately, in most countries, policy makers have a very poor understanding of health research, and frequently health researchers have a similarly poor understanding of the role and function of policy makers. A variety of useful mechanisms that would assist in communication between decision makers and researchers are implemented in some countries. Health planning units may have responsibility for regularly reviewing, and even funding, health systems research. Other mechanisms include *ad hoc*, or regular, seminars at the Ministry level. A more comprehensive approach can be achieved through national health policy or epidemiology boards, such as those in Thailand, Mexico and the Cameroons. These boards are composed of scientists, government policy makers, leaders in non-governmental organizations and often lay people, and have the responsibility to review and fund important public health research activities. Whether this mechanism or some other be used, it is of critical importance to have a way of effectively and speedily translating research results into public health action.

Many health systems in developing countries are moving towards devolving responsibility for health care systems down to the district level. Thus, health intervention research should be part of the district health plan (or, at least, should be mentioned in the plan, even if the research itself is not undertaken by the district health team but by a specialized research group). This will ensure regular review of the state, and of the implications, of the research. Decentralization offers an excellent opportunity to link research with public health practice.

2.2 Introduction into operational control programmes

Before a newly proven intervention can be put into operation, the Ministry must consider at least two further factors that relate to its effectiveness. Sometimes, interventions with newly demonstrated effectiveness must be fitted into an ongoing control programme based on other interventions. For example, malaria vaccines, when developed, will have to be added to whatever is the existing malaria control strategy, which may include vector control and case detection and treatment measures. An overall integrated strategy for control will have to be developed and this might require trials of various combinations of interventions to determine the optimal mix.

A second important issue that the Ministry must consider is that the efficacy of an intervention measured in the circumstances of a trial can rarely be attained when the intervention is implemented under routine circumstances. Community effectiveness (coverage and efficacy as actually achieved by the routine health service), rather than trial effectiveness, is the measure of relevance for the Ministry (Tugwell *et al.* 1985). Demonstration of high levels of efficacy under field trial conditions is important but, by itself, is not necessarily sufficient to justify the widespread introduction of the intervention without further studies directly relevant to its implementation. Practical examples of this approach are given by Tanner *et al.* (1993).

2.3 Managing the implementation

The importance of understanding the setting and circumstances in which the intervention will be used in a public health programme must be understood both by policy makers and researchers. When the public health importance of an intervention is being assessed, managerial constraints must be considered that may make it impossible to achieve useful levels of efficacy. The principles and methods of continuous quality improvement management, with its emphasis on making sure that the right things get done in the right way at the right time, is proving to be a useful approach to the management of health systems in developing countries. Such approaches may help ensure that the efficacy as demonstrated under trial conditions can be approached under routine conditions (F. Omaswa, personal communication).

2.4 Costs

The costs of introducing a new intervention must also be analysed and assessed in relation to other uses of the resources. Ideally, the benefits (healthy life gained) per unit expenditure required for adding the intervention to the health system would be compared with benefits that could be gained by expenditure on another health programme. In practice, no developing country at this time has its health information in such a form that explicit comparisons of this kind can be made meaningfully. But efforts to build the capacity in developing countries for country-specific health research that would provide the skills for improved health-related decision making are receiving increased attention (Commission on Health Research for Development 1990). An important step was taken in this direction with the publication of the World Bank report *Investing in health* (World Bank 1993a) which strongly advocated the use of burden of disease measures in making decisions concerning resource allocation for health. By combining losses due to morbidity and mortality into a single indicator, comparisons can be made of the relative disease burdens due to different causes or in different populations. The composite measure also shows promise for use as a common denominator in assessing the comparative benefits to be gained by alternative interventions, and thus it may become a useful tool for aiding decision makers in their choices (World Bank 1993b). Investigators in several countries are now working towards making such measures available for practical use by health planners. These further kinds of study concerning improved management methods and better tools for health planning decisions have not been discussed in this manual, but it is important that investigators appreciate that decisions about disease control interventions must be put into the context of these broader concerns.

REFERENCES

Commission on Health Research for Development (1990). *Health research: essential link to equity in development.* Oxford University Press, New York.

Tanner, M., Lengeler, C. and Nicolaus, L. (1993). From the efficacy of disease control tools to community effectiveness. *Transactions of the Royal Society of Tropical Medicine and Hygiene*, **87**, 518–23.

Tugwell, P., Bennett, K.J., Sackett, D.L. and Haynes, R.B. (1985). The measurement iterative loop: a framework for the critical appraisal of need, benefits and costs of health interventions. *Journal of Chronic Diseases*, **38**, 339–51.

World Bank (1993a). *World development report, 1993: investing in health.* Oxford University Press, New York.

World Bank (1993b). *Disease control priorities in the developing world.* (ed Jamieson, D.T., Mosley, W.H., Measham, A.R. and Bobadilla, J.L.) Oxford University Press, New York.

Index